Best Practice Protocols for Physique Assessment in Sport

Patria A. Hume • Deborah A. Kerr
Timothy R. Ackland

Editors

Best Practice Protocols for Physique Assessment in Sport

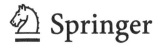

Springer

Editors
Patria A. Hume
Sport Performance Research Institute
New Zealand
Auckland University of Technology
Auckland, New Zealand

Deborah A. Kerr
School of Public Health
Curtin University
Perth, West Australia, Australia

Timothy R. Ackland
School of Sport Science, Exercise and
Health
The University of Western Australia
Perth, West Australia, Australia

ISBN 978-981-10-5417-4   ISBN 978-981-10-5418-1   (eBook)
https://doi.org/10.1007/978-981-10-5418-1

Library of Congress Control Number: 2017960953

Printed on acid-free paper

This Springer imprint is published by Springer Nature
The registered company is Springer Nature Singapore Pte Ltd.
The registered company address is: 152 Beach Road, #21-01/04 Gateway East, Singapore 189721, Singapore

We dedicate this book to our body composition mentors and thank them for passing their technical and academic expertise onto us, for providing inspiration and encouragement and for leading by excellent example.

Professor J.E. Lindsay Carter, Ph.D., Dr.H.C., Professor Emeritus, San Diego State University, USA.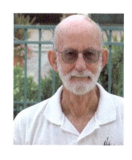
Lindsay graduated from the University of Otago (1950–1952) and Auckland Teachers College (1953). He held teaching and research positions at the School of Physical Education (UO) in 1954–1955 and again in 1960–1962. From 1956 to 1959, he was a Fulbright Scholar at the University of Iowa, Iowa City, where he obtained his M.A. and Ph.D. degrees. From 1962 to 1992, he was a professor in the Department of Physical Education at San Diego State University, San Diego, California, USA, where he taught applied anatomy and

*kinesiology, biomechanics, adaptive physical
education, growth and development and
kinanthropometry. He received the
Outstanding Faculty Award (1983) and the
Exceptional Merit Service Award (1984).
Currently he is professor emeritus in the
School of Exercise and Nutritional Sciences
at San Diego State University and continues
his research in kinanthropometry, along with
consulting, workshops and invited
presentations. In addition to other honours,
Lindsay received honorary doctorate degrees
from universities in Hungary (1998) and
Belgium (2005). He was elected to the
Inaugural Wall of Fame at the School of
Physical Education, University of Otago,
New Zealand, in May 2006. Lindsay's
research work has focused on the structure
and function of athletes and non-athletes. He
is the co-developer of the Heath-Carter
somatotype method which is presently the
most widely used in body build research. He
has published over 130 articles and chapters
and has been author or editor of nine books.
He was a key investigator in
kinanthropometric studies of Olympic and
World Championship athletes in Mexico City
(1968), Montreal (1976), Perth (1991),
Uruguay (1995) and Zimbabwe (1995). He
has served as a consultant or co-investigator
for studies in 18 countries. In addition, he
has given invited presentations and/or
workshops in many countries. Lindsay has
been a mentor to Patria for body composition
projects and teaching. He provided funding
and support to enable the J.E. Lindsay
Carter Kinanthropometry Laboratory to be
established at Auckland University of*

Technology (AUT), New Zealand, in 2004. In 2012, AUT opened the J.E. Lindsay Carter Kinanthropometry Clinic and Archive at AUT Millennium in honour of Lindsay.

Professor Bill Ross, Ph.D., Emeritus Professor, Canada.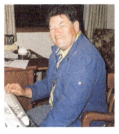
Dr. William (Bill) D. Ross, formerly a professor at Simon Fraser University, is a life member of ISAK. Bill was a postdoctoral research fellow at the Institute of Child Health, London. He was given an Award for Distinguished Service by the British Columbia Recreation Association for leadership in working with health, fitness and lifestyle enhancement professionals. In 1988, he was the first Canadian awarded the internationally prestigious Philip Noel-Baker Research Prize for new models and approaches for the study of human proportionality, dimensionality and body composition and for his leadership in kinanthropometry. In 1992 Magyar Testnevelési Egyetem (now Semmelweis University in Hungary) awarded him an honorary doctorate for his international scientific leadership. Bill served ISAK as chairman of its International Working Group on Scholarship, Awards and Curriculum until 1999. Bill is currently the scientific director for Rosscraft Innovations Incorporated, a company manufacturing and marketing instruments and teaching materials. Bill has numerous publications including a DVD movie on anthropometry technique which is

used in ISAK courses. Bill and his wife Mary have dedicated their working life to training and mentoring anthropometrists worldwide. Bill was Deborah A. Kerr's master of science supervisor at Simon Fraser University where he introduced her to kinanthropometry—the study of human size, shape, proportion, composition, maturation and gross function. Bill inspired Deborah to appreciate the history of science. She continues to train anthropometrists as he trained her—with rigour, fairness and an appreciation that anthropometry is a team sport.

Professor John Bloomfield, Ph.D., AM Cit. WA, Emeritus Professor, The University of Western Australia.
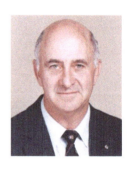
John was the foundation professor at Australia's first university-based Department of Physical Education at UWA and is viewed by many as the father of sports and exercise science in Australia. He has published over 100 peer-reviewed papers and book chapters, has authored or coauthored six books and has lectured and consulted on sports science topics in over 23 countries. Together with colleagues Professor Brian Blanksby, Professor Bruce Elliott and Professor Timothy R. Ackland, John was a co-chief investigator for the UWA Growth and Development Study. John has had a profound influence on Australian sport, having served as president of the Australian

Sports Medicine Federation (now Sports Medicine Australia) and chair of the Australian Sports Commission, and was one of the driving forces behind the establishment of the Australian Institute of Sport. John's many accomplishments were recognised in 2011 when he was inducted into the Sport Australia Hall of Fame. John was one of Tim's Ph.D. supervisors and career mentors, having first inspired him through the study of applied anatomy and sports performance at UWA during the 1970s and 1980s.

Professor Patria A. Hume

Associate Professor Deborah A. Kerr

Professor Timothy R. Ackland

Foreword

In a world of constant scientific advancement, it is not surprising that new technologies have emerged in the field of physique assessment. Where previously only few methods existed, new devices such as dual-energy X-ray absorptiometry, impedance technologies (bioelectrical impedance analysis, multi-frequency bioelectrical impedance analysis, bioelectrical impedance spectroscopy), ultrasound, 3D photometry and air-displacement plethysmography (i.e. Bod Pod) are now readily available. Practitioners, all over the world, are employing these new technologies to measure and monitor change in body size, shape and composition for the purposes of health management and sports performance.

Traditionally amongst sports science practitioners, surface anthropometry has been used to assess body composition through a standardised and internationally recognised methodology (ISAK). However, it is now common for practitioners to incorporate additional body composition measurements using these new technologies. The accuracy and reliability of these measures are critical in a field where tracking small changes in an athlete's physique is important.

When athletes have their body composition measured across multiple technologies in a non-standardised manner, they often receive varying results which can be confusing and, in some cases, distressing. Currently, no reference or model exists for the standardisation of many of these new devices. There is often a lack of established protocols to ensure best practice in physique assessment.

This textbook will serve as a valuable resource for practitioners as it brings together eminent experts in the discipline who understand the importance of providing athletes with accurate, reliable and comparable body composition information to guide their daily training regimes. The authors have produced guidelines that represent current best practice standards for each assessment method by covering important aspects such as subject presentation and preparation, body positioning, equipment calibration and interpretation of results.

As manager of the National Sport Science Quality Assurance Program, I am delighted to recommend this book to all practitioners wanting to provide the highest-quality servicing in athlete physique assessment.

Belconnen, ACT, Australia   Kate Fuller

Preface

This book outlines best practice protocols for physique assessment of competitive and recreational athletes. We provide guidance on the use of new technologies for body composition analysis. While surface anthropometry has traditionally been used to assess body composition through the internationally recognised methodology of the International Society for the Advancement of Kinanthropometry (ISAK), the commercialisation of devices providing bioelectrical impedance analysis, dual-energy X-ray absorptiometry, magnetic resonance imaging, 3D photometry (3D scanning), air-displacement plethysmography (i.e. Bod Pod), ultrasound techniques and dilution techniques (doubly labelled water) has led to the adoption of new and often non-standardised measurement techniques.

We detail standardisation procedures for each technology in terms of athlete preparation, equipment calibration, test protocols, data reporting and data interpretation. Each chapter covers a different technology/tool and outlines how it works, what it is used to measure and what the issues are surrounding its validity, practicality and reliability. This book provides an essential reference for device technicians and sport practitioners, ensuring that high-performance athletes are afforded accurate and comparable body composition information to guide their training routines. Chapters also address commonly asked questions by coaches, such as how often body composition should be assessed, how body composition can be used to select athletes for performance or to monitor athletes' growth and development and how to select and set up equipment used during sport in relation to the athletes and to assess the effectiveness of their training and dietary interventions.

Part I of the book focuses on why physique is measured. Chapters include discussion of physique assessment in youth sports for talent identification and development; monitoring of developing athlete's anthropometry, growth and health; and optimising of anthropometry for sports performance and anthropometry for sports equipment design and fit.

Part II of the book focuses on how to use the selected method and report the data to your athlete and coach.

Chapters include discussion of athlete considerations for measurement, non-imaging methods (surface anthropometry, air-displacement plethysmography,

3D scanning, doubly labelled water, bioelectrical impedance, new innovations) and imaging methods (dual-energy X-ray absorptiometry, ultrasound, computed tomography and magnetic resonance imaging). Each chapter in Part II describes:

- Why you measure physique using the techniques and technologies. A description of how the technique allows measurement of physique is provided. Precision and accuracy, validity, practicality and sensitivity to monitor change of physique are described. Current issues surrounding the advantages and disadvantages of the technique are provided.
- What the techniques and technologies are. The hardware, software and skills required are described, and equipment selection, calibration, training and accreditation systems are outlined.
- How you use the selected technique for athletes. The technical specifics on how to conduct the assessment and analyse and report the data are outlined. Athlete presentation and preparation protocols are described.
- What the technique is used to measure. Key variables gained from the technique and what is useful for monitoring athletes are outlined.

Part III of the book focuses on applications of physique assessment in athletes. Chapters include discussion on physique assessment in practice, large-scale sampling of athletes, anthropometry profiles for types of sport, body image for athletes and training and accreditation systems.

Auckland, New Zealand   Patria A. Hume
Perth, WA, Australia   Deborah A. Kerr
Perth, WA, Australia   Timothy R. Ackland

Acknowledgements

We acknowledge the academic colleagues, athletes and coaches, who have enabled our reflections on best practice protocols for physique assessment in sport.

Contents

List of Abbreviations[1]

%BF	Percentage body fat
3D	Three-dimensional
AEE	Activity energy expenditure
BIA	Bioelectrical impedance analysis
BIS	Bioelectrical impedance spectroscopy
BMI	Body mass index
CI	Confidence intervals
CT	Computed tomography
DLW	Doubly-labelled water
DXA	Dual energy X-ray absorptiometry
FTIR	Fourier transform infrared spectroscopy
IAEA	International Atomic Energy Agency
IOC	International Olympic Committee
IRMS	Isotope ratio mass spectrometer
ISAK	International Society for the Advancement of Kinanthropometry
MRI	Magnetic resonance imaging
PAL	Physical activity level
PET	Positron emission tomography
REE	Resting energy expenditure
RMR	Resting metabolic rate
SD	Standard deviation
TBW	Total body water
TBW	Total body water
TEE	Total energy expenditure
TEF	Thermic effect of food

---

[1] We have tried to avoid using abbreviations given it makes reading content harder for those unfamiliar with physique assessment. However, we have provided a list of commonly used abbreviations in the area to help readers.

TEM   Technical error of measurement
WHO   World Health Organisation
WHR   Waist-to-hip ratio
WHtR   Waist-to-height ratio
WTR   Waist-to-thigh ratio

Editors and Contributors

Editors

Patria A. Hume, Ph.D., MSc (Hons), BSc, ISAK4 Sport Performance Research Institute New Zealand, Auckland University of Technology, Auckland, New Zealand

Deborah A. Kerr, Ph.D., MSc, GradDipDiet, BAppSc, ISAK4 School of Public Health, Curtin University, Perth, West Australia, Australia

Timothy R. Ackland, Ph.D., F.A.S.M.F., F.R.S.B. School of Sport Science, Exercise and Health, The University of Western Australia, Perth, West Australia, Australia

Contributors[2]

Jacqueline A. Alderson, Ph.D., F.I.S.B.S. School of Sport Science, Exercise and Health, Faculty of Science, University of Western Australia, Crawley, WA, Australia

J. Hans de Ridder, Ph.D., I.S.A.K.4. School of Human Movement Sciences, Faculty of Health Sciences, North-West University—Potchefstroom Campus, Potchefstroom, South Africa

Kagan J. Ducker, Ph.D., BSc (Hons), ESSAM, ISAK3 Curtin University, Bentley, WA, Australia

---

[2]Authors contributing chapters to this book, and the online video material that supports this book, are leading researchers and practitioners in fields that use physique assessment for athletes.

Kate Fuller, B.Sc. (H.M.S.), I.S.A.K.3. Manager, National Sport Science Quality Assurance Program, Australian Sports Commission, Belconnen, ACT, Australia

Stephen C. Hollings, Ph.D., M.Phil., Dip.Ed. Sports Performance Research Institute New Zealand (SPRINZ), Faculty of Health and Environmental Sciences, Auckland University of Technology, Auckland, New Zealand

Masaharu Kagawa, Ph.D., BSc (Hons), ISAK3 Institute of Nutrition Sciences, Kagawa Nutrition University, Sakado, Saitama, Japan

Justin W.L. Keogh, Ph.D., B.H.M.S. (Hons.) Bond Institute of Health and Sport, Faculty of Health Sciences and Medicine, Bond University, Robina, QLD, Australia

Ava Kerr, B.Sc., M.Sc., A.E.S., C.S.C.S. Faculty of Science, Health, Education and Engineering, University of the Sunshine Coast, Maroochydore DC, QLD, Australia

Stephven Kolose, M.Sc., P.G.Dip.Erg., B.Sc. Operations Analysis and Human Systems Group, Defence Technology Agency, New Zealand Defence Force, Auckland, New Zealand

Anna V. Lorimer, Ph.D., BSc (Hons), ISAK3 Sports Performance Research Institute New Zealand (SPRINZ), Faculty of Health and Environmental Sciences, Auckland University of Technology, Auckland, New Zealand

Duncan J. Macfarlane, B.Sc. (Hons.), B.Ph.Ed. Flora Ho Sports Centre, The University of Hong Kong, Pokfulam, Hong Kong

Kristen L. MacKenzie-Shalders, Ph.D., A.P.D., I.S.A.K.3. Bond Institute of Health and Sport, Faculty of Health Sciences and Medicine, Bond University, Robina, QLD, Australia

Wolfram Müller, Ph.D., Mag.rer.nat. Institute of Biophysics, Medical University of Graz, Graz, Austria

Alisa Nana, Ph.D., A.P.D., A.S.D. College of Sports Science and Technology, Mahidol University, Salaya, Nakhon Pathom, Thailand

Clinton O. Njoku, M.Sc. (Hons.), B.Sc. Department of Anatomy, Faculty of Medicine—Preclinicals, Ebonyi State University, Abakaliki, Nigeria

Helen O'Connor, Dip.N.D., B.Sc., Ph.D. Faculty of Health Sciences, University of Sydney, Lidcombe, NSW, Australia

Elaine C. Rush, Ph.D., M.Sc. (Hons.), M.N.Z.M. Faculty of Health and Environmental Sciences, Auckland University of Technology, Auckland, New Zealand

Greg Shaw, B.H.Sc. (Nutr. & Diet.), I.S.A.K.3. AIS Sports Nutrition, Australian Institute of Sport, Australian Sports Commission, Canberra, ACT, Australia

Kelly R. Sheerin, MHSc, BHSc (Hons), BSc, ISAK3 Sports Performance Research Institute New Zealand (SPRINZ), Faculty of Health and Environmental Sciences, Auckland University of Technology, Auckland, New Zealand

Gary Slater, Ph.D., M.Sc., B.Sc., A.P.D., I.S.A.K.3. School of Health and Sport Sciences, Faculty of Science, Health, Education and Engineering, University of the Sunshine Coast, Maroochydore DC, QLD, Australia

Arthur D. Stewart, Ph.D., I.S.A.K.4. School of Health Sciences, Robert Gordon University, Aberdeen, UK

Editor's Biography

Patria A. Hume Patria A. Hume is professor of human performance at the Faculty of Health and Environmental Sciences, Auckland University of Technology, New Zealand. Patria has a Ph.D. in sports injury biomechanics and an M.Sc. (Hons.) and B.Sc. in exercise physiology and sports psychology. Patria was the inaugural director of the Sports Performance Research Institute New Zealand (SPRINZ) from 2000 to 2009 and is director of the SPRINZ J.E. Lindsay Carter Kinanthropometry Clinic and Archive. Patria was the associate dean of research for the Faculty of Health and Environmental Sciences (2013–2015). Patria's research 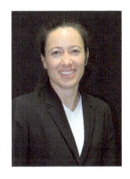 focuses on improving sports performance using sports biomechanics and sports anthropometry and reducing sporting injuries by investigating injury mechanisms and using injury prevention methods and sports epidemiology analyses. In 2000, Patria was a co-investigator for the Sydney Olympics anthropometry project. Patria served as director of the International Society for the Advancement of Kinanthropometry (2006–2009) and is an editor of several journals including *Sports Medicine*. Patria received the 2016 Geoffrey Dyson Award from the International Society for Biomechanics in Sports and the 2016 AUT Research Medal. Patria provides surface anthropometry and ultrasound body composition analysis to athletes and conducts research using body composition techniques.

Deborah A. Kerr Associate Professor Deborah A. Kerr is a research academic with a Ph.D. in exercise and bone health and master of science in body composition. Deborah is an accredited practising dietitian and a fellow of Sports Dietitians Australia and an internationally recognised expert in body composition and physique assessment.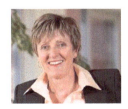

Deborah is the only Level 4 ISAK-accredited anthropometrist in Australia and one of 16 appointed by ISAK worldwide which qualifies her to conduct accredited training courses in anthropometry. Deborah's research focuses on improving sports performance using sports nutrition and sports anthropometry, and she has been an investigator on several large sports anthropometry projects. In 2000, Deborah was a co-investigator for the Sydney Olympics anthropometry project. She has published numerous book chapters and journal publications in body composition and physique assessment. Deborah served as director of the International Society for the Advancement of Kinanthropometry (ISAK) and for Sports Dietitians Australia.

Timothy R. Ackland Tim Ackland is professor of applied anatomy and biomechanics and was head of the School of Sport Science, Exercise and Health, at the University of Western Australia. He has research interests in the mechanics of human movement with themes spanning exercise rehabilitation, high-performance sport and human performance in industry. Professor Ackland has published over 130 peer-reviewed papers, 5 academic books and 30 book chapters. He has served as a director of Sports Medicine Australia and was a member of the IOC Medical Commission's Working Party on Body Composition, 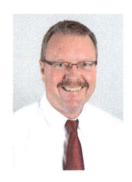 Health and Performance. Tim also chaired the Scientific Programme Committee for the 5th IOC World Congress on Sport Sciences for the 2000 Olympics and was conference co-chair for Sports Medicine Australia in Perth in 2001. In 2000, Tim was a principal researcher for the Sydney Olympics anthropometry project. Tim has been an ISAK4 kinanthropometrist.

Author's Biography

Jacqueline A. Alderson Jacqueline Alderson is an associate professor in the Faculty of Science at the University of Western Australia. Her current research interests include biomechanical modelling and technological innovation in biomechanics, with specific research groups working in the areas of sports injury prevention, markerless motion capture, application of novel measurement techniques and adopting of 'big data' techniques to advance the sports sciences (machine learning, deep neural networks). She has authored 100+ peer-reviewed textbooks, book chapters, research papers and conference proceedings and is a pas-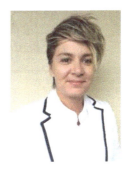
sionate advocate for the promotion of science in schools. She was a member of the Sydney Olympics biomechanics research team and is a fellow and former director of the International Society of Biomechanics in Sport (ISBS).

J. Hans de Ridder Professor Hans de Ridder is director of the School of Human Movement Sciences at the North-West University in Potchefstroom, South Africa. He is the senior vice-president of the International Society for the Advancement of Kinanthropometry (ISAK) and an ISAK-accredited Level 4 criterion anthropometrist. Hans has taught ISAK courses for many years which form part of the ISAK accreditation system that has operated worldwide since 1996. Hans received life membership from ISAK in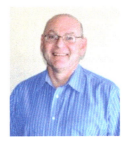
2014, being the fifth person to receive this prestigious award. He was awarded the 2002 Stals Prize and the 2011 Albert Strating Prize for exceptional contribution to science and health by the S.A. Academy for Science and Art. Hans is the assistant editor of the *African Journal for Physical Health Education, Recreation and Dance* and also the founding secretary-general of the BRICS Council of Exercise and Sports Science in 2015.

Kagan J. Ducker Dr. Kagan Ducker is one of the sports and exercise physiologists who work in the School of Physiotherapy and Exercise Science at Curtin University. He is an Exercise and Sports Science Australia (ESSA) Level 2 accredited sports scientist (ASpS2) and is also an International Society for the Advancement of Kinanthropometry (ISAK) Level 3 (instructor) anthropometrist. He comes from a background of working with and researching on elite athletes, and this continues to be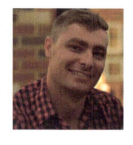
his predominant research and teaching focus. Kagan has previously completed a body of research on the effects of ergogenic aids on the performance of rowers, runners and team-sport athletes. He is currently exploring research in ergogenic aids, anthropometry and body composition in sports, the effect of mental toughness and resilience on physical activity and exercise performance issues in elite field hockey.

Kate Fuller Kate Fuller is the manager of the Australian Institute of Sport's National Sport Science Quality Assurance (NSSQA) Program. The NSSQA Program assumes a national leadership role in overseeing quality assurance in the delivery of sports science services to athletes and coaches through the national network involved in the assessment of Olympic-, national- and state-level athletes in Australia. The NSSQA accreditation programmes help to promote continuous improvement in testing stan-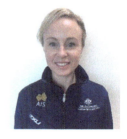
dards and ensure that services provided by 'accredited' laboratories/facilities are of the highest quality and test results are reliable and accurate. Kate joined the NSSQA Program in 2006 and took on the managerial role in 2014. Kate is an ISAK Level 3 anthropometrist and has an extensive background working as a physiologist in the elite sport sector, corporate health industry and sleep disorders field.

Stephen C. Hollings Dr. Stephen Hollings is a research associate with Sports Performance Research Institute New Zealand (SPRINZ), Auckland University of Technology, New Zealand. Stephen's research focuses on performance progression and athlete transition. Stephen was previously a lecturer in physical education at the University of Liverpool (UK), before moving to New Zealand to become director of physical recreation at the University of Auckland.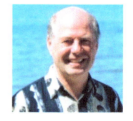
Stephen was the J.E. Lindsay Carter Kinanthropometry Clinic and Archive sports science educator for 2013–2014, with responsibility for the maintenance of archive materials. Steve is a British Olympian (Munich 1972 in 3000 m steeplechase). He was director of coaching and director of high performance for Athletics New Zealand and is currently their statistician. Stephen was the senior manager for coach and officials education with the International Association of Athletics Federations (IAAF) at their headquarters in Monaco, returning to New Zealand in 2003 to become the director of the IAAF's Oceania High Performance Training Centre.

Masaharu Kagawa Masaharu Kagawa is associate professor of the Institute of Nutrition Sciences at Kagawa Nutrition University in Japan. Masa was awarded his Ph.D. in public health from Curtin University of Technology, Australia. Masa is a registered public health nutritionist of the Nutrition Society of Australia (NSA) and the first Japanese Level 3 (instructor) anthropometrist accredited by the International Society for the Advancement of Kinanthropometry (ISAK). Masa's research interests include all topics associated with anthropometry and body composition assessments in the fields of public health and nutrition, particularly in relation to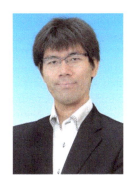
obesity and health screening, body image, maternal and child health and sports science. Masa has been involved in a number of cross-ethnic, cross-cultural studies, including international multi-centred collaborative projects on childhood obesity and assessments of elite athletes at the Sydney 2000 Olympic Games. Masa was appointed deputy director of the Institute of Nutrition Sciences in 2015. He has also been appointed as an adjunct professor of the Faculty of Public Health at Mahidol University in Thailand, a visiting associate professor of the School of Public Health at Curtin University in Australia, an adjunct associate professor of the School of Exercise and Nutrition Sciences and a member of the Institute of Health and Biomedical Innovation (IHBI) at Queensland University of Technology (QUT) in Australia.

Justin W.L. Keogh Justin Keogh is an associate professor in the Faculty of Health Sciences and Medicine, Bond University, Australia. Justin's research focuses on using the disciplines of biomechanics and skill acquisition to obtain greater insight into the acute effects and chronic adaptations resulting from resistance training and ways to improve the transfer of resistance and skill-based training to competitive performance. A recent emphasis of this research has been in strongman competitions and the AFL. Justin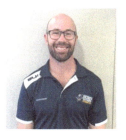
was the head coach of the Paralympic New Zealand powerlifting team from 2006 to 2009. He is currently the coordinator of the master of sports science programme at Bond University. Justin is a fellow of the International Society of Biomechanics in Sport as well as the Australian Association of Gerontology. Justin is a member of the Exercise and Sports Science Australia Research Committee and the Australian Strength and Conditioning Association Conference Committee. He is currently on the editorial board of several journals including the *Journal of Strength and Conditioning Research* and *PeerJ*.

Ava Kerr Ava Kerr is the manager of Health, Sport and Exercise Science Facilities at the University of the Sunshine Coast. She leads a technical services team to support delivery of teaching and research activities within sports and exercise science and nutrition and dietetics programmes. Ava is completing her Ph.D. on body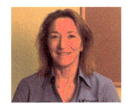

composition assessment methods and is passionate about best practice and quality control strategies to minimise measurement error. Ava is an accredited exercise scientist with Exercise and Sports Science Australia, an ISAK3 instructor and an Australian and New Zealand Bone and Mineral Society clinical densitometry technician. Ava is a Level 2 strength and conditioning coach with the Australian Strength and Conditioning Association and a certified strength and conditioning coach with the National Strength and Conditioning Association.

Stephven Kolose Stephven is a human factors researcher for Defence Technology Agency, New Zealand Defence Force (NZDF). He has developed and implemented NZDF's first tri-service anthropometry survey. Stephven is also enrolled in a Ph.D. programme at SPRINZ, Auckland University of Technology. His thesis is designed to examine the literature on 3D body scanning in large-scale military anthropometric surveys, review international survey protocols and measurement validation procedures and then apply this knowledge to the New Zealand Defence Force survey 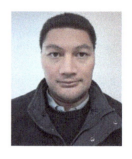 and potential applications for temporal trends, clothing fit and other kinanthropometric characteristics.

Anna V. Lorimer Dr. Anna Lorimer is a researcher within the Sports Performance Research Institute New Zealand (SPRINZ), Auckland University of Technology, New Zealand. Anna is the webmaster for the J.E. Lindsay Carter Kinanthropometry Clinic and Archive. Anna, as a long-distance triathlete, coach and biomechanist, is able to use anthropometry to monitor the effectiveness of training and dietary interventions.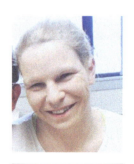

Duncan J. Macfarlane Having gained his double-major B.Sc. (physiology and biochemistry; first-class honours in physiology) and B.Ph.Ed. at Otago University, Duncan Macfarlane was a Commonwealth scholar at University College, Oxford, where he obtained his D.Phil. in respiratory physiology. He held the post of lecturer in the School of Physical Education at the University of Otago from 1986 to 1993. He then joined the University of Hong Kong in 1994 and is currently associate professor and head of ser- 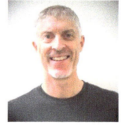 vice (Centre for Sports and Exercise)—having previously been the director of the Institute of Human Performance. His research focuses on quantifying precise/novel measurements of physical activity and body composition, including body image. He is an editorial board member of the *Journal of Sports Sciences* and the *International Journal of Behavioral Nutrition and Physical Activity*, a fellow of the American College of Sports Medicine and a Level 3 accredited anthropometrist with ISAK (International Society for the Advancement of Kinanthropometry).

Kristen L. MacKenzie-Shalders Dr. Kristen MacKenzie-Shalders currently leads the sports nutrition component of the master of nutrition and dietetics practice programme at Bond University (Australia). She is an accredited practising dietitian, advanced sports dietitian and accredited sports scientist who has worked within, and consulted to, elite sport programmes for over a decade. Her Ph.D. thesis was entitled 'Energy and Protein Intake in Developing Male Football Players: Nutritional Solutions for Optimal Performance and Body Composition Outcomes', and her 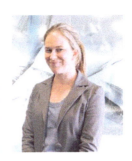 research interests include energy metabolism, protein metabolism, body composition, applied sports nutrition, athlete development, weight management and technological advances in nutrition/athlete monitoring. Kristen has completed her Level 3 ISAK accreditation and has technical and research expertise in a range of body composition assessment methods.

Wolfram Müller Wolfram Müller is professor of medical physics and biophysics at the Department of Biophysics, Medical University of Graz, Austria. His research fields include biophysics, medical physics, development of measurement techniques, body composition and anthropometry, sports medicine and exercise physiology, training sciences, 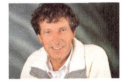 biomechanics, sport physics and sport aerodynamics. Wolfram was founding president of the International Association of Sciences in Medicine and Sports, coordinator of the IOC Working Group on Body Composition, Health and Performance (2009–2015), director of the Centre of Human Performance Research Graz (2007–2011), research leader of the IOC Prize Award Project Underweight Problems in Sports (2002 Olympic Games, UT, USA) and visiting professor at the Department of Bioengineering and at the Cardiovascular Research and Training Institute at the University of Utah (2000–2001). He has supported elite athletes and Olympic medallists (alpine skiing, ski jumping, Nordic combined, bobsleigh, sailing, gymnastics), was coach of the Austrian National Skiing Team (1980–1983), has worked as a coach in artistic gymnastics and has developed physical exercise programmes for the general public.

Alisa Nana Alisa Nana completed her Ph.D. through RMIT University in 2013. Her Ph.D. research was undertaken at the Australian Institute of Sport (AIS) and examined the reliability of dual-energy X-ray absorptiometry in assessing body composition in elite athletes. Alisa then became the Physique and Fuel Centre dietitian at the AIS and was the main dual-energy X-ray absorptiometry technician who has undertaken over a thousand bone mineral density and body composition scans in athletes. Alisa is currently a lecturer in sports nutrition at the College of Sports Science and Technology at Mahidol University, Thailand. She is an 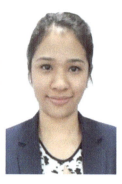 accredited practising dietitian and an accredited sports dietitian and is currently one of the main consulting sports dietitians at the Sports Authority of Thailand.

Clinton O. Njoku Clinton Ogbonnaya Njoku is a senior lecturer in the Department of Anatomy at Ebonyi State University, Abakaliki, Nigeria. His research interest borders on osteology, body composition and obesity which he assesses using varieties of body composition techniques. He was recently trained for assessing body composition through air-displacement plethysmography (Bod Pod), 3D photonic scanning and ultrasound between May 2015 and June 2016 at Robert Gordon University, Aberdeen, UK, under the supervision of Dr. Arthur D. Stewart. He is in charge of the Anatomical Measurement and Body Composition Unit of the College of Health Sciences, Ebonyi 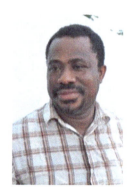 State University, Abakaliki, Nigeria. Clinton is a member of professional bodies of anatomy and body composition.

Helen O'Connor Helen O'Connor is an associate professor in sports nutrition. Her current research interests include metabolism and weight management, particularly in young women and in using novel exercise interventions for metabolic syndrome and fatty liver disease. Helen is also researching the impact of iron deficiency and obesity on cognition. As an ISAK Level 3 anthropometrist, Helen also has an interest in body composition and anthropometry. In the area of nutrition for sports performance, Helen's research focuses on hydration and thermoregula- 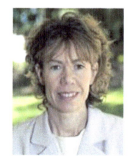 tion and interventions to minimise nutritional risk in elite athletes. Helen coordinates four units of study in nutrition for the Faculty of Health Science and is course director for the combined and double degree in exercise science and nutrition and dietetics, both of which are across faculty programmes with the Faculties of Health Science and Science. Themes of research include exercise, health and performance.

Elaine C. Rush Elaine Rush, MNZM, is professor of nutrition at the Faculty of Health and Environmental Sciences, Auckland University of Technology. Elaine has been involved in health and education for all her working career, and in 2014 she was appointed as a member of the New Zealand Order of Merit for services to health. Her diverse research expertise in the measurement of body 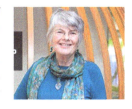 composition, energy expenditure, physical activity, nutrition and risk factors for disease and interest in ethnic differences in health and involvement in programmes and actions that will make a difference particularly for the health of Māori, Pacific and South Asian New Zealand people across the lifecycle have led to over 150 publications. The projects she is involved in include Energize in preschools and primary schools reaching more than 70,000 children, the health and growth of children whose mothers had gestational diabetes and the longitudinal Pacific Island Family study which is tracking over 1000 Pacific children from birth. She is scientific director of the New Zealand Nutrition Foundation.

Greg Shaw Greg Shaw is a senior sports dietitian at the Australian Institute of Sport, Canberra, Australia. He has worked with a range of elite and age group athletes, monitoring their growth and maturation and designing nutrition programmes to help them develop a performance physique. Greg is a Level 3 anthropometrist who works with staff and students to maintain skills in kinanthropometry. He is particularly interested in the numerous techniques and technologies available to monitor changes in an athlete's physique.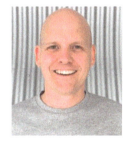

Kelly R. Sheerin Kelly Sheerin is lecturer in the Faculty of Health and Environmental Sciences and a researcher within the Sports Performance Research Institute New Zealand (SPRINZ), Auckland University of Technology, New Zealand. Kelly has an M.H.Sc. (Hons.), a B.Sc. in sports and exercise science and psychology and a B.H.Sc. in physiotherapy. Kelly is a clinically active physiotherapist and sports scientist who heads the Sports Performance Clinics and is also deputy director of the SPRINZ J.E. Lindsay Carter Kinanthropometry Clinic and Archive. Kelly's broad research focus is on the impact of injury prevention interventions on a 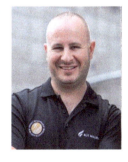 wide range of sporting disciplines. Kelly is currently undertaking his Ph.D. bringing together injury prevention, anthropometry, sports biomechanics and cutting-edge technology to provide real-time gait retraining to reduce tibial stress injury risk in runners.

Gary Slater Gary Slater is an advanced accredited sports dietitian and sports physiologist who has been working in elite sport since 1996. Gary currently splits his time between coordinating a master's degree in sports nutrition at the University of the Sunshine Coast and his role as national performance nutrition coordinator for the Australian Rugby Union. He also consults to professional teams, including the Queensland Reds and Queensland Academy of Sport, and an array of individual elite and recreational athletes, focusing on nutrition strategies that are performance driven. His professional interests relate primarily to enhancing sports performance. Gary is particularly passionate about 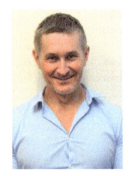 factors influencing muscle protein metabolism and muscle hypertrophy/atrophy, nutritional recovery strategies, ergogenic aids and the influence of body composition on sports performance. Gary is an International Society for the Advancement of Kinanthropometry (ISAK) Level 3 instructor and Australian and New Zealand Bone and Mineral Society (ANZBMS) clinical densitometry technician.

Arthur D. Stewart Dr. Arthur Stewart is a reader in health sciences at Robert Gordon University. Arthur's research encompasses anatomical body measurement in relation to human performance, health and the working environment, using a wide range of techniques. These have traditionally included anthropometry, dual-energy X-ray absorptiometry and magnetic resonance imaging but more recently have focused on ultrasound and 3D photonic scanning and related body size to ergonomics and safety. With over 33 years in academia, he has authored over 100 publica- 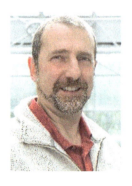 tions involving studies with international athletes, eating-disordered and obese patients and healthy adults and specific occupational groups. He remains a criterion anthropometrist of the International Society for the Advancement of Kinanthropometry and was vice-president from 2008 to 2014, was formerly the editor of the *Journal of Sports Sciences* Kinanthropometry and Body Composition section (2006–2012) and is a member of the Ad Hoc Working Group on Body Composition, Health and Performance for the International Olympic Committee's Medical and Scientific Commission.

Part I

Why Measure Physique?

Sport performance and sport injury risk may be affected by physique. Selection for sport may be enhanced using physique. Monitoring growth may help reduce injury risk. The effectiveness of training and nutrition programmes may be assessed via changes in physique. Physique characteristics of elite athletes may be an indicator of success in sport. There are gender and ethnic differences in physique. Sports-specific differences in body composition exist. These are some of the reasons why physique is measured as outlined in part I chapters which include discussion of physique assessment in youth sports for talent identification and development, monitoring developing athlete's anthropometry, growth and health, optimising anthropometry for sport performance and anthropometry for sports equipment design and fit.

Chapter 1
Physique Assessment in Youth Sports for Talent Identification and Development

Patria A. Hume and Arthur D. Stewart

Abstract Kinanthropometry can be useful in youth sports for talent development and improving sports performance. We consider the relationship between structure (as measured by anthropometry), physiology, psychology and skill for talent identification and how using these factors in isolation may risk overlooking potential champions. There must be care in predicting future adult performances based on adolescent testing because of the varied stability of physical traits during growth, especially surrounding adolescence. Segment breadths remain stable in relation to stature throughout adolescence and can be used for predictive purposes; however, segment lengths are unstable and should not be used as prediction criteria in talent identification programmes. Proportionality can be an important self-selector for sports. We outline how to predict adult size and proportions from the growing child, how there can be optimal size and proportions for the ideal performance (morphological optimisation) in sport and how athletes can tailor soft tissue for maximum functional effectiveness by training, tapering, etc. (morphological prototype). We examine how performance might be enhanced or retarded by biological maturity and how biological maturity is affected by energy balance in the young athlete—delaying maturation in some groups. Early maturers are often taller, heavier, more powerful and faster than their counterparts during the early to mid-teenage years, which has often led to selection biases in sporting competitions grouped by chronological age. Coaches need to consider anthropometric characteristics to avoid biasing their athlete selection.

P.A. Hume (✉)
Sport Performance Research Institute New Zealand,
Auckland University of Technology, Auckland, New Zealand
e-mail: patria.hume@aut.ac.nz

A.D. Stewart
Robert Gordon University, Aberdeen, UK
e-mail: a.d.stewart@rgu.ac.uk

© Springer Nature Singapore Pte Ltd. 2018
P.A. Hume et al. (eds.), *Best Practice Protocols for Physique Assessment in Sport*,
https://doi.org/10.1007/978-981-10-5418-1_1

Keywords Kinanthropometry • Youth sports • Talent development • Potential champions • Predicting • Physical traits • Growth • Adolescence • Proportionality Morphological optimisation • Morphological prototype • Biological maturity Energy balance • Maturation • Chronological age • Anthropometric characteristics Athlete selection

1.1   Optimal Size and Proportions for the Ideal Performance (Morphological Optimisation)

Sports performance generally involves maximising force, acceleration, speed or mechanical efficiency. In fulfilment of these biomechanical imperatives, there are optimal size and proportions underpinning the ideal performance in sport, referred to as *morphological optimisation*. Some sports have morphology-related limiting factors that prevent players from reaching elite levels (e.g. gymnastics, weightlifting, court sports and contact sports), while other sports seem to have few morphology-related limiting factors (e.g. racquet sports, mobile field sports and set field sports).

Morphology-related limiting factors are prevalent in elite competitors in gymnastics, diving and power sports, where performance may be limited by angular acceleration. Gymnasts and divers are typically the smallest and lightest of all sports people, with a high ratio of sitting height to stature caused by shorter than average lower limb lengths. Historically, world-class performances have been achieved in these sports in children still to attain adult stature. Weightlifters and powerlifters have a high ratio of sitting height to stature caused by shorter than average upper and lower limb lengths and low crural and brachial indexes (i.e. a short distal segment) (Keogh et al. 2009). Distance runners are short and light athletes with relatively short lower limbs and a high crural index and a low brachial index. A low skelic index appears characteristic of female strength athletes, while a low brachial index is typical of female endurance and strength athletes. These findings are congruent with biomechanical imperatives to maximise force and/or minimise energy expenditure offering sports-specific advantage (Stewart et al. 2010).

In athletic field events such as discus and javelin, competitors are generally tall and possess a high brachial index. Jumpers have a high relative lower limb length and a high crural index which provide a mechanically advantageous lever system for jumping. Court sports, such as basketball, netball and volleyball, have athletes that rely on jumping prowess and must have a linear physique and a high relative lower limb length. These athletes typically have a low ratio of sitting height to stature caused by longer than average lower limb lengths. These ratios vary significantly according to team position (e.g. in basketball players). Contact field sports such as rugby and football are affected by body size with several specialist positions requiring tall stature and increased body mass, where absolute rather than relative power is paramount.

Several morphology-related limiting factors exist for aquatic sports. Elite sprint and slalom paddlers generally possess a high brachial index which delivers greater leverage. World championship performance in swimming is influenced by tall stature and absolute limb lengths and the size of hands and feet. Tall, linear physiques provide some advantage for tennis players on certain playing surfaces, but smaller more agile players can be more successful on the slower clay court. Tall, linear physiques are an advantage for fast bowlers in cricket to increase the lever length in ball delivery. Tall, linear physiques may also be an advantage for soccer players in certain playing positions such as in goal-scoring opportunities from a goal kick, while smaller more agile soccer players tend to be more successful in other roles. Combative sports vary in their ideal physiques, by counterpoising the advantage offered by reach and a linear physique (as in taekwondo) with that offered by a low centre of mass and consequent stability of a broader physique (as in wrestling and judo) (Ackland et al. 2009).

Taken together, these structural advantages offered by skeletal factors which do not respond to athletic training have implications for selectivity of sports in which athletes are likely to excel. This does not preclude success of anatomically disadvantaged individuals; it merely requires that some physiological or psychological factors can negate the disadvantage resulting from morphological factors. Knowledge of the morphology-related limiting factors can be useful for selection criteria for youth athletes when entering a sport—as long as the measurements are stable during youth and adolescence or valid prediction methods are available based on sound research including longitudinal data analyses.

1.2 Tailoring Soft Tissue for Maximum Functional Effectiveness by Training (Morphological Prototype)

With the essential skeletal framework largely determined genetically, how can athletes fine-tune the physique for optimal performance? Bodily tissues can be theoretically grouped as 'active' or 'ballast' whether they enhance or retard force generation. Extra muscle for strength must be 'worth its own weight', and relative strength has been shown to scale to mass raised to the power 0.69, with composition assumed to be constant. Some muscle groups are rate limiters for force production, while others are merely passive. Altering strength in one group alters length-tension relationships and inertial properties and may destabilise joints and lead to injury. With current emphasis on core stability for several sports, in others, such as flat racing or time trial cycling, adding mass to the upper body may be considered a disadvantage.

In contrast to the law of specificity of training affecting muscle, adipose tissue responds to the body's energy balance in a more general way. Excess adipose tissue stored as an energy surplus will adversely affect performance in most sports. However, viewed as an endocrine organ responsible for the production of biomolecules implicated in our general health, we should be careful to ensure the athlete's health (and in female athletes, specifically reproductive health) is not threatened as a result of training which seeks to optimise sports performance. However, an athlete's physique responds to the periodisation in a training programme in a dynamic way, by adjusting adipose tissue, muscle tissue, glycogen stores and water balance. This phenomenon was first described in relation to the proximity to Olympic competition in ice skaters as *morphological prototype*. Anthropometric tools have been used in profiling athletes' trajectory, thereby optimising the trainable parameters at times when they mattered most. This has important implications for weight category sports, where athletes may be at risk of employing unsafe weight control practices in order to 'make weight'.

1.3 Anticipating Adult Morphology in the Growing Child

We have considered factors which prevail concerning adult performance, each exerting its independent influence, so now we consider factors affecting morphology and the potential for growth at any time point before adulthood. This is not straightforward as there needs to be consideration of predicting adult size, in addition to biological maturation, each with consequences for performance.

Skeletal age assessment—perhaps the most reliable of maturation indices—incurs X-ray exposure and ethical issues. Assessment of secondary sex characteristics is considered intrusive, and self-assessment may be unreliable, and serial measurements of stature required to identify peak height velocity may not be possible or valid. Although females generally mature earlier than males, large individual variability confounds easy prediction of final stature. A viable alternative involves a validated equation by Mirwald et al. (2002) based on the mean peak height velocity (~13.45 years in boys and ~11.77 years in girls in their sample) and its relation to sitting height and leg length and their interaction. A maturity offset regression predicts the time from peak height velocity in cross-validated gender-specific regressions, so final stature can be anticipated, knowing the likelihood of the remaining growth trajectory. Such an estimate can then be coupled with morphological optimisation prospectively in talent identification.

Sexual maturation profoundly affects morphology and sports performance. In school sports settings, early maturers may excel in team sports as a result of size and speed advantages, and sexual dimorphism alters the power to weight ratio during adolescence positively in males and usually negatively in females, with consequences for power sports. Because it may take 4 or more years for 95% of children to pass the same maturation 'milestone', it is unsurprising that the process may disguise athletic talent, with the result that early-maturing females and late-maturing males are easily overlooked.

1.4 Kinanthropometry and Talent Identification and Development for Sports Performance

Talent *identification* describes the scientific process used to identify talent. Talent *detection* is the process used to identify talent from outside the sport, and talent *selection* allows the identification of talent from within the sport. Talent *development* is where those with identified talent are provided with opportunity to achieve full potential. Kinanthropometry can be useful in youth sports for talent detection, selection and development programmes.

Comparisons between the best athletes and the rest of the athletes have shown anthropometric differences that may be useful for talent identification. Normative data (e.g. body mass, height and fat) for athletes in a form that may be used to develop profiles are useful in the processes of talent identification and body composition modification.

Examples of elite athlete cross-sectional profile data are from the 1976 Montreal Summer Olympics (Carter et al. 1982), 2000 Sydney Olympic rowing (Hebbelinck et al. 1981) and slalom canoe and kayak (Ridge et al. 2007), and winter Olympic sports (Stanula et al. 2013). Some studies have provided multi-year comparisons, while other studies have provided longitudinal data to enable descriptions of body characteristics over time with the changing nature of sport. For example, in the Sydney 2000 study of kayak paddlers, the male slalom paddlers were older, lighter, shorter, and leaner than previously reported slalom paddlers. Female slalom paddlers were taller, lighter, older, and less fat than those reported previously. Changes to the technical aspect of the events and to competition rules, and the nature and approach to training, can be reasons for body composition changes over time (Ridge et al. 2007). Historical changes in the size and age of 14 US women's Olympic gymnastic teams (a total of 106 team members) from 1956 to 2008 have shown that since 1956, height, mass, age, body mass index and team Olympic rank have been declining (Sands et al. 2012). However, in the last four Olympic Games, the size of the US women's gymnasts increased. The minimum-age rule modifications may have played a role in gymnast size changes. Given there are changes in body composition over time, it is important to look at recent body composition data in relation to performance and therefore talent identification.

Often in an attempt to determine anthropometric characteristics that may be useful for screening youth athletes, comparisons are made between youth and elite athletes or athlete and nonathletes. For example, morphological analyses of 6 female and 18 male youth tennis players compared to their nonsport peers showed that the majority of youth tennis players were taller and had longer lower limbs and lower amounts of adipose tissue and larger arm circumferences compared to their nonsport peers (Bojzan et al. 2008). Prediction functions have been developed for variables that distinguish best between talented and less talented team sports players aged 11–16 years in rugby, soccer, field hockey and netball (Spamer and Coetzee 2002). While these types of comparisons are useful in tracking youths towards elite performance, the individual variability in growth, lack of stability of measures throughout adolescence and limited predictability of performance from unidimensional data mean that their utility is limited.

1.5 Biological Maturity and Effects on Performance

Performance can be enhanced or retarded by biological maturity. Biological maturity is affected by energy balance in the young athlete delaying maturation in some groups. Early maturers are often taller, heavier, more powerful and faster than their counterparts during the early to mid-teenage years which has often led to selection biases in sporting competitions grouped by chronological age. Anderson and Ward (2002) proposed a classification system for youth sports that is maturation based, using the anthropometric prediction of vertical jump impulse potential. Impulse was calculated for children between 8 and 18 years from vertical jump height ($I = m[2gh]^{0.5}$). Equations were developed that accounted for differences in muscle tissue development while utilising variables easily measured in both males and females, including age and measures of height, forearm girth and calf girth. Using restricted ranges of impulse scores, males and females could be classed into appropriate groups for competition and sport, competing together until the age of 14. At and beyond this age, females had a similar capacity to generate impulse and could compete in one group, while restricted impulse categories could be useful for males until the age of 18 years.

Coelho e Silva et al. (2003) assessed physical growth and maturation-related variation in 112 Portuguese young male soccer players. The effect of chronological age on body size was evident within the 11–12-year group and 13–14-year group, while the effect of maturational status on motor performance was only significant within the older group. The reduced variation in older boys reflects approaching maturity in late adolescence.

Hirose (2009) examined physical and maturational differences between 332 adolescent elite soccer players who were considered to have high potential to play soccer at a professional level as decided subjectively by coaches. There was a bias according to the month of birth which influenced differences in individual skeletal age and body size. The height of players born in the last quarter of the year was significantly smaller than that of players born in the first quarter of the year when data were adjusted for maturation. Hirose recommended that individual biological maturation should be considered when selecting adolescent soccer players.

1.6 Predicting Future Adult Performances Based on Adolescent Testing

Caution is advised when predicting future adult performances based on adolescent testing because of the varied stability of physical traits during adolescent growth. Segment breadths remain relatively stable throughout adolescence and can be used for predictive purposes; however, segment lengths are usually unstable and should not be used as prediction criteria for talent identification. However, this variability (e.g. a 6% change in leg length to sitting height ratio) can form the basis for a final stature prediction based on the maturity offset (Mirwald et al. 2002).

Changing morphology of the growing athlete and the skill level acquired are inevitably interlinked, so models which combine dimensional measures with skill are warranted. A multidisciplinary selection model for youth soccer was developed by Vaeyens et al. (2006) based on analyses of relationships between physical (anthropometry and maturity status), sport-specific performance characteristics and level of skill in elite, sub-elite, and nonelite youth soccer players in four age groups between 12 and 16 years. Characteristics that discriminated successful youth soccer players varied with competitive age levels. The clear implication is that talent identification models should be flexible and provide opportunities for changing parameters in a long-term developmental context.

1.7 The Relationship Between Structure, Physiology, Psychology and Skill for Talent Identification

Complex and dynamic interrelationships between anatomical structure, physiology, psychology and skill prevail in sport. If any of these factors are used for talent identification in isolation, there is a risk of overlooking potential winners; an important principle that the scientific and coaching communities have been slow to appreciate. A range of relevant anthropometric factors can be considered which are subject to strong genetic influences (e.g. stature) or are largely environmentally determined and susceptible to training effects. Consequently, anthropometric profiling can generate a useful database against which talented groups may be compared. However, anthropometric measurement alone does not provide a representative assessment of a player's physical capabilities in sports where open skills are influential. There may be marked individual differences in anthropometric and physiological characteristics among elite performers. For example, top-class soccer players have to adapt to the physical demands of the game, which are multifactorial. Players may not need to have an extraordinary capacity within any of the areas of physical performance but must possess a reasonably high level within all areas (Reilly et al. 2000).

Assessing body composition in the growing and developing individual is fraught with difficulty due to a range of issues. Increasing energy expenditure can reduce fat, while fat-free body mass can be maintained. However, the dual metabolic challenges of exercise and growth deplete the same reserve, violating methodological assumptions concerning stability of the fat-free body mass and rendering change detection problematic. Even though a range of methods suitable for children is available, including anthropometry and body density, accuracy in predicting fat and fat-free mass can be worse than assumed. In addition, individual variability is such that the threshold of performance impairment due to chronic depletion of energy reserves will tend to differ between individuals. In this context, the pragmatic solution is to align anthropometric data with those of performance, fatigue and general health. Coaches are best placed to do this after a full dialogue with both the athlete and the sports scientist.

1.8 Summary

The nature of talent identification is holistic. Coaches need to consider performance, skill and psychological factors and anthropometric factors which are growth related and training related and which anticipate adult morphology. Alignment of morphology to performance, and recognition of the wide individual variability in maturation rate, will help avoid biasing athlete selection or overlooking talented individuals with potential to excel.

References

Ackland TR, Kerr DA, Newton RU (2009) Modifying physical capacities. In: Ackland TA, Elliot BC, Bloomfield J (eds) Applied anatomy and biomechanics in sport, 2nd edn. Human Kinetics, Champaign, IL, pp 227–276

Anderson GS, Ward R (2002) Classifying children for sports participation based upon anthropometric measurement. Eur J Sport Sci 2(3):1–13

Bojzan A, Pietraszewska J, Migasiewicz J, Tomaszewski W, Bach W (2008) Selected anthropometric parameters of young tennis players in the context of the usefulness for this sports discipline and motor organ contusion prophylaxis. Med Sport 24(5):337–347

Carter JEL, Ross WD, Aubry SP, Hebbelinck M, Borms J (1982) Physical structure of Olympic athletes. Part 1: The Montreal Olympic games anthropological project. S. Karger, Basel

Coelho e Silva M, Figueiredo A, Malina RM (2003) Physical growth and maturation related variation in young male soccer athletes. Acta Kinesiol Univ Tartuensis 8:34–50

Hebbelinck M, Ross WD, Carter JE, Borms J (1981) Body build of female Olympic rowers. In: Borms J, Hebbelinck M, Venerando A (eds) Female athlete: a socio-psychological and kinanthropometric approach. Basel, S. Karger, pp 201–205

Hirose N (2009) Relationships among birth-month distribution, skeletal age and anthropometric characteristics in adolescent elite soccer players. J Sports Sci 27(11), 1159–1166

Keogh JWL, Hume PA, Mellow P, Pearson SN (2009) Can absolute and proportional anthropometric characteristics distinguish stronger and weaker powerlifters? J Strength Cond Res 23(8):2256–2265

Mirwald RL, Baxter-Jones ADG, Bailey DA, Beunen GP (2002) An assessment of maturity from anthropometric measurements. Med Sci Sports Exerc 34(4):689–694

Reilly T, Bangsbo J, Franks A (2000) Anthropometric and physiological predispositions for elite soccer. J Sports Sci 18(9):669–683

Ridge BR, Broad E, Kerr DA, Ackland TR (2007) Morphological characteristics of Olympic slalom canoe and kayak paddlers. Eur J Sport Sci 7(2):107–111

Sands WA, Slater C, McNeal JR, Murray SR, Stone MH (2012) Historical trends in the size of us olympic female artistic gymnasts. Int J Sports Physiol Perform 7(4):350–355

Spamer EJ, Coetzee M (2002) Variables which distinguish between talented and less talented participants in youth sport - a comparative study. Kinesiology 34(2):141–152

Stanula A, Roczniok R, Gabryś T, Szmatlan-gabryś U, Maszczyk A, Pietraszewski P (2013) Relations between BMI, body mass and height, and sports competence among participants of the 2010 winter Olympic games: does sport metabolic demand differentiate? Percept Mot Skills 117(3):837

Stewart AD, Benson PJ, Olds T, Marfell-Jones M, MacSween A, Nevill AM (2010) Self selection of athletes into sports via skeletal ratios. In: Lieberman DC (ed) Aerobic exercise and athletic performance: types, duration and health benefits. Nova Science Publishers, New York, NY

Vaeyens R, Malina RM, Janssens M, Van Renterghem B, Bourgois J, Vrijens J, Philippaerts RM (2006) A multidisciplinary selection model for youth soccer: the Ghent Youth Soccer Project. Br J Sports Med 40(11):928–934

Chapter 2
Anthropometry and Health for Sport

Masaharu Kagawa

Abstract This chapter describes current applications of anthropometry for the assessment of health and nutritional status, to monitor adequate growth and to screen for and diagnose lifestyle-related diseases. A healthy body is required if sport performance is to be maximized. Anthropometric measurements need to be undertaken by trained anthropometrists with appropriate knowledge in order to provide meaningful information on health and nutritional status of individuals and the target population.

Keywords Kinanthropometry • Health • Nutritional status • Monitoring • Growth • Screening • Lifestyle-related diseases • Body mass index • Obesity • Energy balance • Fat distribution • Metabolic syndrome • Waist circumference

2.1 Double Burden of Malnutrition: Malnourishment and Obesity

The World Health Organization defines health as a state of complete physical, mental, and social well-being and not merely the absence of disease or infirmity (World Health Organization 2006). Health is the fundamental component for growth, daily living, improved productivity, and the quality of life. A significant global health problem is the double burden of malnutrition that includes both under- and overnutrition. The World Health Organization reported that undernutrition was associated with 54% or 10.8 million child deaths in 2001 (Blössner and de Onis 2005), and also more than one billion adults in the world were estimated to be overweight and at least 300 million as clinically obese (World Health Organization 2002). Poor

M. Kagawa
Kagawa Nutrition University, Sakado, Japan
e-mail: mskagawa@eiyo.ac.jp

© Springer Nature Singapore Pte Ltd. 2018
P.A. Hume et al. (eds.), *Best Practice Protocols for Physique Assessment in Sport*,
https://doi.org/10.1007/978-981-10-5418-1_2

nutrition in utero leads to intrauterine growth restriction, resulting in low birth weight and greater risk of both physical and cognitive development. In addition, according to the developmental origin of health and disease theory (Gillman et al. 2007), the low birth weight infants may be at an increased risk of developing obesity-related chronic health problems, including cardiovascular diseases, type II diabetes mellitus, and various types of cancers later in life.

Maintenance of health is crucial in optimizing performance in physical activity, exercise, and in sports settings. Severely malnourished status may increase a risk of developing a number of health problems. As the phenomenon is common among female athletes, particularly those who participate in sports with an aesthetic component and different weight categories, it has been known as the female athlete triad (Morgenthal 2002). However, a number of studies have reported that male athletes also experience energy and nutrient deficiencies (Papadopoulou et al. 2012; Cole et al. 2005; Kagawa et al. 2014) and the International Olympic Committee (IOC) proposed in 2014 a concept of relative energy deficiency in sport (Mountjoy et al. 2014).

Excessive fat accumulation from positive energy balance is also known to affect physical performance. Subcutaneous adipose tissue as measured by skinfold thickness is associated with better performance in female athletes (Claessens et al. 1999; Kerr et al. 2007), and obesity is associated with biomechanical functions, including gait and balance (Wearing et al. 2006a, b; Del Porto et al. 2012). Both underweight and obesity also increase risk of injuries (Yard and Comstock 2011). Assessments of health status are therefore important for prevention and treatment of illness and for maintenance of physical fitness and to determine factors influencing physical performance.

2.2 Anthropometry as a Tool for Health Assessments

Anthropometry, including stature, body mass, skinfolds, and circumference measurements, provides an inexpensive, portable, convenient, and simple technique for individual health assessments and mass screening. Unlike imaging techniques, anthropometry cannot provide body composition and visceral fat distribution without using population-specific prediction equations. However, when conducted by individuals with appropriate skills using a standardized protocol, anthropometry and anthropometry-derived indices are suitable for large-scale screening.

2.2.1 Application of Stature and Body Mass in Health Assessments

Stature and body mass are associated with a wide range of health conditions. Inadequate energy and nutritional intake will result in retarded growth. Either together with or independent of genetic factors, nutritional status may influence dysfunctions of growth-related hormones (e.g., growth hormone, thyroid hormone, insulin-like growth factors, and estrogen). Hormonal dysfunctions are associated with conditions that have symptoms of abnormally short or tall stature, such as acromegaly, gigantism, dwarfism, and cretinism. Previous studies including systematic review and meta-analyses reported that tall stature is associated with the development of different types of cancers (Gunnell et al. 2001; Green et al. 2011; Kabat et al. 2013; Murphy et al. 2013). Assessment of stature and body mass is therefore a useful variable in identifying overall health status. Common approaches of utilizing stature and body mass include application of growth charts and calculation of relative weight-for-height and weight-to-height ratios.

Application of gender-specific curves for stature and body mass may be the most commonly used tools for assessment and monitoring of growth in children and adolescents. Inadequate state of growth has been described as stunting, wasting, underweight, and overweight, depending on differences in comparison variables. The term stunting is defined as a short stature in relation to the average of the same age and gender group, whereas underweight is defined as a small in body mass relative to the same age and gender group. The terms undernutrition and malnutrition were proposed (Waterlow 1972) to distinguish between weight-for-height (current nutritional status) and weight-for-age (past energy and nutritional history). The most commonly applied growth charts where local standards are not available are provided by the Center for Health Statistics and Centers for Disease Control task force (Hamill 1977) and by the World Health Organization (World Health Organization and United Nations Children's Fund 2009; Bloem 2007). These charts were revised in 2000 and 2006, respectively, and the United Nations Children's Fund (UNICEF) and the World Health Organization defined each condition of malnutrition for infants and children under 5 years (see Table 2.1) based on the proposed percentiles and z-scores. Adolescents and adults use different diagnostic criteria for severe malnutrition. For adolescents aged above 10 years, body mass index-for-age (below <5th percentile) or height-for-age (below <2nd percentile or -2 SD of the Center for Health Statistic/World Health Organization reference) has been used, whereas body mass index below 16 kg/m^2 and presence of edema have been used for adults (World Health Organization 1999).

Table 2.1 Diagnostic criteria for different conditions of malnutrition

Category	Definition
Stunting	2 SD below the height-for-age of the gender-matched population
Underweight	2 SD below the weight-for-age of the gender-matched population
Wasting	2 SD below the weight-for-height of the age- and gender-matched population
Overweight	2 SD above the weight-for-height of the age- and gender-matched population

Cited from United Nations Children's Fund et al. (2012)
SD standard deviation

A relative weight-for-height can be calculated as actual weight/reference weight × 100 and expressed as a percentage. A desirable weight using the table is usually set between 90% and 110% of the midpoint weight-for-height of a medium-framed individual by gender. Values below 90% are used to define underweight, between 110% and 120% as overweight, and above 120% as obese (Dalton 1997). The relative weight-for-height involves a number of considerations in its application. One major consideration is that the chart is limited to the year and study cohort at the time when the standard was developed. Therefore, it is important to consider that body size or the balance between body mass and stature of the population living today may be different from the time when the standard was developed. Also an increase in mortality (at a population level) for those who were outside of the normal or recommended range does not mean that individuals have high total or visceral body fat accumulation.

Among many weight-to-height ratios, including the ponderal index and the Kaup index, the body mass index may be the most common index. While body mass index was proposed in 1972 (Keys et al. 1972), the equation—mass (kg)/stature (m)^2—was originally proposed in 1832 and named the Quetelet index (Eknoyan 2008). In 1997, the World Health Organization chose to utilize body mass index as an index to assess overweight and obesity in adults (World Health Organization 1997), and the international classification scheme in Table 2.2 was proposed. Application of body mass index to children and adolescents has been considered inappropriate as their proportion changes as they grow. However, in order to allow international comparison for childhood obesity, the World Health Organization has established the International Obesity Task Force classification that provides gender- and age-specific body mass index cutoff points for lean, overweight, and obese categories (Cole et al. 2000; Cole et al. 2007).

Although body mass index was not originally proposed to identify obesity, body mass index has a quadratic relationship with percentage body fat in both genders (Jackson et al. 2002). Several large-scale epidemiological studies reported that body mass index is positively associated with a number of obesity-related chronic diseases, including cardiovascular diseases and type II diabetes mellitus (Boffetta et al. 2011; Global Burden of Metabolic Risk Factors for Chronic Diseases Collaboration

Table 2.2 The body mass index classification proposed by the World Health Organization for adults

Classification		Body mass index (kg/m^2)
Underweight	Severe underweight	<16.00
	Moderate underweight	16.00–16.99
	Mild underweight	17.00–18.49
Normal range		18.50–24.99
Overweight	Pre-obese	25.00–29.99
	Obese class I	30.00–34.99
	Obese class II	35.00–39.99
	Obese class III	≥40.00

Cited from World Health Organization (2000), WHO expert consultation (2004)

(BMI Mediated Effects) et al. 2014). A recent study using data from the National Health Interview Survey reported that the body mass index-mortality relationship is also quadratic (U-shape for men and J-shape for women) (Wong et al. 2011).

While body mass index has been utilized in assessments of overweight and obesity, it is important to appreciate that it is simply a measure of heaviness, not of fatness, as it does not use any measures of body composition. A classic study by Garn suggested three limitations of body mass index: (1) body mass index is stature dependent and in different directions at different points in the life cycle; (2) body mass index may be affected by relative leg length or relative sitting height; and (3) body mass index may reflect both lean and fat tissues to a comparable degree (Garn et al. 1986). Many studies have reported misclassification of individuals and variability in the relationship between body mass index and percentage body fat due to these limitations (Ross et al. 1988; Wang et al. 1994; Deurenberg et al. 1998; Kagawa et al. 2006; Rush et al. 2007). Such limitations are also applicable to other weight-to-height ratio, and therefore it is important to use these indices with caution, particularly when the index was applied to individuals and special population. For a better use of body mass index to different racial groups, the World Health Organization expert consultation proposed new cutoff points (i.e., 23 kg/m², 27.5 kg/m², 32.5 kg/m², and 37.5 kg/m²) as public health action points in 2004 (WHO expert consultation 2004).

2.2.2 Application for Assessment of Fat Distribution

The fat distribution pattern is affected by race, gender, age, genetic components, and lifestyle factors (Cornier et al. 2011). The effect of regional fat distribution was first reported in 1947 with terms android and gynoid used to differentiate individuals with upper-body fat accumulation and those with lower-body fat accumulation (Vague 1996). Later, four types of obesity that differ in fat accumulation pattern were defined (Bouchard 1991), thereby affecting the physique of individuals (see Table 2.3). Type II and type III obesity are often called the central obesity. Although fat distribution pattern is affected by a number of factors, women are more likely to develop gynoid-type obesity (Lemieux et al. 1993).

Table 2.3 Four types of obesity differed by fat distribution pattern

Type of obesity	Description
Type I	Excess body mass or percent fat without any particular concentration of fat in a given area of the body
Type II	Excess subcutaneous fat on the trunk, particularly in the abdominal area (android or apple-shaped obesity)
Type III	Excess abdominal visceral fat
Type IV	Excess fat on the truncal-abdominal or the gluteo-femoral area (gynoid or pear-shaped obesity)

Cited from Bouchard (1991)

Health risk differs between fat distribution patterns. Compared to type IV obesity, or gynoid obesity, the central obesity with a large amount of visceral fat accumulation has been associated with a number of metabolic abnormalities, including hypertension, hyperinsulinemia, and hyperlipidemia (Rasouli et al. 2007; Arsenault et al. 2012). These metabolic abnormalities increase the risk of developing cardiovascular diseases and type II diabetes mellitus (Arsenault et al. 2012), a condition generally known as metabolic syndrome (International Diabetes Federation 2006). In addition to an abdominal visceral fat, there are lipids that accumulate directly onto organs such as liver, heart, pancreas, and skeletal muscle tissues. These lipids are called ectopic fat and are considered as another risk factor for metabolic abnormalities (Rasouli et al. 2007; Arsenault et al. 2012).

Skinfold measurement is useful for assessment of subcutaneous fat distribution pattern. It was first used by Czech anthropologist Jindřich Matiegka in 1921 (Brozek and Prokopec 2001) and considered as a noninvasive, portable, and cost-effective approach that provides indication of both regional and overall subcutaneous fatness. Determining total body fatness and fat distribution using skinfold assessment may be useful in health assessments as approximately 40–60% of total body fat is considered to be accumulated subcutaneously (Wang et al. 2000). Studying 1410 participants aged 9–49 years, the amount and distribution of subcutaneous adipose tissue (SAT) and somatotype were important predictors of coronary heart diseases (Katzmarzyk et al. 1999). However, many reported correlations between indices from skinfolds and metabolic biomarkers were low to moderate (de Jongh et al. 2006; Tresaco et al. 2009). There are no international diagnosis criteria for overweight and obesity and for excessive visceral fat accumulation based on skinfolds that can be utilized to identify metabolic abnormalities. Skinfold values can be used to estimate body composition by using prediction equations. However, the estimated values should be handled with care as all prediction equations are population-specific.

Circumferences measure the size of a body region of interest that is composed of bone, lean, adipose, and residual tissues. With assumption of constant thickness of skin and subcutaneous adipose tissue accumulations surrounding lean tissues, a greater circumference for individuals of the same body size may indicate a greater visceral adipose tissue accumulation or a greater lean tissue development. Common circumference sites include the mid-upper arm circumference and waist circumference.

2.2.2.1 Mid-Upper Arm Circumference

The mid-upper arm circumference has been used widely as an indicator of protein-energy malnutrition. In 1966, mid-upper arm circumference was proposed as a useful surrogate parameter to assess nutritional status of children and provide a gender-specific reference for children aged between 1 and 60 months (Jelliffe 1966). Later, a classification for mid-upper arm circumference was proposed to distinguish a level of malnutrition for children (Shakir and Morley 1974). The classification has been commonly applied to children aged between 1 and 5 years as it has been considered that arm circumference remains relatively constant in this age range (Myatt et al. 2006). In their updated guideline, the World Health Organization proposed mid-upper arm circumference <115 mm and ≥125 mm as one of the conditions for immediate management of severe acute malnutrition and discharge from treatment, respectively, for infants and children aged between 6 and 59 months (World Health Organization 2013). In addition to infants and children, the mid-upper arm circumference has been utilized as part of the Mini Nutrition Assessment study for elderly aged above 60 years (Vellas et al. 1999; Vellas et al. 2006). Furthermore, a recent study has suggested that mid-upper arm circumference may be useful in screening for obesity among children aged 9–11 years (Chaput et al. 2016).

Measured mid-upper arm circumference can be utilized to calculate indices to estimate the amount of adipose and lean tissues in the region. Common indices include upper arm muscle diameter, muscle arm circumference or mid-arm muscle circumference, and upper arm fat and muscle areas (Jelliffe 1966; Frisancho and Garn 1971; Lukaski 1987; Gurney and Jelliffe 1973; Gurney 1969; Frisancho 1981). Calculation of these indices requires triceps skinfold. The indices are based on several assumptions that will affect estimation error. Gender is also an important variable in the calculation of anthropometric indices as gender-specific arm muscle area equations reduce average estimation errors by 7–8% when compared with data from computed tomography scans (Heymsfield et al. 1982).

2.2.2.2 Waist Circumference

Waist and abdominal circumferences are frequently used as surrogate measures of central obesity and visceral fat accumulation. While there are many anthropometric indices for assessing patterns of fat accumulation, waist circumference has become widely adopted due to its simplicity compared to other indices that require measurements at multiple sites and, more importantly, its better association with abdominal fat accumulation than other indices. In 1992, associations between computerized tomography and anthropometric variables including body mass index, waist circumference, and waist-to-hip ratio were examined using 28 obese participants (15 men and 13 women) and 33 normal weight or slightly overweight participants (23 men and 10 women) (Busetto et al. 1992). While waist circumference had moderate to strong correlations with total, visceral, and subcutaneous fat cross-sectional areas, regardless of gender, waist-to-hip ratio had weaker correlations, particularly among obese women. Although waist circumference is more strongly associated with abdominal subcutaneous adipose tissue rather than visceral adipose tissue (VAT) (Bosy-Westphal et al. 2010), waist circumference explains a large percentage of the variance in intra-abdominal adipose tissue (IAAT), a key risk factor for metabolic abnormalities and development of chronic diseases, among adults and children (Benfield et al. 2008; Berentzen et al. 2012).

Due to its strong association with fat accumulation and related metabolic abnormalities, waist circumference has been included in many diagnostic criteria of the metabolic syndrome, including those proposed by the European Group for the Study of Insulin Resistance (EGIR) and the National Cholesterol Education Program—Third Adult Treatment Panel (NCEP ATP III) (Alberti et al. 2006). These criteria are commonly adopted for global studies, though nation-specific diagnostic criteria (e.g., for Japanese) also exist (The Metabolic syndrome diagnostic criteria examination committee 2005). The International Diabetes Federation proposed international diagnostic criteria in 2006 (International Diabetes Federation 2006), and Table 2.4 presents a summary of differences between diagnostic criteria. Compared to adults, there is a dearth of research on appropriate waist circumference cutoff points compared for children and adolescents. Therefore, the International Diabetes Federation has proposed the use of the 90th percentile as the cutoff, instead of an absolute waist circumference value until further evidence became available (International Diabetes Federation 2007).

While waist circumference has been a key component of existing diagnostic criteria for metabolic syndrome, the criteria also indicate differences in waist circumference cutoff points. Several factors may contribute to these differences, including (1) the definition of waist used in the criteria, (2) differences in body size of the target population, and (3) racial differences in the association between waist circumference and VAT or metabolic pathways. Since waist circumference may be also influenced by posture, respiratory phase, meal time, and biological variables such as age, gender, and ethnicity, and consequently affects its association with metabolic biomarkers, most authors recommend standardizing the protocol for waist circumference (Agarwal et al. 2009; World Health Organization 2011).

Like mid-upper arm circumference, waist circumference can be utilized to compute a number of indices such as the waist-to-hip ratio, the waist-to-height ratio, and the waist-to-thigh ratio. While these indices are associated with chronic health problems and increase in body fat (Yusuf et al. 2005; Dalton et al. 2003; Welborn et al. 2003; Taylor et al. 2010; Kagawa et al. 2007; Lu et al. 2010; de Carvalho Vidigal et al. 2013), values obtained from these indices may be affected by the definition and protocol of the waist measurement. There is a lack of knowledge of differences in values and their associations with metabolic biomarkers and fat accumulations between circumference ratios using circumferences with different definitions (Kagawa et al. 2008).

2.3   Summary

This chapter describes current applications of anthropometry for the assessment of health and nutritional status. Understanding health and nutritional status is important in order to monitor adequate growth, to screen for and diagnose lifestyle-related diseases, and to optimize physical fitness and performance. Most anthropometric indices are noninvasive, cost-effective, convenient, and readily applicable in field and clinical settings. However, these indices do not directly measure body composition and metabolic markers, and therefore their validity and accuracy relative to the

Table 2.4 Differences in diagnostic criteria for the metabolic syndrome

Variables		WHO (1999)	EGIR (1999)	NCEP ATP III (2001)	Japanese criteria (2005)[a]	IDF (2006)
Key conditions		Impaired glucose intolerance (IGT) or diabetes and/or insulin resistance	Insulin resistance defined as hyperinsulinaemia	–	Central obesity defined as waist circumference[b]	Central obesity defined as waist circumference with ethnicity specific values[c]
Additionally diagnosed complications		Two or more	Two	Three or more	Two or more	Two or more
Obesity (Central obesity)	Body mass index	>30.0 kg/m²	–	–	–	>30.0 kg/m²
	Waist-to-hip ratio	Male: >0.90 Female: >0.85	–	–	–	–
	Waist circumference	–	Male: ≥94 cm Female: ≥80 cm	Male: >102 cm Female: >88 cm	Male: ≥85 cm Female: ≥90 cm	Ethnic- and gender-specific values[d]
Triglyceride		≥150 mg/dl	>178 mg/dl or treatment	≥150 mg/dl	≥150 mg/dl	≥150 mg/dl or specific treatment for this lipid abnormality
HDL cholesterol		Male: <35 mg/dl Female: <39 mg/dl	<39 mg/dl or treatment	Male: <40 mg/dl Female: <50 mg/dl	<40 mg/dl	Male: <40 mg/dl Female: <50 mg/dl or specific treatment for this lipid abnormality
Blood pressure		Systolic: ≥140 mm Hg Diastolic: ≥90 mm Hg	Systolic: ≥ 140 mm Hg Diastolic: ≥ 90 mm Hg or treatment	Systolic: ≥130 mm Hg Diastolic: ≥ 85 mm Hg	Systolic: ≥130 mm Hg Diastolic: ≥85 mm Hg	Systolic: ≥130 mm Hg Diastolic: ≥85 mm Hg or treatment of previously diagnosed hypertension

(continued)

Table 2.4 (continued)

Variables	WHO (1999)	EGIR (1999)	NCEP ATP III (2001)	Japanese criteria (2005)[a]	IDF (2006)
Fasting blood glucose	–	>110 mg/dl but non-diabetic	≥100 mg/dl[c]	≥110 mg/dl	≥100 mg/dl or diagnosed type II diabetes mellitus
Microalubuminuria	Urinary albumin excretion rate ≥ 20 µg/min or Albumin: creatinine ratio ≥ 30 mg/g	–	–	–	–

Cited from Alberti et al. (2006), the Metabolic syndrome diagnostic criteria examination committee (2005), and International Diabetes Federation (2006)
WHO World Health Organization, *EGIR* the European Group for the Study of Insulin Resistance, *NCEP ATP III* the National Cholesterol Education Program—Third Adult Treatment Panel, *IDF* the International Diabetes Federation

[a]These criteria were proposed by the Japan Society for the Study of Obesity, Japan Atherosclerosis Society, Japan Diabetes Society, Japanese Society of Hypertension, Japanese Circulation Society, Japanese Society of Nephrology, Japanese Society on Thrombosis and Hemostasis, and Japanese Society of Internal Medicine

[b]It is preferred to conduct visceral fat assessment using computer tomography (CT) or similar methods. Waist circumference was measured at the level of the umbilicus while standing and during expiration

[c]If the participant had body mass index > 30.0 kg/m^2, a central obesity can be assumed and thus the waist circumference does not need to be measured

[d]Europids: ≥94 cm for males and ≥80 cm for females; South Asians, Chinese, and Japanese: ≥90 cm for males and ≥80 cm for females; For sub-Saharan Africans, Eastern Mediterranean, and Middle East (Arab) populations, use European data until more specific data are available; For Ethnic South and Central Americans, use South Asian recommendations until more specific data are available

[e]The criteria for fasting blood glucose was modified in 2004 from ≥110 mg/dl

target variable may vary between populations of interest. It is important to confirm the relationship and applicability of these indices prior to administration. Care is required with the measurement protocol, site definitions, and equipment used, in order to allow comparison between studies or samples. Most importantly, accuracy and reliability of anthropometry is largely dependent upon the skill of the anthropometrist. Therefore, anthropometric measurements need to be undertaken by trained anthropometrist with appropriate knowledge in order that obtained variables and calculated indices provide meaningful information on health and nutritional status of individuals and the target population.

References

Agarwal SK, Misra A, Aggarwal P, Bardia A, Goel R, Vikram NK, Wasir JS, Hussain N, Ramachandran K, Pandey RM (2009) Waist circumference measurement by site, posture, respiratory phase, and meal time: implications for methodology. Obesity (Silver Spring, MD) 17(5):1056–1061

Alberti KGMM, Zimmet P, Shaw J (2006) Metabolic syndrome - a new world-wide definition. A Consensus Statement from the International Diabetes Federation. Diabet Med 23(5):469–480

Arsenault BJ, Beaumont EP, Després JP, Larose E (2012) Mapping body fat distribution: a key step towards the identification of the vulnerable patient? Ann Med 44(8):758–772

Balkau B, Charles MA (1999) Comment on the provisional report from the WHO consultation. European Group for the Study of Insulin Resistance (EGIR). Diabetic Medicine 16(5): 442–443.

Benfield LL, Fox KR, Peters DM, Blake H, Rogers I, Grant C, Ness A (2008) Magnetic resonance imaging of abdominal adiposity in a large cohort of British children. Int J Obes (Lond) 32(1):91–99

Berentzen TL, Ängquist L, Kotronen A, Borra R, Yki-Järvinen H, Iozzo P, Parkkola R, Nuutila P, Ross R, Allison DB, Heymsfield SB, Overvad K, Sørensen TI, Jakobsen MU (2012) Waist circumference adjusted for body mass index and intra-abdominal fat mass. PLoS One 7(2):e32213

Bloem M (2007) The 2006 WHO child growth standards. Br Med J 334(7596):705–706

Blössner M, de Onis M (2005) Malnutrition - quantifying the health impact at national and local levels. Environmental Burden of Disease Series, No. 12. World Health Organization, Geneva

Boffetta P, McLerran D, Chen Y, Inoue M, Sinha R, He J, Gupta PC, Tsugane S, Irie F, Tamakoshi A, Gao YT, Shu XO, Wang R, Tsuji I, Kuriyama S, Matsuo K, Satoh H, Chen CJ, Yuan JM, Yoo KY, Ahsan H, Pan WH, Gu D, Pednekar MS, Sasazuki S, Sairenchi T, Yang G, Xiang YB, Nagai M, Tanaka H, Nishino Y, You SL, Koh WP, Park SK, Shen CY, Thornquist M, Kang D, Rolland B, Feng Z, Zheng W, Potter JD (2011) Body mass index and diabetes in Asia: a cross-sectional pooled analysis of 900,000 individuals in the Asia cohort consortium. PLoS One 6(6):e19930

Bosy-Westphal A, Booke CA, Blöcker T, Kossel E, Goele K, Later W, Hitze B, Heller M, Glüer CC, Müller MJ (2010) Measurement site for waist circumference affects its accuracy as an index of visceral and abdominal subcutaneous fat in a Caucasian population. J Nutr 140(5):954–961

Bouchard C (1991) Heredity and the path to overweight and obesity. Med Sci Sports Exerc 23(3):285–291

Brozek J, Prokopec M (2001) Historical note: early history of the anthropometry of body composition. Am J Hum Biol 13(2):157–158

Busetto L, Baggio MB, Zurlo F, Carraro R, Digito M, Enzi G (1992) Assessment of abdominal fat distribution in obese patients: anthropometry versus computerized tomography. Int J Obes Relat Metab Disord 16(10):731–736

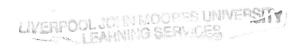

Chaput JP, Katzmarzyk PT, Barnes JD, Fogelholm M, Hu G, Kuriyan R, Kurpad A, Lambert EV, Maher C, Maia J, Matsudo V, Olds T, Onywera V, Sarmiento OL, Standage M, Tudor-Locke C, Zhao P, Tremblay MS, ISCOLE Research Group (2016) Mid-upper arm circumference as a screening tool for identifying children with obesity: a 12-country study. Pediatr Obes. https://doi.org/10.1111/ijpo.12162

Claessens AL, Lefevre J, Beunen G, Malina RM (1999) The contribution of anthropometric characteristics to performance scores in elite female gymnasts. J Sports Med Phys Fitness 39(4):355–360

Cole CR, Salvaterra GF, Davis JEJ, Borja ME, Powell LM, Dubbs EC, Bordi PL (2005) Evaluation of dietary practices of national collegiate athletic association division I football players. J Strength Cond Res 19(3):490–494

Cole TJ, Bellizzi MC, Flegal KM, Dietz WH (2000) Establishing a standard definition for child overweight and obesity worldwide: international survey. Br Med J 320(7244):1240–1124

Cole TJ, Flegal KM, Nicholls D, Jackson AA (2007) Body mass index cut offs to define thinness in children and adolescents: international survey. Br Med J 335(7612):194–201

Cornier MA, Després JP, Davis N, Grossniklaus DA, Klein S, Lamarche B, Lopez-Jimenez F, Rao G, St-Onge MP, Towfighi A, Poirier P, American Heart Association Obesity Committee of the Council on Nutrition, Physical Activity and Metabolism, Council on Arteriosclerosis, Thrombosis and Vascular Biology, Council on Cardiovascular Disease in the Young, Council on Cardiovascular Radiology and Intervention, Council on Cardiovascular Nursing, Council on Epidemiology and Prevention, Council on the Kidney in Cardiovascular Disease and Stroke Council (2011) Assessing adiposity: a scientific statement from the American Heart Association. Circulation 124(18):1996–2019

Dalton M, Cameron AJ, Zimmet PZ, Shaw JE, Jolley D, Dunstan DW, Welborn TA, AusDiab Steering Committee (2003) Waist circumference, waist-hip ratio and body mass index and their correlation with cardiovascular disease risk factors in Australian adults. J Intern Med 254(6):555–563

Dalton S (1997) Overweight and weight management: the health professional's guide to understanding and treatment. Aspen Publishers, Inc., Philadelphia, PA

de Carvalho Vidigal F, Paez de Lima Rosado LE, Paixão Rosado G, de Cassia Lanes Ribeiro R, do Carmo Castro Franceschini S, Priore SE, Gomes de Souza EC (2013) Predictive ability of the anthropometric and body composition indicators for detecting changes in inflammatory biomarkers. Nutr Hosp 28(5):1639–1645

de Jongh RT, Ijzerman RG, Serné EH, Voordouw JJ, Yudkin JS, de Waal HA, Stehouwer CD, van Weissenbruch MM (2006) Visceral and truncal subcutaneous adipose tissue are associated with impaired capillary recruitment in healthy individuals. J Clin Endocrinol Metabol 91(12):5100–5106

Del Porto HC, Pechak CM, Smith DR, Reed-Jones RJ (2012) Biomechanical effects of obesity on balance. Int J Exerc Sci 5(4):301–320

Deurenberg P, Yap M, van Staveren WA (1998) Body mass index and percent body fat: a meta analysis among different ethnic groups. Int J Obes (Lond) 22(12):1164–1171

Eknoyan G (2008) Adolphe Quetelet (1796-1874) - the average man and indices of obesity. Nephrol Dial Transplant 23(1):47–51

Expert Panel on Detection, Evaluation, and Treatment of High Blood Cholesterol In Adults (Adult Treatment Panel III) (2001) Executive Summary of the Third Report of The National Cholesterol Education Program (NCEP). JAMA 285(19):2486–2497

Frisancho AR (1981) New norms of upper limb fat and muscle areas for assessment of nutritional status. Am J Clin Nutr 34(11):2540–2545

Frisancho AR, Garn SM (1971) Skin-fold thickness and muscle size: implications for developmental status and nutritional evaluation of children from Honduras. Am J Clin Nutr 24(5):541–546

Garn SM, Leonard WR, Hawthorne VM (1986) Three limitations of the body mass index. Am J Clin Nutr 44(6):996–997

Gillman MW, Barker D, Bier D, Cagampang F, Challis J, Fall C, Godfrey K, Gluckman P, Hanson M, Kuh D, Nathanielsz P, Nestel P, Thornburg KL (2007) Meeting report on the 3rd International Congress on Developmental Origins of Health and Disease (DOHaD). Pediatr Res 61(5 Pt 1):625–629

Global Burden of Metabolic Risk Factors for Chronic Diseases Collaboration (BMI Mediated Effects), Lu Y, Hajifathalian K, Ezzati M, Woodward M, Rimm EB, Danaei G (2014) Metabolic mediators of the effects of body-mass index, overweight, and obesity on coronary heart disease and stroke: a pooled analysis of 97 prospective cohorts with 1·8 million participants. Lancet 383(9921):970–983

Green J, Cairns BJ, Casabonne D, Wright FL, Reeves G, Beral V, Million Women Study collaborators (2011) Height and cancer incidence in the Million Women Study: prospective cohort, and meta-analysis of prospective studies of height and total cancer risk. Lancet Oncol 12(8):785–794

Gunnell D, Okasha M, Smith GD, Oliver SE, Sandhu J, Holly JM (2001) Height, leg length, and cancer risk: a systematic review. Epidemiol Rev 23(2):313–342

Gurney JM (1969) Field experience in Abeokuta, Nigeria (with special reference to differentiating protein and calorie reserves). J Trop Pediatr 15(4):225–232

Gurney JM, Jelliffe DB (1973) Arm anthropometry in nutritional assessment: nomogram for rapid calculation of muscle circumference and cross-sectional muscle and fat areas. Am J Clin Nutr 26(9):912–915

Hamill PVV (1977) NCHS growth curves for children, vol (PHS) 78-1650. United States. National Center for Health Statistics. Vital and health statistics, vol No. 165. DHEW Publication, Hyattsville, MD

Heymsfield S, McManus C, Smith J, Stevens V, Nixon DW (1982) Anthropometric measurement of muscle mass: revised equations for calculating bone-free arm muscle area. Am J Clin Nutr 36(4):680–690

The IDF consensus worldwide definition of the metabolic syndrome (2006) http://www.idf.org/webdata/docs/IDF_Meta_def_final.pdf. Accessed 18 Mar 2008

International Diabetes Federation (2007) The IDF consensus definition of the metabolic syndrome in children and adolescents. IDF, Brussels

Jackson A, Stanforth PR, Gagnon J, Rankinen T, Leon AS, Rao DC, Skinner JS, Bouchard C, Wilmore JH (2002) The effect of sex, age and race on estimating percentage body fat from body mass index: the heritage family study. Int J Obes Relat Metab Disord 26(6):789–796

Jelliffe DB (1966) The assessment of the nutritional status of the community (with special reference to field surveys in developing regions of the world). Monogr Ser World Health Organ 53:3–271

Kabat GC, Heo M, Kamensky V, Miller AB, Rohan TE (2013) Adult height in relation to risk of cancer in a cohort of Canadian women. Int J Cancer 132(5):1125–1132

Kagawa M, Byrne NM, Hills AP (2008) Comparison of body fat estimation using waist to height ratio (WHtR) using different "waist" measurements in Australian adults. Br J Nutr 100(5):1135–1141

Kagawa M, Hills AP, Binns CW (2007) The usefulness of the waist-to-height ratio to predict trunk fat accumulation in Japanese and Australian Caucasian young males living in Australia. Int J Body Compos Res 5(2):57–63

Kagawa M, Kerr D, Uchida H, Binns CW (2006) Differences in the relationship between BMI and percentage body fat between Japanese and Australian-Caucasian young men. Br J Nutr 95(5):1002–1007

Kagawa M, Kobata T, Ishida R, Nakamura K (2014) Physical and nutritional status of professional Japanese futsal players. Austin J Nutr Food Sci 2(6):1–5

Katzmarzyk PT, Malina RM, Song TMK, Bouchard C (1999) Physique, subcutaneous fat, adipose tissue distribution, and risk factors in the Québec Family Study. Int J Obes Relat Metab Disord 23(5):476–484

Kerr DA, Ross WD, Norton K, Hume P, Kagawa M, Ackland TR (2007) Olympic lightweight and open-class rowers possess distinctive physical and proportionality characteristics. J Sports Sci 25(1):43–53

Keys A, Fidanza F, Karvonen MJ, Kimura N, Taylor HL (1972) Indices of relative weight and obesity. J Chronic Dis 25(6):329–343

Lemieux S, Prud'homme D, Bouchard C, Tremblay A, Déprés JP (1993) Sex differences in the relation of visceral adipose tissue accumulation to total body fatness. Am J Clin Nutr 58(4):463–467

Lu B, Zhou J, Waring ME, Parker DR, Eaton (2010) Abdominal obesity and peripheral vascular disease in men and women: a comparison of waist-to-thigh ratio and waist circumference as measures of abdominal obesity. Atherosclerosis 208(1):253–257

Lukaski HC (1987) Methods for the assessment of body composition: traditional and new. Am J Clin Nutr 46(4):537–556

Morgenthal AP (2002) Female athlete triad. J Chiroprac Med 1(3):97–106

Mountjoy M, Sundgot-Borgen J, Burke L, Carter S, Constantini N, Lebrun C, Meyer N, Sherman R, Steffen K, Budgett R, Ljungqvist A (2014) The IOC consensus statement: beyond the Female Athlete Triad--Relative Energy Deficiency in Sport (RED-S). Br J Sports Med 48(7):491–497

Murphy F, Kroll ME, Pirie K, Reeves G, Green J, Beral V (2013) Body size in relation to incidence of subtypes of haematological malignancy in the prospective Million Women Study. Br J Cancer 108(11):2390–2398

Myatt M, Khara T, Collins S (2006) A review of methods to detect cases of severely malnourished children in the community for their admission into community-based therapeutic care programs. Food Nutr Bull 27(3 Suppl):S7–S23

Papadopoulou SK, Gouvianaki A, Grammatikopoulou MG, Maraki Z, Pagkalos IG, Malliaropoulos N, Hassapidou MN, Maffulli N (2012) Body composition and dietary intake of elite cross-country skiers members of the Greek national team. Asian J Sports Med 3(4):257–266

Rasouli N, Molavi B, Elbein SC, Kern PA (2007) Ectopic fat accumulation and metabolic syndrome. Diabetes Obes Metab 9(1):1–10

Ross WD, Crawford SM, Kerr DA, Ward R (1988) Relationship of the Body Mass Index with skinfolds, girths, and bone breadths in Canadian men and women aged 20-70 years. Am J Phys Anthropol 77(2):169–173

Rush EC, Goedecke JH, Jennings C, Micklesfield L, Dugas L, Lambert EV, Plank LD (2007) BMI, fat and muscle differences in urban women of five ethnicities from two countries. Int J Obes (Lond) 31(1):1–8

Shakir A, Morley D (1974) Letter: measuring malnutrition. Lancet 1(7860):758–759

Taylor AE, Ebrahim S, Ben-Shlomo Y, Martin RM, Whincup PH, Yarnell JW, Wannamethee SG, Lawlor DA (2010) Comparison of the associations of body mass index and measures of central adiposity and fat mass with coronary heart disease, diabetes, and all-cause mortality: a study using data from 4 UK cohorts. Am J Clin Nutr 91(3):547–556

The Metabolic syndrome diagnostic criteria examination committee (2005) Definition and diagnostic criteria of metabolic syndrome [in Japanese]. J Jpn Soc Int Med 94(4):794–809

Tresaco B, Moreno LA, Ruiz JR, Ortega FB, Bueno G, González-Gross M, Wärnberg J, Gutiérrez A, García-Fuentes M, Marcos A, Castillo MJ, Bueno M, AVENA Study Group (2009) Truncal and abdominal fat as determinants of high triglycerides and low HDL-cholesterol in adolescents. Obesity (Silver Spring, MD) 17(5):1086–1091

United Nations Children's Fund, World Health Organization, The World Bank (2012) Levels and trends in child malnutrition: UNICEF-WHO-The World Bank joint child malnutrition estimates. WHO, Geneva

Vague J (1996) Sexual differentiation. A determinant factor of the forms of obesity. 1947. Obes Res 4(2):201–203

Vellas B, Guigoz Y, Garry PJ, Nourhashemi F, Bennahum D, Lauque S, Albarede JL (1999) The Mini Nutritional Assessment (MNA) and its use in grading the nutritional state of elderly patients. Nutrition 15(2):116–122

Vellas B, Villars H, Abellan G, Soto ME, Rolland Y, Guigoz Y, Morley JE, Chumlea W, Salva A, Rubenstein LZ, Garry P (2006) Overview of the MNA--its history and challenges. J Nutr Health Aging 10(6):456–463

Wang J, Thompson JC, Russel M, Burastero S, Heymsfield S, Pierson RN Jr (1994) Asians have lower body mass index (BMI) but higher percent body fat than do whites: comparisons of anthropometric measurements. Am J Clin Nutr 60(1):23–28

Wang J, Thornton JC, Kolesnik S, Pierson RN Jr (2000) Anthropometry in body composition. An overview. Ann N Y Acad Sci 904:317–326

Waterlow JC (1972) Classification and definition of protein-calorie malnutrition. Br Med J 3(5826):566–569

Wearing SC, Hennig EM, Byrne NM, Steele JR, Hills AP (2006a) The biomechanics of restricted movement in adult obesity. Obes Rev 7(1):13–24

Wearing SC, Hennig EM, Byrne NM, Steele JR, Hills AP (2006b) Musculoskeletal disorders associated with obesity: a biomechanical perspective. Obes Rev 7(3):239–250

Welborn TA, Dhaliwal SS, Bennett SA (2003) Waist-hip ratio is the dominant risk factor predicting cardiovascular death in Australia. Med J Aust 179(11-12):580–585

WHO expert consultation (2004) Appropriate body-mass index for Asian populations and its implications for policy and intervention strategies. Lancet 363(10):157–163

Wong ES, Wang BC, Garrison LP, Alfonso-Cristancho R, Flum DR, Arterburn DE, Sullivan SD (2011) Examining the BMI-mortality relationship using fractional polynomials. BMC Med Res Methodol 11:175

World Health Organization (1997) Obesity epidemic puts millions at risk from related diseases. WHO, Geneva

World Health Organization (1999) Management of severe malnutrition: a manual for physicians and their other senior health workers. WHO, Geneva

World Health Organization (1999) Definition, Diagnosis and Classificatin of Diabetes Mellitus and its Complications. Report of a WHO consultation. WHO, Geneva.

World Health Organization (2000) Obesity: preventing and managing the global epidemic. WHO technical report series. WHO, Geneva

World Health Organization (2002) The World health report 2002: reducing risks, promoting healthy life. WHO, Geneva

World Health Organization (2006) Constitution of the World Health Organization. In: Basic documents, 45th edn. WHO, Geneva

World Health Organization (2011) Waist circumference and waist-hip ratio: report of a WHO Expert Consultation. WHO, Geneva

World Health Organization (2013) Guideline: updates on management of severe acute malnutrition in infants and children. WHO, Geneva

World Health Organization, United Nations Children's Fund (2009) WHO child growth standards and the identification of severe acute malnutrition in infants and children. WHO, Geneva

Yard E, Comstock D (2011) Injury patterns by body mass index in US high school athletes. J Phys Act Health 8(2):182–191

Yusuf S, Hawken S, Ounpuu S, Bautista L, Franzosi MG, Commerford P, Lang CC, Rumboldt Z, Onen CL, Lisheng L, Tanomsup S, Wangai PJ, Razak F, Sharma AM, Anand SS, INTERHEART Study Investigators (2005) Obesity and the risk of myocardial infarction in 27,000 participants from 52 countries: a case-control study. Lancet 366(9497):1640–1649

Chapter 3
Optimising Physique for Sports Performance

Gary Slater, Helen O'Connor, and Ava Kerr

Abstract Physical morphology or physique, including body mass or composition, size and shape, is important to optimise athletic performance in many sports. Routine monitoring of body composition amongst athletic populations remains a common practice and provides insight into growth, diet and training adaptations not otherwise available. Examples provided include weightlifting and bodybuilding, sprinting, combat and aesthetic sports. Characteristics such as body mass, lean mass and fat mass are plastic and are able to be manipulated.

Keywords Physique • Physical morphology • Body mass • Body composition Size • Shape • Optimise athletic performance • Monitoring • Growth • Diet • Training adaptations • Weightlifting • Bodybuilding • Sprinting • Combat sport • Aesthetic sport • Lean mass • Fat mass

3.1 Introduction

Many factors ranging from skill and metabolic capacity through to psychological attributes contribute to athletic success. However, physical morphology or physique, including body mass or composition, size and shape, is important to optimise athletic performance in many sports. The impact of physique varies across sports and competition levels, but specific and often extreme morphological characteristics are critical

G. Slater (✉) • A. Kerr
University of the Sunshine Coast, Maroochydore DC, QLD, Australia
e-mail: gslater@usc.edu.au; akerr@usc.edu.au

H. O'Connor
University of Sydney, Lidcombe, NSW, Australia
e-mail: helen.oconnor@sydney.edu.au

© Springer Nature Singapore Pte Ltd. 2018

P.A. Hume et al. (eds.), *Best Practice Protocols for Physique Assessment in Sport*,
https://doi.org/10.1007/978-981-10-5418-1_3

to success at the elite level in some sports (e.g. professional bodybuilders, sumo wrestlers), whereas a wider variety of morphologies are acceptable in others (e.g. netball, soccer, softball). This can often be explained by playing role or position in team sports (e.g. prop forward or linesmen versus a winger or quarterback in football) or a competition rule in others (e.g. weight category sports such as lightweight rowing, combat sport or jockeys). However, in individual sports where physique attributes are diverse (e.g. archery, golf, lawn or ten-pin bowling), success may be more closely linked to skill or psychological attributes than anthropometric characteristics. Practitioners working with athletes who wish to manipulate physique traits must have an appreciation of the influence of variance in these character traits on competitive success, given any intent to change morphology should always be motivated by performance enhancement. While there is evidence to support the optimisation of body composition in some sports, the specific physique traits to emphasise may vary with the sport and potentially specific playing position. Therefore, it is imperative to recognise that physique is just one of an array of 'fitness traits' that may contribute to the overall success of an athlete. The association between physique traits and competitive success should not be overemphasised, but the routine monitoring of body composition amongst athletic populations remains a common practice and provides insight into growth, diet and training adaptations not otherwise available.

3.2 The Relationship Between Competitive Success and Physique Traits

A relationship between competitive success and physique traits has been identified in an array of sports, including football codes (Olds 2001), aesthetically judged sports (Claessens et al. 1999), swimming (Siders et al. 1993), track and field events (Claessens et al. 1994), plus skiing (White and Johnson 1991; Stoggl et al. 2010; Larsson and Henriksson-Larsen 2008) and lightweight (Rodriguez 1986) and heavyweight rowing (Shephard 1998). The specific physique traits associated with competitive success vary with the sport. For athletes participating in aesthetically judged sports, maintenance of low body fat levels is associated with positive outcomes (Claessens et al. 1999; Fry et al. 1991; Faria and Faria 1989). A similar relationship exists in sports where frontal surface area, power-to-weight ratio and/or thermoregulation are important (Norton et al. 1996). However, in sports demanding high force production, muscle mass may be more closely associated with performance outcomes (Olds 2001; Siders et al. 1993; Brechue and Abe 2002; Kyriazis et al. 2010; Stoggl et al. 2010), with specific distribution of muscle mass also important (Stoggl et al. 2010; Larsson and Henriksson-Larsen 2008). Likewise, in sports such as rowing, other physique traits like a shorter sitting height (relative to stature) and longer limb lengths are related to competitive success (DeRose et al. 1989) with such information used successfully in talent identification (Hahn 1990). Less is known about the unique population of athletes with a disability in whom the condition impacts on physique traits, such as those with spinal cord injuries, cerebral palsy and short stature and amputees, but there is at least some evidence confirming physique traits do impact performance in this population (Ide et al. 1994). Because of these relationships, it has become a common practice to monitor physique traits of athletes in response to growth, training and/or dietary interventions (Meyer et al. 2013).

Support for the contribution that specific physique characteristics make to athletic success is often difficult to substantiate from the scientific literature. This is mainly because it can be challenging to design studies sensitive and powerful enough to evaluate the impact of subtle physique changes on sports performance outside of training adaptations and across time, especially when competition success is decided by very small margins. However, there are several lines of evidence demonstrating how and why physique matters to athletic performance. Some of this evidence comes from longitudinal data on groups of successful athletes, including competition gradients revealing selection of more extreme and homogenous morphologies at the elite level (Norton et al. 1996). Comparison of athletes to the relevant source population often also demonstrates how they possess unique physique characteristics as a group and that these remain almost unchanged despite strong secular trends in the opposing direction. For example, marathon runners and professional jockeys remain short and light despite secular increases in stature and mass (O'Connor et al. 2007). Physiology, particularly the influence of body size on the energy cost of movement (Larsen 2003), heat production and thermoregulation (Dennis and Noakes 1999), also supports why athletes with high energy expenditures and heat exposure, such as long-distance runners, tend to be smaller and lighter in physique. This explains, at least in part, the Kenyan dominance of long-distance running (Larsen 2003).

Mathematical modelling of performance has also been undertaken to infer the impact of physique traits amongst track cyclists (Waldron et al. 2016), including a prediction of performance implications from any change in athlete morphology (Olds et al. 1993). Such information can be particularly valuable for practitioners working with athletes as there is less longitudinal data available on the performance implications of physique manipulation. Gains in lean body mass amongst elite youth rugby league players from one season to the next are associated with improvements in lower body speed and power (Waldron et al. 2014), with comparable outcomes noted in cyclists (Ronnestad et al. 2010). Similarly, gains in upper body muscle mass in team sport athletes throughout a season are associated with improvements in upper body strength performance (Bilsborough et al. 2016). Collectively, these data confirm that changes in physique traits do influence performance variables and thus warrant both monitoring and, potentially, manipulation, in the hope of optimising an athlete's morphology for their sport and specific position/role.

3.2.1 Sport-Specific Challenges to Athletes

Sports vary widely in the specific challenges they present to athletes. Modern pentathlon is an interesting sport to explore the association between physique traits and competitive success given the diversity of modalities, including skill-focused (shooting and fencing), aquatic (200 m freestyle) and weight-bearing (2000 m cross-country running and show jumping) events. Perhaps not surprisingly, physique traits play little role in skilled performance but do impact swim performance, with more marked impacts on the weight-bearing disciplines of show jumping and cross-country (Claessens et al. 1994). Body weight is carried over a distance in endurance sports, and this results in a significant energy cost and increased heat production. Low body mass, the result of low body fat, smaller stature and lean mass, is a distinct advantage for endurance sports such as distance running as it reduces the energy cost of locomotion (Larsen 2003) and minimises heat production (Dennis and Noakes 1999). From a thermoregulatory viewpoint, low body fat and a higher ratio of body surface area to mass promote superior heat loss (O'Connor et al. 2007). Amongst triathletes, this lower endomorphy and increased ectomorphy rating also enhances performance, with the greatest impact on the run leg (Kandel et al. 2014). While the impact of physique traits on competitive success in triathlon is not always evident (Knechtle et al. 2007), it does align with the changing morphology of elite junior triathletes (Landers et al. 2013).

3.2.1.1 Weightlifting and Bodybuilding

Within the lifting events, physique traits influence performance in several ways. While the expression of strength has a significant neural component, lifting performance is closely associated with skeletal muscle mass (Brechue and Abe 2002). Excluding the open-weight category, weightlifters also tend to have low body fat levels, enhancing development of strength per unit body mass (Keogh et al. 2007). Successful weightlifters also have a higher sitting height-to-stature ratio with shorter limbs, creating a biomechanical advantage (Keogh et al. 2009). An association between physique traits and competitive success in the Olympic throwing events has been recognised for some time, with successful athletes heavier and taller than their counterparts (Khosla 1968) and growth in size at a rate well in excess of population secular trends (Norton and Olds 2001). In contrast to other strength sports, bodybuilding is unique in that competitive success is judged purely on the basis of the size, symmetry and definition of musculature. Not surprisingly, bodybuilders are the most muscular of all the strength athletes (Huygens et al. 2002). Successful bodybuilders have lower body fat, yet are taller and heavier with wider skeletal proportions, especially the ratio of biacromial to bi-iliocristal breadths (Fry et al. 1991).

3.2.1.2 Sprinting

Similarly, successful sprinters have physique traits that predispose them to excellence. Some of these traits are responsive to training stimuli and nutritional interventions, including skeletal muscle fibre type and area (Dowson et al. 1998), fascicle area and length (Aagaard et al. 2001; Abe et al. 2001) plus low adiposity (Dowson et al. 1998), while other architectural features such as stature, toe, foot and lower leg length are not (Lee and Piazza 2009). The available literature clearly reflects an emphasis on the importance for sprinters to maximise skeletal muscle mass to enhance power. However, this may not be appropriate for all sprinters with skeletal muscle hypertrophy possibly resulting in adverse adaptations, including a transition away from fast-twitch glycolytic fibres and slower contraction velocity characteristics (Alway et al. 1988) if inappropriately prescribed. Rather than absolute power output, acceleration in sprinting is also a function of power to weight. Greater muscle strength and power are usually accompanied by an increase in muscle cross-sectional area, but the ability to generate force also requires improved neuromuscular recruitment. In a study comparing heavier, more muscular adult to adolescent sprinters, higher muscularity and mass were reported to explain slower sprint start dynamics (Aerenhouts et al. 2012).

While optimising muscle mass is important for the development of explosive power, especially at the sprint start, training should advance technical skills to facilitate effective transfer of strength benefits. Although most studies report a 'normalised' muscle strength of participants by adjusting for total or lean body mass, this unfortunately fails to adequately account for regional mass differences (e.g. differences in upper to lower body mass) which are likely important for performance. Locating mass closer to the joint centre helps optimise biomechanical efficiency, a concept supported by research showing sprinters with greater deposition of muscle in the upper portion of the quadriceps are faster (Kumagai et al. 2000). Thus muscularity for sprinters needs to be optimised rather than maximised, and, currently, there are insufficient comprehensive morphological data to provide detailed guidance. Similarly, small differences in adiposity on the limbs of sprinters have also been demonstrated to predict performance with relatively small reductions in medial calf skinfold associated with faster run times (Legaz and Eston 2005). This suggests that subtle differences in the distribution of mass influence performance, possibly the result of increased muscular effort and energy expenditure associated with heavier lower limbs when running.

3.2.1.3 Combat Sports

One group of sports which has received relatively little investigation into the relationship between physique traits and competition success is the Olympic combat sports, including boxing, taekwondo, judo and wrestling. This is surprising given each sport has specified weight divisions, established to create equity by matching athletes of similar size. Despite this, athletes typically aim to reduce their natural body mass to compete in a lower weight category, via a combination of both acute and chronic weight loss strategies, presumably to obtain a size or leverage advantage over smaller opponents. Indeed, there is some evidence that heavier athletes are more successful within a specified weight category (Reale et al. 2016a; Wroble and Moxley 1998); however, this remains a contentious issue and may vary depending on the specific sport and level of competition (Wroble and Moxley 1998; Horswill et al. 1994; Kazemi et al. 2011; Reale et al. 2016b). Although often grouped together, Olympic combat sports can be broadly categorised into striking (boxing and tae-kwondo) and grappling sports (judo and wrestling). In striking sports, athletes uti-lise movement and distance, attempting to land blows on their opponents with their hands as is the case in boxing, or with their feet/legs, the predominant scoring strikes in taekwondo. In the grappling sports, the objective is to manipulate the opponent's body to throw them to the ground, pin the opponent or force the oppo-nent to submit via a chokehold or joint manipulation technique. These strategic differences may alter the physique characteristics associated with performance advantages. Understanding the differences in morphological optimisation between combat sport athletes may provide value for talent identification programmes or for talent transfer between combat sports. This information also provides a benchmark for working with individual combat sport athletes, assisting in the identification of ideal weight divisions or the manipulation of body composition within a weight division (Reale et al. 2016a).

3.2.1.4 Aesthetic Sports

Specific physique characteristics are sometimes required for aesthetic reasons, and coaches and athletes are aware that failure to attain the right appearance will result in lower scores for artistic impression in sports like artistic (Claessens et al. 1999) and rhythmic gymnastics (Di Cagno et al. 2009; Douda et al. 2008), with similar associations likely in other sports like figure skating and diving (Benardot et al. 2014). These scores come down to the 'trained eye' of the judge who likely experi-enced similar evaluation during their own athletic careers. Sometimes the extreme leanness desired is driven largely by appearance rather than performance enhance-ment, but opinion and culture within the sport are often entrenched and difficult to change. In recent years, the need for athletes to appear physically attractive is also driven by sponsorship opportunities which help to fund if not completely outstrip the financial rewards of successful competition. The desired physique may be dic-tated by societal attractiveness rather than athletic performance (O'Connor and Catterson 2010).

3.3   What Physique Characteristics Can Be Manipulated for Sport?

Clearly, physique characteristics impact performance and this is more important for some sports than others. Characteristics such as stature, skeletal lengths and breadths are not adaptable, but body mass, lean mass and fat mass are more plastic and are able to be manipulated. Practitioners working with athletes wishing to manipulate physique traits must have an appreciation of the influence of variance in these physique traits on competitive success, given any intent to change morphology should always be motivated by performance enhancement. While there is evidence to support the optimisation of body composition in some sports, the specific physique traits to emphasise may vary with the sport and, potentially, the specific playing position. Recognition must be given to the fact that implementation of strategies to achieve an extreme physique is rarely necessary, and such aggressive interventions may result in impaired training adaptations and ultimately impaired performance (Mountjoy et al. 2014). Thus the regular monitoring of physique traits is strongly advocated, in conjunction with performance or indirect indices of performance, to assist in the identification of an ideal morphology for the specific athlete. This recognises the influence of an athlete's genetic profile, which not only impacts on their presenting morphology but also their responsiveness to interventions (Ivey et al. 2000) and the associated physique capacity (Kouri et al. 1995).

It is imperative to recognise that physique is just one of an array of 'fitness traits' that may contribute to the overall success of an athlete, and the association between physique traits and competitive success should not be overemphasised. However, the routine monitoring of physique traits amongst athletic populations can offer insight into their adaptations to training and/or dietary interventions and help establish an individual database to assist the practitioner and athlete to make an informed opinion on what may be considered morphological optimisation for that individual within their respective sport.

3.4 Summary

Optimising physique for sports performance is possible. Monitoring of body composition enables evaluation of the effectiveness of interventions for athlete's training and diet.

References

Aagaard P, Andersen JL, Dyhre-Poulsen P, Leffers AM, Wagner A, Magnusson SP, Halkjaer-Kristensen J, Simonsen EB (2001) A mechanism for increased contractile strength of human pennate muscle in response to strength training: changes in muscle architecture. J Physiol 534(Pt. 2):613–623

Abe T, Fukashiro S, Harada Y, Kawamoto K (2001) Relationship between sprint performance and muscle fascicle length in female sprinters. J Physiol Anthropol Appl Human Sci 20(2):141–147

Aerenhouts D, Delecluse C, Hagman F, Taeymans J, Debaere S, Van Gheluwe B, Clarys P (2012) Comparison of anthropometric characteristics and sprint start performance between elite adolescent and adult sprint athletes. Eur J Sport Sci 12(1):9–15

Alway SE, MacDougall JD, Sale DG, Sutton JR, McComas AJ (1988) Functional and structural adaptations in skeletal muscle of trained athletes. J Appl Physiol 64(3):1114–1120

Benardot D, Zimmermann W, Cox GR, Marks S (2014) Nutritional recommendations for divers. Int J Sport Nutr Exerc Metab 24(4):392–403

Bilsborough JC, Greenway K, Livingston S, Cordy J, Coutts AJ (2016) Changes in anthropometry, upper-body strength, and nutrient intake in professional Australian football players during a season. Int J Sports Physiol Perform 11(3):290–300

Brechue WF, Abe T (2002) The role of FFM accumulation and skeletal muscle architecture in powerlifting performance. Eur J Appl Physiol 86(4):327–336

Claessens AL, Hlatky S, Lefevre J, Holdhaus H (1994) The role of anthropometric characteristics in modern pentathlon performance in female athletes. J Sports Sci 12(4):391–401

Claessens AL, Lefevre J, Beunen G, Malina RM (1999) The contribution of anthropometric characteristics to performance scores in elite female gymnasts. J Sports Med Phys Fitness 39(4):355–360

Dennis SC, Noakes TD (1999) Advantages of a smaller bodymass in humans when distance-running in warm, humid conditions. Eur J Appl Physiol Occup Physiol 79(3):280–284

DeRose EH, Crawford SM, Kerr DA, Ward R, Ross WD (1989) Physique characteristics of Pan American Games lightweight rowers. Int J Sports Med 10(4):292–297

Di Cagno A, Baldari C, Battaglia C, Monteiro MD, Pappalardo A, Piazza M, Guidetti L (2009) Factors influencing performance of competitive and amateur rhythmic gymnastics--gender differences. J Sci Med Sport 12(3):411–416

Douda HT, Toubekis AG, Avloniti AA, Tokmakidis SP (2008) Physiological and anthropometric determinants of rhythmic gymnastics performance. Int J Sports Physiol Perform 3(1):41–54

Dowson MN, Nevill ME, Lakomy HK, Nevill AM, Hazeldine RJ (1998) Modelling the relationship between isokinetic muscle strength and sprint running performance. J Sports Sci 16(3):257–265

Faria IE, Faria EW (1989) Relationship of the anthropometric and physical characteristics of male junior gymnasts to performance. J Sports Med Phys Fitness 29(4):369–378

Fry AC, Ryan AJ, Schwab RJ, Powell DR, Kraemer WJ (1991) Anthropometric characteristics as discriminators of body-building success. J Sports Sci 9(1):23–32

Hahn A (1990) Identification and selection of talent in Australian rowing. Excel 6(3):5–11

Horswill C, Scott JR, Dick RW, Hayes J (1994) Influence of rapid weight gain after the weigh-in on success in collegiate wrestlers. Med Sci Sports Exerc 26(10):1290–1294

Huygens W, Claessens AL, Thomis M, Loos R, Van Langendonck L, Peeters M, Philippaerts R, Meynaerts E, Vlietinck R, Beunen G (2002) Body composition estimations by BIA versus anthropometric equations in body builders and other power athletes. J Sports Med Phys Fitness 42(1):45–55

Ide M, Ogata H, Kobayashi M, Tajima F, Hatada K (1994) Anthropometric features of wheelchair marathon race competitors with spinal cord injuries. Paraplegia 32(3):174–179

Ivey FM, Roth SM, Ferrell RE, Tracy BL, Lemmer JT, Hurlbut DE, Martel GF, Siegel EL, Fozard JL, Jeffrey Metter E, Fleg JL, Hurley BF (2000) Effects of age, gender, and myostatin genotype on the hypertrophic response to heavy resistance strength training. J Gerontol A Biol Sci Med Sci 55(11):M641–M648

Kandel M, Baeyens JP, Clarys P (2014) Somatotype, training and performance in Ironman athletes. Eur J Sport Sci 14(4):301–308

Kazemi M, Rahman A, De Ciantis M (2011) Weight cycling in adolescent Taekwondo athletes. J Can Chiropr Assoc 55(4):318–324

Keogh JW, Hume PA, Pearson SN, Mellow P (2007) Anthropometric dimensions of male power-lifters of varying body mass. J Sports Sci 25(12):1365–1376

Keogh JW, Hume PA, Pearson SN, Mellow PJ (2009) Can absolute and proportional anthropometric characteristics distinguish stronger and weaker powerlifters? J Strength Cond Res 23(8):2256–2265

Khosla T (1968) Unfairness of certain events in Olympic Games. Br Med J 4(5623):111

Knechtle B, Knechtle P, Andonie JL, Kohler G (2007) Influence of anthropometry on race performance in extreme endurance triathletes: World Challenge Deca Iron Triathlon 2006. Br J Sports Med 41(10):644–648

Kouri EM, Pope HG Jr, Katz DL, Oliva P (1995) Fat-free mass index in users and nonusers of anabolic-androgenic steroids. Clin J Sport Med 5(4):223–228

Kumagai K, Abe T, Brechue WF, Ryushi T, Takano S, Mizuno M (2000) Sprint performance is related to muscle fascicle length in male 100-m sprinters. J Appl Physiol 88(3):811–816

Kyriazis T, Terzis G, Karampatsos G, Kavouras S, Georgiadis G (2010) Body composition and performance in shot put athletes at preseason and at competition. Int J Sports Physiol Perform 5(3):417–421

Landers GJ, Ong KB, Ackland TR, Blanksby BA, Main LC, Smith D (2013) Kinanthropometric differences between 1997 World championship junior elite and 2011 national junior elite triathletes. J Sci Med Sport 16(5):444–449

Larsen HB (2003) Kenyan dominance in distance running. Comp Biochem Physiol A Mol Integr Physiol 136(1):161–170

Larsson P, Henriksson-Larsen K (2008) Body composition and performance in cross-country skiing. Int J Sports Med 29(12):971–975

Lee SS, Piazza SJ (2009) Built for speed: musculoskeletal structure and sprinting ability. J Exp Biol 212(Pt 22):3700–3707

Legaz A, Eston R (2005) Changes in performance, skinfold thicknesses, and fat patterning after three years of intense athletic conditioning in high level runners. Br J Sports Med 39(11):851–856

Meyer NL, Sundgot-Borgen J, Lohman TG, Ackland TR, Stewart AD, Maughan RJ, Smith S, Muller W (2013) Body composition for health and performance: a survey of body composition assessment practice carried out by the Ad Hoc Research Working Group on Body Composition, Health and Performance under the auspices of the IOC Medical Commission. Br J Sports Med 47(16):1044–1053

Mountjoy M, Sundgot-Borgen J, Burke L, Carter S, Constantini N, Lebrun C, Meyer N, Sherman R, Steffen K, Budgett R, Ljungqvist A (2014) The IOC consensus statement: beyond the Female Athlete Triad--Relative Energy Deficiency in Sport (RED-S). Br J Sports Med 48(7):491–497

Norton K, Olds T (2001) Morphological evolution of athletes over the 20th century: causes and consequences. Sports Med 31(11):763–783

Norton K, Olds T, Olive S, Craig N (1996) Anthropometry and sports performance. In: Norton K, Olds T (eds) Anthropometrica. University of New South Wales Press, Sydney, pp 287–364

O'Connor H, Catterson I (2010) Weight loss and the athlete. In: Burke L, Deakin V (eds) Clinical Sports Nutrition, 4th edn. McGraw Hill, North Ryde, pp 116–148

O'Connor H, Olds T, Maughan RJ, International Association of Athletics F (2007) Physique and performance for track and field events. J Sports Sci 25(Suppl 1):S49–S60

Olds T (2001) The evolution of physique in male rugby union players in the twentieth century. J Sports Sci 19(4):253–262

Olds TS, Norton KI, Craig NP (1993) Mathematical model of cycling performance. J Appl Physiol 75(2):730–737

Reale R, Cox GR, Slater G, Burke LM (2016a) Regain in body mass after weigh-in is linked to success in real life judo competition. Int J Sport Nutr Exerc Metab 26(6):525–530

Reale R, Cox GR, Slater G, Burke LM (2016b) Weight re-gain not linked to success in a real life multi-day boxing tournament. Int J Sports Physiol Perform 11:1–26, 2016

Rodriguez FA (1986) Physical structure of international lightweight rowers. In: Reilly T, Watkins J, Borms J (eds) Kinanthropometry III. E and F.N. Spon Ltd, London, pp 255–261

Ronnestad BR, Hansen EA, Raastad T (2010) Effect of heavy strength training on thigh muscle cross-sectional area, performance determinants, and performance in well-trained cyclists. Eur J Appl Physiol 108(5):965–975

Shephard RJ (1998) Science and medicine of rowing: A review. J Sports Sci 16:603–620

Siders WA, Lukaski HC, Bolonchuk WW (1993) Relationships among swimming performance, body composition and somatotype in competitive collegiate swimmers. J Sports Med Phys Fitness 33(2):166–171

Stoggl T, Enqvist J, Muller E, Holmberg HC (2010) Relationships between body composition, body dimensions, and peak speed in cross-country sprint skiing. J Sports Sci 28(2):161–169

Waldron M, Gray A, Furlan N, Murphy A (2016) Predicting the sprint performance of adolescent track cyclists using the 3-minute all-out test. J Strength Cond Res 30(8):2299–2306

Waldron M, Worsfold P, Twist C, Lamb K (2014) Changes in anthropometry and performance, and their interrelationships, across three seasons in elite youth rugby league players. J Strength Cond Res 28(11):3128–3136

White AT, Johnson SC (1991) Physiological comparison of international, national and regional alpine skiers. Int J Sports Med 12(4):374–378

Wroble RR, Moxley DP (1998) Acute weight gain and its relationship to success in high school wrestlers. Med Sci Sports Exerc 30(6):949–951

Chapter 4
Physique Assessment for Sports Ergonomics Applications

Patria A. Hume and Justin W.L. Keogh

Abstract Physique assessment is important for many sports ergonomics applications. Examples from sports including cycling, rowing, tennis and golf and shoe and clothing design for able-bodied athletes are initially provided. The final section focuses on athletes with a disability to illustrate the use of athlete dimensions for sports ergonomics applications to optimise performance in adults and child athletes.

Keywords Physique • Ergonomics • Equipment • Apparel • Footwear • Smart clothing • Disability • Paralympics

4.1 Introduction

Anthropometry uncovers the relationships between different body dimensions, and these relationships can be used in the design and/or optimisation of products or spaces for activities of daily living and sports participation. Anthropometry enables us to develop standards and specific requirements against which equipment and working environments can be assessed for their suitability with the user population. To assess anatomical body measurement in relation to sports performance and the athlete environment (i.e. ergonomics), a wide range of techniques are available including surface anthropometry, dual X-ray absorptiometry and magnetic resonance

P.A. Hume (✉)
Sport Performance Research Institute New Zealand,
Auckland University of Technology, Auckland, New Zealand
e-mail: patria.hume@aut.ac.nz

J.W.L. Keogh
Bond University, Robina, QLD 4226, Australia
e-mail: jkeogh@bond.edu.au

© Springer Nature Singapore Pte Ltd. 2018   37
P.A. Hume et al. (eds.), *Best Practice Protocols for Physique Assessment in Sport*,
https://doi.org/10.1007/978-981-10-5418-1_4

imaging, ultrasound and 3D photonic scanning. Custom fitting of apparel is now becoming available due to 3D scanning machines. Examples of the use of ergonomics applications in sport such as the development of novel sports apparel, footwear and equipment are reported in journals such as *Sports Engineering*, *The Journal of Sports Engineering and Technology* and *Prosthetics and Orthotics International*.

4.2 Equipment Set-Up, Footwear and Apparel Design and Selection with Respect to Athlete Physique

In competition, marginal gains can represent the difference between success and failure. Dimensions of physique are important when considering sports equipment design and fit.

The benefits of anatomical and biomechanical screening of competitive cyclists before positional set-up to gain competitive advantage have been described (Dinsdale and Dinsdale 2011; Bini et al. 2014). Efficient, injury-free cycling is reliant on pedalling symmetry, which is reliant on efficient lower-limb biomechanics, correct foot function and a stable, level pelvis. Leg-length inequality must be clearly differentiated into anatomical and functional and then addressed appropriately to achieve a successful outcome. The cycling biomechanist needs to measure anthropometric dimensions accurately to enable correct bike set-up related to the athlete's body dimensions. When using the length of body segments to configure the saddle height, the distance from the greater trochanter to the floor, the distance from the pubis to the floor and the distance from the ischial tuberosity to the floor have all been used (Bini et al. 2011).

Rowing is a sport with an ergonomic relationship between the athletes and the boat set-up. Scaling rigging set-up according to rower's body dimensions and strength has been deemed important for Australian elite single scullers (Barrett and Manning 2004) and New Zealand elite rowers (Soper and Hume 2004). Adjustment of the rowing skiff foot-stretcher position based on lower limb segment lengths and range of motion can optimise the work angle of the knees and ankles to obtain maximum efficiency for the leg drive (Hume et al. 2000).

Children's access to many sports can be restricted because equipment is often not designed to suit a child's physique and capabilities. The design and development of sports equipment for children were investigated for golf and tennis equipment by assessing the ability of children to generate reasonable strokes to propel the balls (Stanbridge et al. 2004). The same factors (experience, arm span and grip strength) had similar influence on equipment fitting in both sports. In particular, significant predictors of tennis racket length were arm span and elbow to wrist length. Racket balance was predicted by elbow to wrist length, while racket mass was predicted by arm span and hand length. The significant predictors of golf club length were arm span. As lever length increases, so does the force that the child can create to propel the ball further. However, the advantages of this force can only be truly utilised if the child has the strength and ability to control the racket or club during the stroke. Equipment-fitting guidelines are providing valuable information to improve junior equipment.

Correct footwear fit is important for function and to reduce injuries such as blisters. The shoe industry provides shoes of different size and width to account for different dimensions of athletes' feet. Three-dimensional foot scanners are also in use for bespoke shoe creation for elite athletes. At the community athlete level, however, measurement of feet when trying shoes is not readily undertaken, rather athletes try on shoes and see if they feel comfortable. Shoe clinics can provide a more professional shoe fit with foot length and width measurement, and biomechanics running clinics provide functional fit in shoes after taking a series of anthropometric variables into consideration. For example, the AUT Millennium's Running and Cycling Mechanics Clinic measures arch height and several foot dimensions before providing functional shoe fit and analysis using 3D biomechanics gait assessment (https://www.youtube.com/watch?v=iYmcgVx_OmU).

Foot morphology of junior football players (146 soccer and 122 rugby players) was measured to determine implications for football shoe design (Soper et al. 2001). Given there were differences between right and left foot sizes in length and width in many players, it was recommended that shoe companies sell shoes with the option of different sizes for each foot. A similar approach is available for women's underwear to take account of the differences in bra size versus underpants size. However, this approach has yet to be translated to the shoe industry. Additional research into the potential performance and/or injury risk benefits that may result from using shoes matched to the length and width of each foot may be required to encourage the shoe industry to provide different shoe sizes for each foot to their customers.

Athletic clothing needs to fit well for comfort but also performance. Advances in competitive swimsuits and resulting improvements in race times have demonstrated the importance of form-fitting clothing. The development of apparel such as singing shirts or cycling jackets that indicate when you turn is an example of technology that use cloth-printed circuit boards made into interactive garments with inbuilt sensors for touch, light and sound. These items are being developed to aid athlete performance during competition and in many cases to provide feedback during training to improve technique. For examples of clothing knitted to monitor a person's heart rate, breathing and joint movement, see AUT's Colab creative technologies laboratory (https://colab.aut.ac.nz/).

4.3 Ergonomics with Respect to Physique of Athletes with a Disability

Perhaps the one segment of the population who may most benefit from sports ergonomics research and development in improving their sporting performance and reducing their injury risk are athletes with a disability. A number of reviews have been published in the previous decade highlighting the advancements in our under-standing of how the disciplines of sport science and medicine may be used in con-junction with continuing developments in assistive technology to assist these individuals compete to the best of their ability (Burkett 2010; Churton and Keogh 2013; Keogh 2011).

As a result of this increasing scientific and community interest, many more indi-viduals with a disability are beginning to participate and compete in sport from recreational to elite levels. These athletes and the sporting organisations they com-pete in have long ago realised that standard wheelchair or prosthetic devices that individuals use during their regular activities of daily living may not optimise their sporting performance. To satisfy the sporting goals of these athletes, especially those competing at the elite Paralympic level, significant technological advance-ments have occurred in the design of prostheses, throwing frames/chairs and wheel-chairs (Burkett 2010; Frossard et al. 2007; Vanlandewijck et al. 2001). However, in order for these technological advances to improve Paralympic sports performance, a variety of standard anthropometric measures of the athlete have to be taken into account to maximise the fit between each athlete and the specific assistive device (technology). Another issue affecting the way in which sports technology can be used in Paralympic sports is the heterogeneity of athlete anthropometry and func-tional ability that reflects the diversity of each individual athletes' disability. The vast differences in level of disability and function may reflect inter-athlete variation in the site and/or number of limb amputations, level of spinal cord lesion or severity of conditions such as polio or cerebral palsy.

The importance of quantifying the individual Paralympic athletes' anthropome-try to maximise the potential benefit of their assistive technology may be observed in the selection and fitting of the appropriate prosthesis (prosthetic limb) for running and cycling athletes. Specifically, the prosthesis needs to be fitted so that it moves naturally with the intact portion of the limb (stump), with the shear forces acting on the stump surface minimised in magnitude and applied over as large an area as pos-sible so to reduce the potential for pressure sores or blisters. When the prosthesis makes contact with the ground during running or applies force to the pedals during cycling, a greater proportion of the ground reaction force may be transmitted through the prosthesis to the stump-socket interface. For above-knee amputees, this means substantially greater impact/ground reaction forces are likely to be transmit-ted through to the femur than would be experienced by an able-bodied runner/cyclist. This means that any variations in the prosthesis, stump location and the stump-socket interface may alter the magnitude, direction, time and point of appli-cation of these ground reaction on the intact portion of the limb. Such differences may all have implications to athletic performance and injury risk during running and cycling events.

The interaction between the stump and socket of the prosthesis may RR change during a training session or competition as a result of variation in environmental factors such as pressure and humidity as well as the amount of sweat produced by the athlete. As the stump is typically contained in a volume-specific socket, any changes in these environmental factors will result in some alteration to the fit of the prosthesis to the stump which will directly alter the manner in which the forces are transmitted through the stump-socket interface. This has the potential to lead to reduced performance and increased risk of blisters and pressure sores or even impact-related injury. For athletes with unilateral lower limb amputations, there may be considerable asymmetries in the kinematics and kinetics of the intact and prosthetic limb when walking, running or cycling (Childers et al. 2011; Lloyd et al. 2010; Burkett et al. 2003). There is some preliminary evidence that this asymmetry may have a moderate relationship with increased risk of osteoarthritis (Lloyd et al. 2010).

Alterations in the design of throwing frames/chairs for Paralympic sports including the shot-put and discus have been implemented in an attempt to improve sporting performance. While the development of these throwing frames and the optimisation of these frames for individual athlete characteristics are often based on a trial and error approach, a small number of studies have sought to examine the relationship between anthropometry, body positioning in the throwing frames and throwing performance. An initial study in this area reported some moderate relationships between foot position and functional level of 12 Paralympic athletes, although no clear relationships were observed between foot position and distance thrown (O'Riordan et al. 2004). In a large-scale study, the potential relationships between 26 characteristics of the throwing frames to the athlete anthropometric characteristics and the manner in which they position their body on the throwing frame have been evaluated (Frossard et al. 2010). The authors acknowledged that a range of methodological limitations including the relatively low sample size of elite athletes and high number of dependent measures assessed means further research is required to more clearly characterise the optimal way in which the throwing frame needs to be constructed so to accommodate the individual athlete and maximise throwing performance (Frossard et al. 2010). An implication of these two throwing frame studies was that companies that manufacture throwing frames need to ensure these frames are highly adjustable to cater for the variety of functional levels and anthropometric characteristics of athletes with a disability.

Wheelchairs are also commonly used by athletes with a disability in sports such as athletics (from the 100 m sprint to the marathon) and a range of team and individual ball sports including basketball, rugby and tennis. Within each of these sports, the typical wheelchair has been modified to suit some of the unique demands of each sport. For example, racing wheelchairs for the 100 m sprint and longer distance events have evolved into tricycles with the front wheel positioned a large distance in front of the athlete to provide additional anterior-posterior stability when accelerating and improve turning performance. These racing wheelchairs are also typically low and relatively narrow to minimise the air resistance acting on the athlete and wheelchair. The ball sports also typically utilise wheelchairs with an additional small wheel, generally positioned posteriorly that again improves stability and manoeuvrability. The wheelchairs of rugby players have been perhaps most highly modified, with additional reinforced front and side bumper guards to protect the player and wheelchair from frequent high-impact collisions. The chairs used in wheelchair rugby also have a wheel camber in which the lower portion of the wheels is wider than the upper portion. While this alteration reduces the chair's maximum speed and overall economy, its increased base of support provides additional manoeuvrability and stability during contact situations (Mason et al. 2011; Tsai et al. 2012). Beyond the specific sport requirements, further challenges for the design and optimal integration of wheelchair technology into sport ergonomics are the different functional ability and classifications for Paralympic athletes competing in the same sport. Accurate measurement of the athletes' physique dimensions will enable custom wheelchairs to be made.

An example of challenges facing wheelchair designers and Paralympic sport is wheelchair basketball, where players are classified on a 0.5 scale from 1.0 through to 4.5. The lower point players (1.0–2.0) have the greatest physical disability and are unable to actively stabilise their pelvis. This means that the lower point wheelchair basketball players require a wheelchair that provides external mechanical support to their lumbo-pelvic region, with this often achieved by using a seat that is angled downwards from front to back. The higher point players (3.0–4.5) who possess greater pelvic stability require little support from the wheelchair, meaning they can use a chair with a relatively flat seat. A flatter seat provides performance advantages, whereby the wheelchair player can reach higher when attempting to rebound, pass and shoot at goal. Therefore, if additional modifications to the wheelchairs of lower point players can be developed to improve lumbo-pelvic stability without losing chair height by a decline seat, the lower point players may contribute even more effectively to the team's performance.

The diameter of the handrim is another aspect of wheelchair design that has undergone research and development to determine its effect on sporting performance and injury risk. For example, studies involving wheelchair basketball players (Coutts 1990) and wheelchair track athletes (Costa et al. 2009) provide some evidence that increases in the handrim diameter allows for greater propulsive impulses to be generated, which results in improved acceleration and change of direction ability. However, any modification to one aspect of wheelchair design such as the seat height/angle and handrim diameter that may theoretically improve performance and/or reduce injury risk still needs to take into account the individuals' anthropometry and level of physical function. Such an understanding of the potential positive and negative performance changes that may result from altering one aspect of the interaction between a Paralympic athlete and their assistive devices influenced the work of Burkett and Mellifont (2008) who were asked to optimise the bike fit of the six Australian Paralympic cyclists who competed at the 2004 Paralympic Games.

As athletes with a disability may experience greater difficulties and quality of life challenges when injured compared to the able-bodied counterparts (Fagher et al. 2016a), additional research needs to be conducted to identify how assistive eirquipment and technology may need to be fitted to the individual athlete with a disability to reduce the risk of injury. Insight into the athletes with a disability perspectives on their risk and determinants of injury has been provided in a recent qualitative study of 18 Paralympic athletes spanning 10 sports (Fagher et al. 2016a). The results of this qualitative study revealed that Paralympic athletes believe their injury risk is multifactorial, with major injury risk factors including the nature of their disability and their use of potentially unsafe training practices. These Paralympic athletes also acknowledged that their physical preparation and appropriate use of safety and competitive equipment may reduce the risk of injury. As a result of this athlete input, a protocol for a prospective study has been published in which 100 Swedish Paralympic athletes will be monitored for approximately 1 year, with the aim to provide prospective estimates of sports-related injury and explore risk factors and mechanisms for injury and illness (Fagher et al. 2016b). It will be interesting if this study provides any insight into the potential role of assistive technology, as a potential risk or preventative factor for injury and illness in this cohort, and any potential interactions that may be observed between the assistive technology used and the anthropometry and functional ability of the athlete.

4.4   Summary

Physique assessment is important for sports ergonomics applications in a variety of able-bodied and disability sports. Equipment design and set-up, footwear and apparel design and fit all need accurate physique dimensions if the technology is to be effectively used to improve performance and/or reduce the risk of injury. Advancements in the quick and accurate assessment of the athletes' three-dimensional physique characteristics are beginning to allow a greater optimisation of sports ergonomic principles and technology to improving sports performance and/or reducing injury risk in a wide cross-section of athlete groups. Additional research and development is still required to better identify the key determinants of a successful matching of the athletes' characteristics to that of the assistive technology.

References

Barrett RS, Manning JM (2004) Relationships between rigging set-up, anthropometry, physical capacity, rowing kinematics and rowing performance. Sports Biomech 3(2):221–225

Bini RR, Hume PA, Croft J (2011) Effects of saddle height on pedal force effectiveness. Procedia Eng 13:51–55

Bini RR, Hume PA, Kilding A (2014) Optimizing bicycle configuration and cyclists' body position to prevent overuse injury using biomechanical approaches biomechanics of cycling. Adis-Springer, pp 92–107.

Burkett B (2010) Technology in Paralympic sport: performance enhancement or essential for performance? Br J Sports Med 44(3):215–220

Burkett B, Mellifont R (2008) Sport science and coaching in Paralympic cycling. Int J Sports Sci Coach 3(1):95–103

Burkett B, Smeathers J, Barker T (2003) Walking and running inter-limb asymmetry for Paralympic trans-femoral amputees, a biomechanical analysis. Prosthet Orthot Int 27(1):36–47

Childers WL, Kistenberg RS, Gregor RJ (2011) Pedaling asymmetries in cyclists with unilateral transtibial amputation: effect of prosthetic foot stiffness. J Appl Biomech 27(4):314–322

Churton E, Keogh JWL (2013) Constraints influencing sports wheelchair propulsion performance and injury risk. BMC Sports Sci Med Rehabil 5:3

Costa GB, Rubio MP, Belloch SL, Soriano PP (2009) Case study: effect of handrim diameter on performance in a paralympic wheelchair athlete. Adapt Phys Activ Q 26:352–363

Coutts KD (1990) Kinematics of sport wheelchair propulsion. J Rehabil Res 27(1):21–26

Dinsdale N, Dinsdale N (2011) The benefits of anatomical and biomechanical screening of competitive cyclists. SportEX Dyn 28:17–20

Fagher K, Forsberg A, Jacobsson J, Timpka T, Dahlstrom O, Lexell J (2016a) Paralympic athletes' perceptions of their experiences of sports-related injuries, risk factors and preventive possibilities. Eur J Sport Sci 16(8):1240–1249

Fagher K, Jacobsson J, Timpka T, Dahlström Ö, Lexell J (2016b) The Sports-Related Injuries and Illnesses in Paralympic Sport Study (SRIIPSS): a study protocol for a prospective longitudinal study. BMC Sports Sci Med Rehabil 8(1):28

Frossard L, Smeathers J, O'Riordan A, Goodman S (2007) Shot trajectory parameters in gold medal stationary shot-putters during world-class competition. Adapt Phys Activ Q 24(4):317–331

Frossard LA, O'Riordan A, Goodman S (2010) Throwing frame and performance of elite male seated shot-putters. Sports Technol 3(2):88–101

Hume PA, Soper C, Joe GM, Williams TR, Aitchison DR, Gunn S (2000) Effects of foot-stretcher angle on the drive phase in ergometer rowing. In: 2000 Pre-Olympic Congress, Brisbane, Australia, 2000. p 197

Keogh JWL (2011) Paralympic sport: an emerging area for research and consultancy in sports biomechanics. Sports Biomech 10(3):234–253

Lloyd CH, Stanhope SJ, Davis IS, Royer TD (2010) Strength asymmetry and osteoarthritis risk factors in unilateral trans-tibial, amputee gait. Gait Posture 32(3):296–300

Mason B, Van Der Woude L, de Groot S, Goosey-Tolfrey V (2011) Effects of camber on the ergonomics of propulsion in wheelchair athletes. Med Sci Sports Exerc 43(2):319–326

O'Riordan A, Goodman S, Frossard L (2004) Relationship between the parameters describing the feet position and the performance of elite seated discus throwers in Class F33/34 participating in the 2002 IPC World Championships. In: AAESS Exercise and Sports Science Conference, Brisbane, 2004

Soper C, Hume P, Cheung K, Benschop A (2001) Foot morphology of junior football players: implications for football shoe design - abstract. In: Australia SM (ed) Sports Medicine Australia, 2001: a sports medicine odyssey: challenges, controversies and change: Australian Conference of Science and Medicine in Sport Perth, WA, Australia, 2001. Sports Medicine Australia, p 101

Soper C, Hume PA (2004) Towards an ideal rowing technique for performance: the contributions from biomechanics. Sports Med 34(12):825–848

Stanbridge KJ, Mitchell SR, Jones R (2004) Design and development of sports equipment for children. Eng Sport 5(1):291–297

Tsai C-Y, Lin C-J, Huang Y-C, Lin P-C, F-C S (2012) The effects of rear-wheel camber on the kinematics of upper extremity during wheelchair propulsion. Biomed Eng Online 11(1):87

Vanlandewijck Y, Theisen D, Daly D (2001) Wheelchair propulsion biomechanics. Sports Med 31(5):339–367

Part II

How to Use the Selected Method and Report the Data

There are a variety of physique assessment techniques that can be selected by the practitioner including surface anthropometry, bioelectrical impedance analysis, dual energy X-ray absorptiometry, magnetic resonance imaging, three-dimensional photometry (3D scanning), air displacement plethysmography (Bod Pod), ultrasound techniques and dilution techniques (doubly labelled water).

Combinations of these techniques allow measurement of fat, fat-free mass, bone mineral content, total body water, extracellular water, total adipose tissue and its subdepots (visceral, subcutaneous and intermuscular), skeletal muscle, select organs and ectopic fat depots (Lee and Gallagher 2008). Clinicians and scientists can quantify a number of body components and can track changes in physique with the aim of determining efficacy of training, nutritional and clinical interventions.

Selection of technique to assess body physique is dependent upon factors including the validity, reliability, cost, safety, time for data collection and analysis, skill required for the practitioner and accessibility of the technology. These are some of the reasons why part II focuses on how to use selected methods and report data to athletes/coaches. Chapters include discussion of athlete considerations for measurement, non-imaging methods (surface anthropometry, air displacement plethysmography, 3D scanning, doubly labelled water, bioelectrical impedance, new innovations) and imaging methods (dual energy X-ray absorptiometry, ultrasound, computed tomography and magnetic resonance imaging). Each chapter in part II describes:

- Why you measure physique using the techniques and technologies. A description of how the technique allows measurement of physique is provided. Precision and accuracy, validity, practicality and sensitivity to monitor change of physique are described. Current issues surrounding the advantages and disadvantages of the technique are provided.

- What the techniques and technologies are. The hardware, software and skills required are described, and equipment selection, calibration, training and accreditation systems are outlined.
- How you use the selected technique for athletes. The technical specifics on how to conduct the assessment and analyse and report the data are outlined. Athlete presentation and preparation protocols are described.
- What technique is used to measure. Key variables gained from the technique and what is useful for monitoring athletes are outlined.

Reference

Lee SY, Gallagher D (2008) Assessment methods in human body composition. Curr Opin Clin Nutr Metabol Care 11(5):566–572

Chapter 5
Athlete Considerations for Physique Measurement

Gary Slater, Greg Shaw, and Ava Kerr

Abstract Physique traits are one of an array of variables known to influence performance of athletes across a wide range of sports. The routine monitoring of physique traits has become common practice amongst athletic populations, affording an opportunity to objectively assess the impact of training and diet and subsequently adjust these variables to optimise adaptations. An array of techniques is available to assess the physique traits of athletes. When selecting the most appropriate technique, a range of factors should be considered, including technical (safety, validity, precision and accuracy of measurement) and practical issues (availability, financial implications, portability, invasiveness, time effectiveness and technical expertise necessary), including the ability of the technique to accommodate the unique physique traits of athletes. Guidelines to assist with facilitating standardisation of athlete presentation prior to assessments are provided, with application to the majority of physique assessment techniques commonly applied amongst athletic populations such as dual-energy X-ray absorptiometry, air displacement plethysmography (i.e. Bod Pod) and bioelectrical impedance analysis. The exception may be surface anthropometry given results are minimally impacted by athlete presentation.

Keywords Physique traits • Monitoring • Training • Diet • Optimise adaptations Techniques • Safety • Validity • Precision • Accuracy • Availability • Financial implications • Portability • Invasiveness • Time effectiveness • Technical expertise Standardisation Athlete presentation • Dual-energy X-ray absorptiometry • Air displacement plethysmography • Bod Pod • Bioelectrical impedance • Surface anthropometry

G. Slater (✉) • A. Kerr
University of the Sunshine Coast, Maroochydore DC, QLD, Australia
e-mail: gslater@usc.edu.au; akerr@usc.edu.au

G. Shaw
Australian Sports Commission, Canberra, ACT, USA
e-mail: greg.shaw@ausport.gov.au

© Springer Nature Singapore Pte Ltd. 2018
P.A. Hume et al. (eds.), *Best Practice Protocols for Physique Assessment in Sport*,
https://doi.org/10.1007/978-981-10-5418-1_5

5.1   Introduction

One of the major influences of performance across many sports is the size, shape and composition of the human body (Cosgrove et al. 1999; Douda et al. 2008; Fleck 1983; Legaz and Eston 2005; Novak et al. 1968; Olds 2001; Raven et al. 1976; Siders et al. 1993; Sprynarova and Parizkova 1971). Consequently, many athletes at some point in their career will change attributes of their physique. This may occur naturally through growth and maturation or via purposeful interventions to enhance performance, undertaken in collaboration with coaches and sports nutrition experts. The routine monitoring of physique traits by trained professionals therefore becomes essential (Meyer et al. 2013) to further optimise training and/or diet to facilitate maximal responses, favourably impacting motivation and compliance to interventions.

The physique trait changes observed as a consequence of lifestyle interventions amongst individuals reflective of the general community can be substantial (Josse et al. 2011; Josse et al. 2010; Longland et al. 2016; Ahmadi et al. 2011). In contrast, the physique trait changes observed amongst athletic populations, while significant from a performance perspective (Colyer et al. 2017; Bilsborough et al. 2016), are more moderated (Argus et al. 2010; D'Ascenzi et al. 2015; Harley et al. 2011; Silvestre et al. 2006), presumably as they approach morphological optimisation for their chosen sport and/or individual genetic limitations. This highlights the importance of selecting physique assessment methods that are both valid and reliable, ensuring precision of measurement to accurately monitor small but important physique trait changes amongst athletes.

5.2   Considerations Prior To Assessment

An array of techniques is available for the measurement of body composition, including anthropometric, radiographic (computed tomography, magnetic resonance imaging, dual-energy X-ray absorptiometry), densitometric (Bod Pod, hydrodensitometry), imaging (3D scanning, ultrasound), metabolic (creatinine, 3-methylhistidine), nuclear (total body potassium, total body nitrogen), isotope dilution and bioelectrical impedance analysis techniques. Responsibility for body composition measurements falls within different professional realms including the sports scientist and sports dietitian and clinician, depending on resources and expertise available (Sundgot-Borgen et al. 2013). All techniques come with their own assumptions and limitations, and there is no single universally accepted gold standard (Ackland et al. 2012).

When selecting the most appropriate technique, a range of factors should be considered, including technical issues such as the safety, validity, precision and accuracy of measurement. Practical issues must be considered like availability, financial implications, portability, invasiveness, time effectiveness and technical expertise necessary to conduct the procedures. Consideration must be given to the ability of body composition assessment methodologies to accommodate the unique physique trait characteristic of some athletes. Tall, broad and muscular individuals or those with extremely low body fat levels can be more challenging to assess for a variety of reasons. Finally, an understanding of the variables of interest to be assessed is required and an understanding of whether the assessment is a one-off measure or to track changes longitudinally, as occurs most often in athletic populations (Meyer et al. 2013). Table 5.1 provides a summary of the most common physique assessment techniques, the information they provide, plus their strengths and weaknesses for use amongst athletic populations.

When collecting data, the physical and emotional well-being of the athlete must also be considered and should remain a priority. The assessment of body composition amongst athletes, especially female athletes and dancers, has been questioned due to the possibility of assessments promoting anxiety and disordered eating (Carson et al. 2001). When undertaken in conjunction with a suitably designed education programme, evidence suggests physique assessments can be undertaken without promoting adverse affective consequences (Whitehead et al. 2003). Where appropriate, consideration should be given to gender comparability between the technician and athlete, with privacy in data collection and reporting always assured. Sensitivity should be shown to cultural beliefs and tradition. Procedures should be explained to those unfamiliar, with information provided in advance on what testing is to be undertaken, the reason for profiling and what measurements are to be taken. Given the variability in human physiology throughout a day and between days, significant attention must also be given to minimising this and its potential influence on the reliability of physique assessment techniques. This will not only assist in enhancing the precision of measurement but also help reduce stress and anxiety, often associated with physique assessment, particularly in those populations where leanness and appearance are important. Thus, detailed information on any specific requirements such as clothing to be worn, plus any diet or physical activity guidance, should be provided well in advance of assessments and considered an essential element of any physique assessment protocol.

5.3 Precision of Measurement

Irrespective of the physique assessment technique chosen, all have some inherent problems, whether in measurement methodology or in the assumptions they make (Ackland et al. 2012). Any variability of physique assessment results can be divided into two categories: technical and biological error. In an effort to enhance precision of measurement, a best practice protocol for assessment of body composition should be implemented, independent of the technique chosen. Specific components of such a protocol will vary depending on the technique utilised but should include consideration of issues like the implementation of quality control procedures and standardisation of athlete presentation prior to all assessments. Data obtained from such

Table 5.1 The most common physique assessment techniques available, including the attributes they measure, plus their strengths and weaknesses for use amongst athletic populations

Technique; commercial availability	Accuracy; reliability	Regional assessment	Attributes measured	Time commitment; minimum assessment frequency	Athlete friendly; health risk	Skilled technician required
Surface anthropometry; very available	Medium; high	Possible but not recommended	FM (via equation), ΣSF	Moderately quick <15 min; 3 weeks	Very; low	Yes
Bioelectrical impedance analysis/bioelectrical impedance spectroscopy; very available	Low; low	Possible but invalid	FFM, FM, TBW	Very quick <1 min; 4 weeks	Very; low	Ideally
Dual-energy X-ray absorptiometry; available	Medium; high	Possible and reliable	NOL, BM, FM	Quick <10 min; 8 weeks	Very; medium	Yes
Bod Pod: available	Medium; high	Not possible	FFM, FM, TBV	Quick <10 min; 4 weeks	Very; low	Ideally
Ultrasound; hard to find	High; medium	Possible and reliable	mm of fat	Quick; 4 weeks	Very; low	Yes
3D scanning; available	Unknown	Possible	FFM, FM, TBV, SV	Very quick <5 min; 4 weeks	Very; low	Yes
Deuterium dilution; very hard to find	Medium; high	Not possible	TBW, FFM, FM	Very slow ~6 h; 4 weeks	Somewhat; low	Yes
3-compartment methodology; hard to find	High; high	Not possible	FM, NOL, BM	Slow ~1 h; 4 weeks	Somewhat; low	Yes
4-compartment methodology; hard to find	High; high	Not possible	FM, MM, RM, BM	Very slow ~6 h; 8 weeks	Somewhat; medium	Yes

UWW = underwater weighing; BM = bone mineral content; FM = fat mass; FFM = fat-free mass; MM = muscle mass; NOL = non-osseous lean; RM = residual mass; SV = segmental volume; ΣSF = sum of skinfolds; TBV = total body volume; TBW = total body water

tightly controlled assessments ensures a high level of precision while still being practical in an athletic setting.

While issues associated with equipment contributing to measurement error are often beyond the control of technicians, athlete presentation can also contribute to the error of repeat testing across most, if not all, physique assessment techniques. There are numerous factors associated with the athletes' presentation or status that have been shown to influence acute or day-to-day variation in the estimation of physique traits, collectively contributing to the biological error of measurement. The impact of these factors will vary depending on the specific physique trait, plus the technique being utilised. For example, failing to account for the time of day, and thus ad libitum food and fluid intake, plus physical activity has a marked impact on the precision of measurement for bioelectrical impedance analysis but little if any impact on subcutaneous skinfold measurements (Kerr et al. 2017). Nuances associated with specific physique assessment techniques should be recognised prior to assessment so that other factors contributing to measurement error are accounted for in testing protocols. For example, male athletes should be clean shaven (Higgins et al. 2001), wearing tight-fitting clothing (Vescovi et al. 2002; Fields et al. 2000) and a silicone swim cap (Peeters and Claessens 2011) during a Bod Pod assessment, while acute exercise-induced water retention can influence magnetic resonance imaging estimates of muscle cross-sectional area for at least 3 days (Kristiansen et al. 2014). In general factors such as time of day, prior food/fluid intake and exercise, body temperature, hydration status and gastrointestinal tract contents should be standardised wherever possible prior to any physique assessment. Fasted early morning assessments following bladder and possibly bowel evacuation may be the most reliable where practical given diurnal variation in body mass.

Implications of client presentation on precision of measurement have been recognised, with the development of best practice protocols of assessment for several physique assessment techniques, including surface anthropometry (Marfell-Jones et al. 2016), dual-energy X-ray absorptiometry (Hangartner et al. 2013; Nana et al. 2015), bioelectrical impedance (Kyle et al. 2004) and ultrasound (Muller et al. 2013), although the implications of client presentation on reliability of the later remain to be explored. Minimising the error or noise associated with a test enhances its reliability, making it easier to identify small but potentially important changes. Reliability of measurement also influences the frequency of assessment, with the most reliable measures given priority when there is a need for frequent review of physique traits. In general, physique assessments should not be undertaken anymore regularly than every 4–8 weeks, depending on the individual athlete and their body composition goals. Practitioners are reminded that frequent assessments, at least in the form of self-weighing, may facilitate the development of disordered eating attitudes and behaviours (Carrigan et al. 2015). A summary of the factors contributing to biological error amongst the most commonly accepted physique assessment techniques is presented in Table 5.2. Details on the specific physique trait(s) impacted and the direction of change are also reported.

Table 5.2 Summary of factors contributing to biological error amongst the commonly used physique assessment techniques for athletes

	Substrate variability	Dehydration	Hot and sweaty	Acute food and fluid intake	Menstrual cycle	Day-to-day variability (% TEM)		Body hair	Clothes
						STD	Non-STD		
Surface anthropometry	–	–	–	–	Monitor	1.0	1.4	–	–
Bioelectrical impedance/ bioelectrical impedance spectroscopy	–	FM ↓	FM ↑	FM and FFM ↑	Monitor	1.5 FFM 14.9 FM	1.2 FFM 9.0 FM	–	–
Dual-energy X-ray absorptiometry	FFM ↓↑	FFM ↓	–	FFM ↑	Monitor	0.7 FFM 3.2 FM	1.1 FFM 3.1 FM	–	FFM ↑
Bod Pod	–	–	FM ↓	FM and FFM ↑	–	0.7 FFM 3.6 FM	0.9 FFM 4.8 FM	FM ↓	FM ↓
Magnetic resonance imaging/ Computed tomography	FFM ↓↑	–	–	–	–	–	–	–	–
Ultrasound	Unknown								
3D scanning	Unknown								

FM = fat mass; FFM = fat-free mass

5.4 Hydration Status

The potential variability in total body water and thus hydration of the fat-free mass may be a particular concern amongst athletic populations, with any significant variance in hydration status influencing interpretation of body composition across most physique assessment techniques, including bioelectrical impedance and hydrodensitometry (Thompson et al. 1991), Bod Pod (Utter et al. 2003; Heiss et al. 2009) and dual-energy X-ray absorptiometry (Rodriguez-Sanchez and Galloway 2015), with surface anthropometry the only exception with hypohydration having little (Rodriguez-Sanchez and Galloway 2015), if any, impact on skinfold values (Kerr et al. 2017). Despite this, only a small proportion of practitioners assess hydration status prior to physique assessment (Meyer et al. 2013).

Total body water content of fat-free mass is often assumed to be set at 73.7% (Brozek et al. 1963) by many physique assessment techniques yet can vary from 67% to 85% (Moore and Boyden 1963). Any deviation from this assumed constant has the potential to impact estimates of body composition across the majority of physique assessment techniques advocated for use within athletic populations. The significance of this impact and the variables that a state of hypohydration or hyperhydration influence will depend on the technique under investigation and possibly the method in which the deviation from a state of euhydration is achieved. For example, any fluid deficit that results from involuntary hypohydration after exercise is identified almost exclusively as lean mass with dual-energy X-ray absorptiometry (Nana et al. 2013) but as fat mass when assessed via bioelectrical impedance. While the impact of exercise on body composition estimates is negated with dual-energy X-ray absorptiometry if a state of euhydration can be maintained, the effect remains with bioelectrical impedance (Rodriguez-Sanchez and Galloway 2015), most likely as a consequence of increased cutaneous blood flow and temperature and skin electrolyte accumulation, which are known to influence electrical conductance and thus precision of bioelectrical impedance measurement (O'Brien et al. 2002). While this sustained impact on physique assessment using bioelectrical impedance may be resolved via a cold shower (Gatterer et al. 2014), this does not account for any concomitant body fluid deficits. Because hydration changes typically involve concomitant changes in fluid and electrolyte content, the interpretation of a change in bioimpedance (and thus body composition) will often be confounded, ensuring uniform change in interpretation of body composition as a consequence of hydration status changes is not possible with bioelectrical impedance (O'Brien et al. 2002). In contrast, while it has been claimed that hypohydration and associated increase in core temperature may promote dilation of peripheral cutaneous arterioles, resulting in substantial increases in subcutaneous skinfold measurements (Jackson and Pollock 1985), there is limited (Rodriguez-Sanchez and Galloway 2015), if any, research supporting this stance, at least when raw data is used (Kerr et al. 2017). Because regression equations used to interpret body composition from subcutaneous skinfolds also use body mass, the reduction in body mass associated with acute hypohydration would result in an underestimation in lean mass with as concomitant overestimation if fat mass.

Any deviation from euhydration amongst athletes is likely to be a state of hypohydration. However, there are situations where fluid overload is evident as a consequence of medical conditions such as renal disease or oedema (Chumlea 2004; Dehghan and Merchant 2008). While such medical conditions are unlikely amongst athletic populations, other issues may need to be considered prior to physique assessment, including training status, dietary intake and female menstrual cycle. Given the impact of variation in hydration status on interpretation of physique traits across many physique assessment techniques, a state of euhydration should be facilitated prior to physique assessment. Given the impact of exercise on hydration status and muscle glycogen stores, consideration should also be given to exercise prior to the assessment of physique traits (Bone et al. 2016). It is recommended that hydration status be confirmed prior to physique assessment (Meyer et al. 2013), with guidance provided the day prior to assessment to assist in facilitating a state of euhydration. While isotope dilution is the reference method of measurement of hydration status (Heymsfield et al. 2015), it is a laborious, time-consuming and expensive process to undertake. Consequently non-invasive biomarkers such as urinary specific gravity, measured either by refractometer or dipstick, are regularly used in practice (Meyer et al. 2013).

5.5 Dietary Intake

Acute food and fluid intake has been shown to influence precision of measurement across the majority of commonly used physique assessment techniques, including dual-energy X-ray absorptiometry, Bod Pod and bioelectrical impedance. The degree of impact, and the variables influenced, differs depending on the method used. The ingestion of a meal or drink prior to a dual-energy X-ray absorptiometry scan can result in a significant increase in lean mass, primarily in the trunk, but not impact on estimates of fat mass or bone mass (Horber et al. 1992). While the ingestion of a light meal with 500 ml fluid was considered to have little impact on results (Horber et al. 1992; Vilaca et al. 2009), subsequent investigations have confirmed the impact of acute food/fluid intake on estimates of lean mass using dual-energy X-ray absorptiometry (Thomsen et al. 1998; Nana et al. 2012). Kerr and colleagues recently assessed the impact of an acute meal (500 g ± 1000 ml water) on physique traits assessed via the most frequently used techniques (Kerr et al. 2017). Aside from the measurement of subcutaneous fat via the skinfold technique, all other physique assessment methods were influenced by the meal. While this consistently increased lean mass estimates via dual-energy X-ray absorptiometry, the compositional impacts varied based on the method. Estimates of both fat mass and fat-free mass were increased with Bod Pod and bioelectrical impedance. Given this, current best practice advice would suggest the assessment of physique traits should be undertaken after an overnight fast. When this is not possible, athletes should be encouraged to standardise their dietary intake prior to each assessment (Colyer et al. 2016).

Alteration in intramuscular solutes, specifically glycogen (Bone et al. 2016; Rouillier et al. 2015; Tinsley et al. 2016) and, to a lesser degree, creatine monohydrate (Safdar et al. 2008; Bone et al. 2016), is another source of biological variation, most likely because of their associated water binding (Olsson and Saltin 1970). This should not come as a surprise as it has previously been shown that changes in cellular substrates achieved by common sports nutrition practices can cause detectable changes in muscle size and mass (Bone et al. 2016). For example, muscle cross-sectional area has been shown to increase using magnetic resonance imaging following a carbohydrate-loading diet (Nygren et al. 2001). Similarly, creatine monohydrate supplementation has been shown to increase lean body mass when assessed by dual-energy X-ray absorptiometry (Safdar et al. 2008). While the impact of intramuscular solutes on other measures of body composition remains to be ascertained, any method impacted by changes in total body water content will likely be impacted by acute variation in intramuscular solutes. Thus, athletes should be provided with direction on how to ensure they arrive for assessment in a state of euhydration with replete muscle glycogen stores. Athletes should be questioned about their supplementation practices prior to each and every assessment.

5.6   Female Menstrual Cycle

It is not well known if the biological variation associated with the female menstrual cycle has a large influence on measures of physique. Theoretically it could be assumed that variations in fluid storage associated with the phase of the menstrual cycle will significantly impact estimates of body composition similar to what variation in hydration status does and therefore should be controlled for (Wenner and Stachenfeld 2012). While body mass does increase during the premenstrual period, the actual body mass change is relatively small (Robinson and Watson 1965), with little impact on interpretation of body composition as inferred via bioelectrical impedance (Gualdi-Russo and Toselli 2002; Gleichauf and Roe 1989). However, given the length, and frequency of menstrual cycles can vary significantly from athlete to athlete, more research is needed to better understand how menstrual cycle can influence the precision of body composition assessment across the spectrum of techniques used commonly to monitor athletes. Until then, the practical recommendation would be to record the phase of the menstrual cycle the athlete is in and attempt to repeat subsequent assessments at a similar time point in the cycle.

5.7   Considerations for Data Capture

A number of physique assessment techniques are supported for use amongst athletic populations. While the development of best practice protocols of assessment has been established for some of these physique assessment techniques, this typically only addresses technical error. In accordance with the Ad Hoc Research Working Group on Body Composition, Health and Performance under the auspices of the IOC Medical Commission, standardised physique assessment protocols should be established that consider all factors associated with measurement error. The implementation of such protocols will optimise precision of measurement, assisting practitioners to further optimise diet and training interventions while limiting athlete anxiety associated with poorly standardised physique assessment. While strategies to minimise technical error vary between physique assessment techniques, biological error primarily comes from factors associated with the presentation status of the athlete and thus can be minimised. Physique assessments undertaken with these issues in mind ensure a high level of precision while still being practical in an athletic setting.

While the impact of time of day, prior food/fluid intake and exercise, body temperature, hydration status and gastrointestinal tract contents will vary depending on the technique used to assess body composition, the following guidelines are recommended to assist in minimising biological error of measurement when undertaking physique assessment of athletes. Further guidance specific to the physique assessment technique may be necessary.

Testing procedures should be explained to those unfamiliar, with information provided in advance on what testing is to be undertaken, the reason for profiling and what measurements are to be taken. Given the variability in human physiology throughout a day and between days, significant attention must also be given to minimising this and its potential influence on the reliability of physique assessment techniques. Detailed information on any specific requirements such as clothing to be worn, plus any diet or physical activity guidance, should be provided well in advance of assessments and considered an essential element of any physique assessment protocol.

Information should be provided in advance of assessment on how to optimise hydration status throughout the day prior to testing. Dietary guidance to facilitate repletion of muscle glycogen stores should also be provided for implementation the day prior to assessment. Assessments should be undertaken first thing in the morning, fasted and rested, with no intense physical activity for at least 12 h. Athletes should arrive at the testing facility via car or public transport, i.e. rested state. While the exact requirements for clothing will vary according to the physique assessment technique, athletes should wear figure hugging but noncompressive clothing that does not contain any metal, which allows ready access to all regions of the body while accommodating athlete privacy and modesty. Athletes need to present in a euhydrated state, with a urine sample collected during evacuation of bladder to confirm hydration status via a measure of urinary specific gravity.

Screening should be implemented prior to all assessments via the use of a questionnaire to assess dietary intake over the past day, including the use of supplements such as creatine monohydrate. Amongst female athletes, phase of menstrual cycle should be documented, with phase ideally standardised between repeat assessments. Assessments should be undertaken in a thermoneutral environment, preferably in a room that affords the athlete (and their data) privacy.

5.8 Summary

The Ad Hoc Research Working Group on Body Composition, Health and Performance of the IOC Medical Commission, recommends standardised physique assessment protocols should be established to enhance the precision of measurement, affording an opportunity to accurately identify small but potentially important changes in physique traits. While issues associated with equipment contributing to measurement error are often beyond the control of technicians, athlete presentation contributes to the error and thus should also be standardised. In general factors such as time of day, prior food or fluid intake, exercise, body temperature, hydration status and gastrointestinal tract contents should be standardised wherever possible prior to any physique assessment. Given the diurnal variation in body mass, fasted early morning assessments following bladder and possibly bowel evacuation may be the most reliable where practical. As hydration status is highly variable amongst athletes, confirmation of hydration status should be sought prior to assessment. The implementation of such protocols will optimise precision of measurement, assisting practitioners to further optimise diet and training interventions while limiting athlete anxiety associated with poorly standardised physique assessment.

References

Ackland TR, Lohman TG, Sundgot-Borgen J, Maughan RJ, Meyer NL, Stewart AD, Muller W (2012) Current status of body composition assessment in sport: review and position statement on behalf of the ad hoc research working group on body composition health and performance, under the auspices of the I.o.C. Medical commission. Sports Medicine 42(3):227–249

Ahmadi N, Eshaghian S, Huizenga R, Sosnin K, Ebrahimi R, Siegel R (2011) Effects of intense exercise and moderate caloric restriction on cardiovascular risk factors and inflammation. Am J Med 124(10):978–982

Argus CK, Gill N, Keogh J, Hopkins WG, Beaven CM (2010) Effects of a short-term pre-season training programme on the body composition and anaerobic performance of professional rugby union players. J Sports Sci 28(6):679–686

Bilsborough JC, Greenway K, Livingston S, Cordy J, Coutts AJ (2016) Changes in anthropometry, upper-body strength, and nutrient intake in professional Australian Football players during a season. Int J Sports Physiol Perform 11(3):290–300

Bone JL, Ross ML, Tomcik KA, Jeacocke NA, Hopkins WG, Burke LM (2016) Manipulation of muscle creatine and glycogen changes DXA estimates of body composition. Med Sci Sports Exerc. 49(5):1029–1035

Brozek J, Grande F, Anderson JT, Keys A (1963) Densitometric analysis of body composition: revision of some quantitative assumptions. Ann N Y Acad Sci 110:113–140

Carrigan KW, Petrie TA, Anderson CM (2015) To weigh or not to weigh? relation to disordered eating attitudes and behaviors among female collegiate athletes. Journal of sport & exercise psychology 37(6):659–665

Carson JD, Bridges E, Canadian Academy of Sport M (2001) Abandoning routine body composition assessment: a strategy to reduce disordered eating among female athletes and dancers. Clin J Sport Med 11(4):280

Chumlea WC (2004) Anthropometric and body composition assessment in dialysis patients. Semin Dial 17(6):466–470

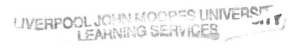

Colyer SL, Roberts SP, Robinson JB, Thompson D, Stokes KA, Bilzon JL, Salo AI (2016) Detecting meaningful body composition changes in athletes using dual-energy x-ray absorptiometry. Physiol Meas 37(4):596–609

Colyer SL, Stokes KA, Bilzon JL, Cardinale M, Salo AI (2017) Physical predictors of elite skeleton start performance. Int J Sports Physiol Perform 12:81–89

Cosgrove MJ, Wilson J, Watt D, Grant SF (1999) The relationship between selected physiological variables of rowers and rowing performance as determined by a 2000 m ergometer test. J Sports Sci 17(11):845–852

D'Ascenzi F, Pelliccia A, Cameli M, Lisi M, Natali BM, Focardi M, Giorgi A, D'Urbano G, Causarano A, Bonifazi M, Mondillo S (2015) Dynamic changes in left ventricular mass and in fat-free mass in top-level athletes during the competitive season. European journal of preventive cardiology 22(1):127–134

Dehghan M, Merchant AT (2008) Is bioelectrical impedance accurate for use in large epidemiological studies? Nutrition journal 7:26

Douda HT, Toubekis AG, Avloniti AA, Tokmakidis SP (2008) Physiological and anthropometric determinants of rhythmic gymnastics performance. Int J Sports Physiol Perform 3(1):41–54

Fields DA, Hunter GR, Goran MI (2000) Validation of the BOD POD with hydrostatic weighing: influence of body clothing. Int J Obes Relat Metab Disord 24(2):200–205

Fleck SJ (1983) Body composition of elite American athletes. Am J Sports Med 11(6):398–403

Gatterer H, Schenk K, Laninschegg L, Schlemmer P, Lukaski H, Burtscher M (2014) Bioimpedance identifies body fluid loss after exercise in the heat: a pilot study with body cooling. PLoS One 9(10):e109729

Gleichauf CN, Roe DA (1989) The menstrual cycle's effect on the reliability of bioimpedance measurements for assessing body composition. Am J Clin Nutr 50(5):903–907

Gualdi-Russo E, Toselli S (2002) Influence of various factors on the measurement of multifrequency bioimpedance. Homo 53(1):1–16

Hangartner TN, Warner S, Braillon P, Jankowski L, Shepherd J (2013) The official positions of the international society for clinical densitometry: acquisition of dual-energy x-ray absorptiometry body composition and considerations regarding analysis and repeatability of measures. J Clin Densitom 16(4):520–536

Harley JA, Hind K, O'Hara JP (2011) Three-compartment body composition changes in elite rugby league players during a super league season, measured by dual energy X-ray absorptiometry. J Strength Cond Res 25(4):1024–1029

Heiss CJ, Gara N, Novotny D, Heberle H, Morgan L, Stufflebeam J, Fairfield M (2009) Effect of a 1 liter fluid load on body composition measured by air displacement plethysmography and bioelectrical impedance. Journal of Exercise Physiology 12(2):1–8

Heymsfield SB, Ebbeling CB, Zheng J, Pietrobelli A, Strauss BJ, Silva AM, Ludwig DS (2015) Multi-component molecular-level body composition reference methods: evolving concepts and future directions. Obes Rev 16(4):282–294

Higgins PB, Fields DA, Hunter GR, Gower BA (2001) Effect of scalp and facial hair on air displacement plethysmography estimates of percentage of body fat. Obes Res 9(5):326–330

Horber FF, Thomi F, Casez JP, Fonteille J, Jaeger P (1992) Impact of hydration status on body composition as measured by dual energy X-ray absorptiometry in normal volunteers and patients on haemodialysis. Br J Radiol 65(778):895–900

Jackson AS, Pollock ML (1985) Practical assessment of body composition. Phys Sportsmed 13(5):76–90

Josse AR, Atkinson SA, Tarnopolsky MA, Phillips SM (2011) Increased consumption of dairy foods and protein during diet- and exercise-induced weight loss promotes fat mass loss and lean mass gain in overweight and obese premenopausal women. J Nutr 141(9):1626–1634

Josse AR, Tang JE, Tarnopolsky MA, Phillips SM (2010) Body composition and strength changes in women with milk and resistance exercise. Med Sci Sports Exerc 42(6):1122–1130

Kerr A, Slater G, Byrne N (2017) Impact of food and fluid intake on technical and biological measurement error in body composition assessment methods in athletes. Br J Nutr. 117:591–601

Kristiansen MS, Uhrbrand A, Hansen M, Shiguetomi-Medina JM, Vissing K, Stodkilde-Jorgensen H, Langberg H (2014) Concomitant changes in cross-sectional area and water content in skeletal muscle after resistance exercise. Scand J Med Sci Sports 24(4):e260–e268

Kyle UG, Bosaeus I, De Lorenzo AD, Deurenberg P, Elia M, Manuel Gomez J, Lilienthal Heitmann B, Kent-Smith L, Melchior JC, Pirlich M, Scharfetter H, MWJS A, Pichard C (2004) Bioelectrical impedance analysis-part II: utilization in clinical practice. Clin Nutr 23(6):1430–1453

Legaz A, Eston R (2005) Changes in performance, skinfold thicknesses, and fat patterning after three years of intense athletic conditioning in high level runners. British Journal of Sports Medicine 39(11):851–856

Longland TM, Oikawa SY, Mitchell CJ, Devries MC, Phillips SM (2016) Higher compared with lower dietary protein during an energy deficit combined with intense exercise promotes greater lean mass gain and fat mass loss: a randomized trial. Am J Clin Nutr 103(3):738–746

Marfell-Jones M, Olds T, Stewart A, Carter L (2016) International standards for anthropometric assessment. ISAK, Potchefstroom

Meyer NL, Sundgot-Borgen J, Lohman TG, Ackland TR, Stewart AD, Maughan RJ, Smith S, Muller W (2013) Body composition for health and performance: a survey of body composition assessment practice carried out by the Ad Hoc Research Working Group on Body Composition, Health and Performance under the auspices of the IOC Medical Commission. Br J Sports Med 47(16):1044–1053

Moore FD, Boyden CM (1963) Body cell mass and limits of hydration of the fat-free body: their relation to estimated skeletal weight. Ann N Y Acad Sci 110:62–71

Muller W, Horn M, Furhapter-Rieger A, Kainz P, Kropfl JM, Maughan RJ, Ahammer H (2013) Body composition in sport: a comparison of a novel ultrasound imaging technique to measure subcutaneous fat tissue compared with skinfold measurement. Br J Sports Med 47(16): 1028–1035

Nana A, Slater GJ, Hopkins WG, Burke LM (2012) Effects of daily activities on dual energy X-ray absorptiometry measurements of body composition in active people. Med Sci Sports Exerc 44(1):180–189

Nana A, Slater GJ, Hopkins WG, Burke LM (2013) Effects of exercise sessions on DXA measurements of body composition in active people. Med Sci Sports Exerc 45(1):178–185

Nana A, Slater GJ, Stewart AD, Burke LM (2015) Methodology review: using dual-energy X-ray absorptiometry (DXA) for the assessment of body composition in athletes and active people. Int J Sport Nutr Exerc Metab 25(2):198–215

Novak LP, Hyatt RE, Alexander JF (1968) Body composition and physiologic function of athletes. Jama 205(11):764–770

Nygren AT, Karlsson M, Norman B, Kaijser L (2001) Effect of glycogen loading on skeletal muscle cross-sectional area and T2 relaxation time. Acta Physiol Scand 173(4):385–390

O'Brien C, Young AJ, Sawka MN, Koulmann N, Jimenez C, Regal D, Bolliet P, Launay JC, Savourey G, Melin B (2002) Bioelectrical impedance to estimate changes in hydration status. Int J Sports Med 23(5):361–366

Olds T (2001) The evolution of physique in male rugby union players in the twentieth century. J Sports Sci 19(4):253–262

Olsson KE, Saltin B (1970) Variation in total body water with muscle glycogen changes in man. Acta Physiol Scand 80(1):11–18

Peeters MW, Claessens AL (2011) Effect of different swim caps on the assessment of body volume and percentage body fat by air displacement plethysmography. J Sports Sci 29(2):191–196

Raven PB, Gettman LR, Pollock ML, Cooper KH (1976) A physiological evaluation of professional soccer players. Br J Sports Med 10(4):209–216

Robinson MF, Watson PE (1965) day-to-day variations in body-weight of young women. Br J Nutr 19:225–235

Rodriguez-Sanchez N, Galloway SD (2015) Errors in dual energy x-ray absorptiometry estimation of body composition induced by hypohydration. Int J Sport Nutr Exerc Metab 25(1):60–68

Rouillier MA, David-Riel S, Brazeau AS, St-Pierre DH, Karelis AD (2015) Effect of an acute high carbohydrate diet on body composition using DXA in young men. Ann Nutr Metab 66(4):233–236

Safdar A, Yardley NJ, Snow R, Melov S, Tarnopolsky MA (2008) Global and targeted gene expression and protein content in skeletal muscle of young men following short-term creatine monohydrate supplementation. Physiological genomics 32(2):219–228

Siders WA, Lukaski HC, Bolonchuk WW (1993) Relationships among swimming performance, body composition and somatotype in competitive collegiate swimmers. J Sports Med Phys Fitness 33(2):166–171

Silvestre R, Kraemer WJ, West C, Judelson DA, Spiering BA, Vingren JL, Hatfield DL, Anderson JM, Maresh CM (2006) Body composition and physical performance during a National Collegiate Athletic Association Division I men's soccer season. J Strength Cond Res 20(4):962–970

Sprynarova S, Parizkova J (1971) Functional capacity and body composition in top weight-lifters, swimmers, runners and skiers. Internationale Zeitschrift fur angewandte Physiologie, einschliesslich Arbeitsphysiologie 29(2):184–194

Sundgot-Borgen J, Meyer NL, Lohman TG, Ackland TR, Maughan RJ, Stewart AD, Muller W (2013) How to minimise the health risks to athletes who compete in weight-sensitive sports review and position statement on behalf of the Ad Hoc Research Working Group on Body Composition, Health and Performance, under the auspices of the IOC Medical Commission. Br J Sports Med 47(16):1012–1022

Thompson DL, Thompson WR, Prestridge TJ, Bailey JG, Bean MH, Brown SP, McDaniel JB (1991) Effects of hydration and dehydration on body composition analysis: a comparative study of bioelectric impedance analysis and hydrodensitometry. J Sports Med Phys Fitness 31(4):565–570

Thomsen TK, Jensen VJ, Henriksen MG (1998) In vivo measurement of human body composition by dual energy X-ray absorptiometry (DXA). The European Journal of Surgery 164(2):133–137

Tinsley GM, Morales FE, Forsse JS, Grandjean PW (2016) Impact of acute dietary manipulations on DXA and BIA body composition estimates. Med Sci Sports Exerc. 49(4):823–832

Utter AC, Goss FL, Swan PD, Harris GS, Robertson RJ, Trone GA (2003) Evaluation of air displacement for assessing body composition of collegiate wrestlers. Med Sci Sports Exerc 35(3):500–505

Vescovi JD, Zimmerman SL, Miller WC, Fernhall B (2002) Effects of clothing on accuracy and reliability of air displacement plethysmography. Med Sci Sports Exerc 34(2):282–285

Vilaca KH, Ferriolli E, Lima NK, Paula FJ, Moriguti JC (2009) Effect of fluid and food intake on the body composition evaluation of elderly persons. J Nutr Health Aging 13(3):183–186

Wenner MM, Stachenfeld NS (2012) Blood pressure and water regulation: understanding sex hormone effects within and between men and women. J Physiol 590(23):5949–5961

Whitehead JR, Eklund RC, Williams AC (2003) Using skinfold calipers while teaching body fatness-related concepts: cognitive and affective outcomes. J Sci Med Sport 6(4):461–476

Chapter 6
Non-imaging Method: Surface Anthropometry

Patria A. Hume, Kelly R. Sheerin, and J. Hans de Ridder

Abstract The International Society for the Advancement of Kinanthropometry (ISAK) protocols should be followed for physical assessment of body size, shape and composition. The advantages of the ISAK surface anthropometry methods are that assessments take approximately 10 min for a restricted profile and up to 30 min for a full profile, and the equipment is readily available and easily calibrated. The methods are valid and reliable if ISAK training is undertaken to ensure correct land-marking is performed. International data are available for comparison of athlete measures for many sports. The disadvantage of the ISAK surface anthropometry technique is that skinfold callipers compress the adipose tissue resulting in variation in measurements. Therefore, a complete data set of the proforma is obtained before repeating the measurements for the second and then third time. This may help to reduce the effects of skinfold compressibility.

Keywords Physique • Equipment • Calliper • Landmarking • Skinfolds • Girths; Breadths; Waist/hip • Waist/height • Circumference • Ratios • Somatotype • Profile International standard

P.A. Hume (✉)
Sport Performance Research Institute New Zealand,
Auckland University of Technology, Auckland, New Zealand
e-mail: patria.hume@aut.ac.nz

K.R. Sheerin
Auckland University of Technology, Auckland, New Zealand
e-mail: kelly.sheerin@aut.ac.nz

J.H. de Ridder
North-West University, Potchefstroom, South Africa
e-mail: hans.deridder@nwu.ac.za

© Springer Nature Singapore Pte Ltd. 2018   61
P.A. Hume et al. (eds.), *Best Practice Protocols for Physique Assessment in Sport*,
https://doi.org/10.1007/978-981-10-5418-1_6

6.1   Introduction

Nutrition and training status is manifest in body size, shape and composition. Clinic/
field techniques for surface physical assessment of body size and shape (girths,
waist-to-hip circumference ratios, waist-to-height ratio, breadths, somatotype) and
body composition (skinfolds) are recommended by the International Society for the
Advancement of Kinanthropometry (ISAK) (Stewart et al. 2011). The ISAK accreditation scheme specifies requirements for conducting ISAK courses and provides
resources for teaching and examining practitioners. An ISAK textbook is provided
to all course participants as part of the course registration fee (Stewart et al. 2011).

6.2   What Is Surface Anthropometry?

The surface anthropometry measures prescribed by ISAK are for a restricted profile
(2 basic measures, 8 skinfolds, 5 girths and 2 breadths) and a full profile (4 basic
measures, 8 skinfolds, 13 girths, 8 lengths and heights, 9 breadths).

6.3   Why Measure Physique Using Surface Anthropometry?

The ISAK surface anthropometry method takes approximately 10 min for a
restricted profile and up to 30 min for a full profile. The methods are valid and reliable if ISAK training is undertaken to ensure correct landmarking is performed. The
equipment is readily available and easily calibrated. However, different equipment
can increase error of measurement, so it is important to source robust and accurate
equipment.

For an assessment test to be of any value, it must be specific enough to be measuring the performance variable of interest and also reliable enough to detect the
relatively small differences in performance that are beneficial to elite athletes. To
minimize technical error of measurement, differences between repeat skinfold measures, measurement sites and measurement techniques have been set out by ISAK.

The importance of accurate skinfold measurement site location using ISAK standard sites was examined in 12 healthy participants (11 male and 1 female;
27.1 ± 6.5 years; 177.3 ± 7.4 cm; 77.8 ± 12.7 kg). Nine measurements, in a 1-cm
grid pattern, centred on each of the eight ISAK-specified skinfold sites, were taken
three times at each grid point by each of two ISAK Criterion (Level 4) measurers
using Harpenden skinfold callipers. Skinfolds taken at the eight peripheral grid
points in a 1-cm grid pattern were generally different (45 out of 64 = 70%) from the
skinfolds taken at the defined ISAK site (the central grid point for this study). There
was an effect by direction (anterior, posterior, superior or inferior). The subscapular
was the most robust skinfold site in terms of little effect with deviation away from

the central ISAK point. All other skinfold sites showed some variation, with most care needed in marking the bicep and tricep skinfold sites. Measuring 1 cm away from a defined ISAK site produced significant differences in the majority of skinfold measurement values obtained. No site was totally free from this variation. Therefore, adherence to identifying, marking and measuring at the defined site is essential (Hume and Marfell-Jones 2008). The international standardization of the ISAK protocols is a strength-enabling data from throughout the world to be combined with confidence.

6.4 How Do You Use Surface Anthropometry for Your Athlete?

6.4.1 Consent to Conduct Measurements

Surface anthropometry body measurement can be stressful for athletes if they are not familiar with the process, so a clear explanation of the measurement process must be outlined. It is recommended that an information sheet be provided to the athlete prior to them attending an assessment session. Explanation of what will happen to the athlete, what they should wear, what measurements will be taken, by whom and approximately how long the measurements will take is needed. Written and verbal informed consent expressed in plain language should be obtained from every athlete, or from their legal parent or guardian, if they are minors or are incapable of making or communicating an informed decision. An informed consent form should be used with contact details for the responsible person and institution. Make it clear that published measurement data will not identify individual athletes without their consent. Also explain to the athlete that he or she is free to withdraw from the measurement procedures at any time without prejudice to themselves.

The anthropometrist should not take any measures which compromise the physical or emotional well-being of the athlete. Every athlete should be offered the option of having a friend or parent as a chaperone. This is particularly important when measuring children. Anthropometrists should also receive training with regard to personal space of athletes, sociocultural aspects of touching and cultural sensitivities to measuring. Athletes should be offered the opportunity of being measured by an anthropometrist of the same sex where possible.

6.4.2 Athlete Clothing for Measurements

For measurements to be made as quickly and efficiently as possible, the athletes should be asked to present themselves in minimal clothing. The clothing worn must be of minimal thickness and follow the natural contours of the body. It must also allow access to bare areas of the skin for skinfolds and other measures. In the matter of dress, anthropometrists should always be sensitive to the cultural beliefs and traditions of the athletes.

6.4.3 General Instructions

Under the ISAK protocol, the right side of the body is normally used for unilateral measurements. If it is impracticable to use the right side due to injury, the left side may be used, where the possible two measurements should be taken at each side. A third measure should be taken where the second measure is not within 5% of the first for skinfolds or within 1% for other dimensions. The mean value is used if two measurements are taken and the median value if three measurements are taken. A complete data set of the proforma (profile) is obtained before repeating the measurements for the second and then third time. This may help reduce the effects of skinfold compressibility. Normally measurements should not be taken after training or competition, swimming or showering, since exercise, warm water and heat can produce dehydration and/or increased blood flow. These may affect body mass, skinfold and girth measurements (Stewart et al. 2011). Ensure the equipment is adequately cleaned after measurement.

6.4.4 Landmarking

Landmarks are identifiable skeletal points which generally lie close to the body's surface and are the 'markers' which identify the exact location of the measurement site or from which a soft tissue site is located (Stewart et al. 2011). Athlete presentation and preparation include wearing appropriate clothing to enable access to the body for marking and measurement. A sound knowledge of anatomy is needed to ensure accurate palpation of bony features to enable ISAK landmarking to occur. Landmarks are found by palpation or measurement, and a quality marking pen is needed to ensure reliable markings on the skin. All landmarks are identified before any measurements are made.

6.4.5 Stretched Stature

Stretched stature (height) is measured on a stadiometer. The athlete stands with the heels together and the heels, buttocks and upper part of the back touching the scale. The clinician aligns the head in the Frankfort plane (technically the lower edge of the eye socket is in the same horizontal plane as the notch superior to the tragus of the ear), and the athlete takes a deep breath in whilst the clinician applies a gentle upwards lift through the mastoid processes (base of the skull) ensuring the athlete heels remain on the stadiometer base and that their head does not tilt posteriorly. The stadiometer headboard is lowered onto the head ensuring the hair is compressed. A loss of approximately 1% in stature is common over the course of the day; therefore, the stretched stature method is used (Reilly et al. 1984). It is therefore important to record the time of day when measurements are made. Measurement of height is necessary to track changes in growth and calculate body mass index (BMI) and waist-to-height ratio. Height should be directly measured using a stadiometer.

6.4.6 Body Mass

Body mass (weight) is measured using calibrated scales (e.g. quality load cell electronic, beam-type, bed scales, chair scales or wheelchair scales). The accuracy of these instruments should be within 50 g. Calibration of scales using calibration weights totalling at least 150 kg should be conducted regularly. The athlete needs to stand on the centre of the scales without support, with their weight distributed evenly on both feet and with the head/eyes facing forwards (not looking down at the feet). Looking down or moving the body weight centre of mass away from the base of support between the feet will result in a different reading than if the correct stance is followed. To monitor changes in body mass over time, use of the same scale is recommended given the variability that can occur between scales. Body mass exhibits variation of about 1 kg in children and 2 kg in adults. It is therefore important to record the time of day when measurements are made.

6.4.7 Arm Span

Arm span is the distance from the tip of the middle finger (dactylion) of one hand to the other. The athlete stands against the wall with feet together, facing the clinician and with their arms raised to the horizontal. The heels, buttocks and upper back, together with dorsal aspects of the arms, should contact the wall. The athlete inspires maximally, and the arms are stretched maximally, whilst arm span is measured. The easiest way to conduct this measurement is to have a chart strip attached to the wall close to a corner where one finger is placed. A non-permanent marker pen is used to mark the distance to the other finger. Note that individuals with a marked kyphosis cannot be measured accurately.

6.4.8 Sitting Height

The distance between the vertex of the head and the inferior aspects of the buttocks when the athlete is seated is measured with a stadiometer. The athlete's hands should be resting on the thighs. The technique is the same as the stretch stature method with the head in the Frankfort plane. Care must be taken to ensure the athlete does not contract the gluteal muscles nor push with the legs.

6.4.9   Girths

The cross-hand technique is used for measuring all girths with a tape. Girths are measured with steel tapes to eliminate tape stretching as may occur with material or plastic tapes. A flexible steel tape of at least 1.5 m in length, calibrated in centimetres with 1 mm gradations, is recommended. The tape should be aligned perpendicular to the length of the limb (e.g. upper arm girth, calf) and should be tight enough, so there are no large gaps against the skin, but not too tight to cause skin indentation.

Two girth measurements that need particular attention are the waist and hip girth. Waist girth should be taken at the minimum girth in the horizontal plane. The athlete needs to be breathing normally, and the measurement is taken at end-tidal breath (end of expiration—but not forced expiration). If the athlete does not have a minimum waist girth, then the measurement is taken half way between the bottom rib and the superior aspect of the iliac crest. Hip girth is taken at the maximum posterior protuberance of the gluteal muscles. If the measurement is taken over clothing, then the tape needs to be pulled more firmly to ensure the measurement is representative of the underlying body structures. Care must be taken when positioning the tape around the athlete as well as removing the tape after the measure to minimize any risk of discomfort or injury.

6.4.10   Lengths and Heights

The segmometer or large sliding calliper can be used to measure segment lengths (e.g. acromiale to radiale) and heights (e.g. tibiale laterale to floor). For the segmometer there are various designs, with general specifications including a steel tape approximately 100 cm long, 15 mm wide, with two straight branches of 8 cm in length attached. During measurement it is important to keep the tape straight and reduce perspective error when reading values off the tape by aligning the eyes perpendicular with the tape scale. For more accurate measurements, the iliospinale height and trochanterion height can also be measured from their respective landmarks to the height of an anthropometric box (exactly 40 cm in height). If the box is used, the height is obtained by adding the box height.

6.4.11   Breadths

Both the large sliding calliper and the small sliding calliper (bone calliper) are used to measure breadths. Bone callipers have sliding branches that allow measurements of small bone breadths. The branches are attached to a rigid scale and must be able to withstand pressure exerted on the bone endpoints. For example, a small sliding calliper used for biepicondylar humerus (elbow) and biepicondylar femur (knee) breadths should have branch lengths of at least 10 cm, an application face width of

1.5 cm, and be accurate to within 0.05 cm. The calliper needs to be held correctly (the pencil grip) so that the fingers can palpate the bony landmarks and the calliper branches can be placed correctly. The underlying soft tissue must be compressed so that the correct bone breadth is measured. The technique for use of large sliding callipers is the same as for the small sliding calliper but requires greater dexterity (see Fig. 6.1 for an example of biacromial breadth measurement). Transverse chest breadth and anterior-posterior chest depth are taken at end-tidal expiration.

6.4.12 Skinfolds

Skinfold thickness describes the amount of subcutaneous fat when the fold is lifted and its thickness measured by specialized callipers. The sum of skinfolds (generally from eight sites in the standard ISAK protocol) provides data for comparison with population norms or for monitoring changes over time within the same individual.

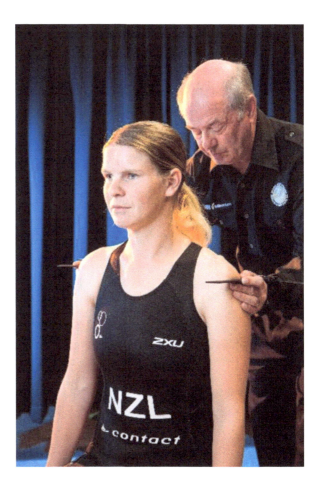

Fig. 6.1 An example of biacromial breadth measurement for an elite iron woman athlete

The ISAK manual contains details of standardized protocols (Stewart et al. 2011) to help minimize the technical error of measurement for repeat skinfold measures at various measurement sites. The standard ISAK protocol for skinfolds requires use of approved skinfold callipers that are regularly calibrated. Skinfold callipers require a constant closing compression of 10 g/mm^2 throughout the range of measurements and should be calibrated to at least 40 mm in 0.2 mm divisions. Eight skinfold sites on the arm, trunk and leg are found using precise bony land marks and girths to address intra- and interindividual differences in subcutaneous fat deposition.

For best practice, mark the athlete using the bony landmarking procedure, take measurements on the right side of the body, raise the skinfold at the landmark, place the calliper 1 cm below the mark, allow the calliper to settle for 2 s and then take the reading. Take one set of measurements at all eight sites and then repeat. Take a third measurement if the first two measurements are outside the tolerance level.

There are several unresolved issues for the skinfold methodology (Ackland et al. 2012), given there is inconsistency in adipose tissue deposition (fat patterning), no fixed relationship between subcutaneous to internal fat, inconsistent compressibility of skinfolds, inconsistent contribution of the skin to the fraction of the skinfold value and inconsistent contributions of lipid and water to the fraction of the adipose tissue.

6.5   How Do You Report the Data to Your Athlete and Coach?

Reports to athletes usually contain a table of the measurements taken and derived variables. Comparisons with international normative data should be provided where possible taking into account the athlete's sport, gender, age and participation level. Some international data are available for comparison of client measures. See J.E. Lindsay Carter Kinanthropometry Clinic and Archive JELCKC archive at jelckca-bodycomp.com.

ISAK supports the reporting of individual skinfold values as well as a simple arithmetic sum of eight skinfolds when monitoring athletes over time or when comparing individual results to normative data. This reporting standard minimizes the aggregation of assumptions and limitations associated with the use of regression equations for predicting a body fat percentage. All body fat regression equations use several raw skinfold values to predict a body fat percentage. The equations are generally derived using another surrogate measure of body fat percentage, such as hydrostatic weighing, air displacement plethysmography or bioelectric impedance, as the dependent variable. However, since these supposed reference measures are neither valid nor reliable, the value of such regression equations is highly questionable.

Devices to measure the thickness of a compressed, double layer of the skin plus the underlying subcutaneous adipose tissue have been used for over 50 years.

Unfortunately, much of the published data cannot be relied upon due to vast differences in calliper specifications, the number and location of skinfold sites and a lack of standardization in operator technique and data treatment. There are over 100 body fat prediction equations derived from skinfold measurements (Lohman et al. 1988), and their inconsistent results stem from differences in the populations that were sampled.

ISAK supports the reporting of individual somatotype which provides quantification of the shape and composition of the human body. Somatotype can be calculated from the restricted ISAK profile items and has useful applications in growth and aging, body image and in sports profiling. The somatotype reduces a large number of measures or visual observations to a simple, three number rating (endomorphy-mesomorphy-ectomorphy) which is independent of size, age and gender. Endomorphy represents relative adiposity of a physique, mesomorphy represents relative musculoskeletal robustness of a physique, and ectomorphy represents relative linearity or slenderness of a physique. Rating values and relative meanings for all three components are 0.5–2.5 = low, 3.0–5.0 = moderate, 5.5–7.0 = high and >7.5 above = extremely high. A novel iPad-based application to rapidly assess body image using somatotype comparisons is now available. It simultaneously assesses body fat, muscle and leanness using realistic quasi-3D images to provide healthcare professionals with an enhanced tool when dealing with body image disorders (Macfarlane et al. 2015).

Waist-to-hip ratio and body mass index are examples of surface anthropometry-derived variables that are not recommended for monitoring in athletes. Central distribution of body fat increases risk for type 2 diabetes, metabolic syndrome, hypertension and coronary heart disease (Klein et al. 2007). Measures of central adiposity include a single circumference or, more commonly, a waist-to-hip ratio. Waist-to-hip ratio correlates well with abdominal fat content and is a predictor of coronary heart disease and type 2 diabetes when using a cut-off ratio of 0.5 as an indicator of risk (Browning et al. 2010). Waist-to-hip ratio can be accurate in children and adults, men and women and across ethnic groups. However, waist-to-hip ratio is not useful as a predictor for sport performance.

Weight for height, known as body mass index (BMI), is calculated as body mass divided by height squared (kg/m^2). The use of body mass index to assess weight for height in individuals reflects recommendations of the National Institutes of Health and World Health Organization (NHLBI Obesity Education Initiative Expert Panel on the Identification Evaluation and Treatment of Overweight and Obesity in Adults 1998). Body mass index correlates with body fat for populations, but there remains considerable variation in body composition among individuals at each level of body mass index. Body mass index may be elevated despite relatively low levels of body fat in those with oedema or in athletes. The relationship between body mass index and body fat differs between sexes, varies among racial and ethnic groups and changes over the life span. A single body mass index classification scheme for the entire adult age range does not reflect the loss of fat-free mass and gain in fat mass that accompany aging. Older (>65 years) men and women have a higher percentage of body fat compared to younger counterparts with the same body mass index.

Women have a higher percentage of body fat compared to men of the same body mass index (Gallagher et al. 1996). Body mass index should only be used as a guide for populations. Both low and high body mass index correlate with morbidity and mortality, although there is ongoing debate regarding issues such as the magnitude of risk for those with body mass index in the overweight range (25–30 kg/m²) and how age modifies risk for morbidity and mortality. Low levels of body mass index are classified as BMI < 17.5 kg/m². It is recommended that body mass index is not used for describing or monitoring athletes.

6.6 Summary

The International Society for the Advancement of Kinanthropometry provides international standards for surface anthropometric assessment, using basic measures, skinfolds, girths, lengths, and breadths. ISAK's mission is to develop a 'best practice' approach to anthropometric measurement and to maintain an international network of colleagues from all associated disciplines.

References

Ackland TR, Lohman TG, Sundgot-Borgen J, Maughan RJ, Meyer NL, Stewart AD, Müller W (2012) Current status of body composition assessment in sport. Sports Med 42(3):227–240

Browning LM, Hsieh SD, Ashwell M (2010) A systematic review of waist-to-height ratio as a screening tool for the prediction of cardiovascular disease and diabetes: 0.5 could be a suitable global boundary value. Nutr Res Rev 23:247–269

Gallagher D, Visser M, Sepulveda D, Pierson RN, Harris T, Heymsfield SB (1996) How useful is body mass index for comparison of body fatness across age, sex, and ethnic groups? Am J Epidemiol 14:3228–3239

Hume P, Marfell-Jones M (2008) The importance of accurate site location for skinfold measurement. J Sports Sci 26(12):1333–1340

Klein S, Allison DB, Heymsfield SB, Kelley DE, Leibel RL, Nonas C (2007) Waist circumference and cardiometabolic risk: a consensus statement from Shaping America's Health: Association for Weight Management and Obesity Prevention; NAASO, the Obesity Society; the American Society for Nutrition; and the American Diabetes Association. Diabetes Care 30:1647–1652

Lohman TG, Roche AF, Martorell R (1988) Anthropometric standardization reference manual. Human Kinetics, Champaign, IL

Macfarlane D, Lee A, Hume PA, Carter JEL (2015) Development and reliability of a novel iPad-based application to rapidly assess body image. In: Am College Sports Med, USA, 2015

NHLBI Obesity Education Initiative Expert Panel on the Identification Evaluation and Treatment of Overweight and Obesity in Adults (1998) Clinical guidelines on the identification, evaluation, and treatment of overweight and obesity in adults: the evidence report. Obes Res 6(Suppl 2):51S–209S

Reilly T, Tyrrell A, Troup TDG (1984) Circadian variation in human stature. Chronobiol Int 1:121–126

Stewart AD, Marfell-Jones MJ, Olds T, de Ridder JH (2011) International standards for anthropometric assessment. ISAK, Lower Hutt

Chapter 7
Non-imaging Method: 3D Scanning

Clinton O. Njoku, Arthur D. Stewart, Patria A. Hume, and Stephven Kolose

Abstract Three-dimensional body scanning is used to determine surface anthro-pometry characteristics such as body volume, segment lengths and girths. Three-dimensional scanning systems use laser, light or infrared technologies to acquire shape and software to allow manual or automatically extracted measures. Body pos-ture during scanning is important to ensure accurate measures can be made from the images. The images vary depending on the configuration, resolution and accuracy of the scanner.

Keywords Three dimensional • Body scanning • Body volume • Segment lengths Girths • Laser • Technologies • Shape • Body posture • Images • Configuration Resolution • Accuracy • Scanner

C.O. Njoku (✉)
Department of Anatomy, Faculty of Medicine–Preclinicals, Ebonyi State University, Abakaliki, Nigeria
e-mail: clinton.njoku@ebsu-edu.net

A.D. Stewart
School of Health Sciences, Robert Gordon University, Aberdeen AB10 7GJ, UK
e-mail: a.d.stewart@rgu.ac.uk

P.A. Hume
Sport Performance Research Institute New Zealand, Auckland University of Technology, Auckland, New Zealand
e-mail: patria.hume@aut.ac.nz

S. Kolose
Operations Analysis and Human Systems Group, Defence Technology Agency, New Zealand Defence Force, Auckland, New Zealand
e-mail: S.Kolose@dta.mil.nz

© Springer Nature Singapore Pte Ltd. 2018   71
P.A. Hume et al. (eds.), *Best Practice Protocols for Physique Assessment in Sport*,
https://doi.org/10.1007/978-981-10-5418-1_7

7.1   Why Measure Physique Using 3D Scanning?

The availability of reliable three-dimensional (3D) whole-body scanners and software-hardware suites capable of rapid measurement, data extraction and analysis has the potential to revolutionise surface anthropometry. The main driver behind 3D scanning has been the apparel industry, envisaging the possibility of garments on demand, tailored to fit each individual perfectly. 3D scanning has parallel applications in human factors, where humanoid manikins can be rescaled using the extracted measurements and animated to interact with the built environment. These techniques are already being employed in military research and in the design of mass transportation and operator workspaces. There are currently only a few examples of 3D anthropometry scanning for applications to health and exercise science (Olds and Rogers 2004) for research purposes. For example, in a study of 85 male participants who completed duel X-ray absorptiometry, Bod Pod and 3D body scanning, the comparisons of body fat percentage showed significant differences between the three methods. Although the 3D body scanner shows promise as a method of evaluating body fat percentage, more refinement is needed before it can be used as a method of assessment (Ryder and Ball 2012). Such differences relate to the physical attribute of the body being measured, and as long as 3D scanning relies on establishing body volume accurately, its body fat prediction will be predicated on the two-compartment model which naïvely assumes a constant density for the fat-free mass and relies on lung volume determination.

7.2   What Is 3D Scanning?

7.2.1   Hardware

Fixed scanners can derive human body shape in several ways, the most common of which uses class 1 (eye-safe) lasers or structured light projected onto the body surface. Multiple digital cameras capture the position of the projected light, and software reconstructs the body contour of the acquired image via a mathematical algorithm which is based on triangulation. Most fixed scanner systems house the cameras in columns which are coordinated to scan the body from head to toe in a co-horizontal plane. In this configuration, three or four columns are enclosed within a booth which reduces ambient light and provides privacy.

A body scan from a fixed scanner typically consists of 500,000–700,000 xyz coordinates referred to as a "point cloud". Each point is joined to their near points to form polygonal meshes. The tiny facets formed by the polygonal mesh can be smoothed, producing a rendered body (the metaphor is that of a plasterer smoothing render over a wire frame). The resulting images vary depending on the accuracy of the scanner and its software and may be enriched with colour and texture data.

Portable scanners are either mounted on a tripod or bench or are hand-held and can be used in a variety of settings. These do not necessarily orient the 3D image in a standard way and thus must be positioned using post-processing tools—a procedure made much easier if a section of horizontal floor is also captured in the scan. Portable scanners generally use structured light, although more recently, depth sensor cameras have been increasingly used. Although their accuracy is improving, depth sensor cameras cannot yet compete with either portable or fixed scanners for accuracy.

7.2.2 Software

Early software approaches were very primitive by today's standards. Body segmentation was first developed using orthogonal only axes. While applications would purport to be able to generate segmental volumes and proportions, close scrutiny of anatomical regions reveals such junctions are invariably oblique rather than orthogonal. Torso-limb segment contact in overweight individuals critically distorts where true boundaries should fall, and extra caution is required for such individuals. Although some users may fail to appreciate these limitations and continue to use orthogonal segmentation, software developments in the last few years have advanced more rapidly than hardware, so more authentic segmentation is now possible using oblique planes. Software tools include basic processing (registration and fusion), mesh simplification, smoothing and even cloud-based storage systems available for the scans. This advancement has been driven by the inadequacy of conventional storage for the massive size of files. For example, a rich mesh acquired using the Artec-L will generate about 20 million data points (~500 MB of data).

7.2.3 Training in 3D Scanning

Unfortunately, there are gaps left by the somewhat haphazard development of the 3D scanning technology. At present, there are no universally recognised training systems for scanning humans, other than manufacturers' own specific guidelines. This process has not been helped by the increasing use of scanning in related fields including engineering, architecture, digital archiving and 3D printing and the cross-disciplinary use of more recent scanners. With such a blurring of boundaries between disciplines, it may be easy to forget that scanning fixed objects and infrastructure can be very different from a living human. In the absence of an agreed, standardised protocol, there is a pressing need for consensus regarding standard participant presentation (clothing), euhydration, fasting (in some cases), breathing cycle, posture and clothing. There are ISO standards which relate to scanning devices, but the nature of the development of the field is so rapid that these standards may date rather quickly. Such standards mostly relate to regulation designed to keep participants and operators safe. Various laws govern the use of class 1 lasers, and structured light scanners can possibly cause photosensitive epilepsy which may occur in about 1 in 2000 adults.

7.3 How Do You Use 3D Scanning for Athletes?

7.3.1 Calibration

Within the scientific field of metrology, different devices scan solid objects of known volume, placed at different distances to provide an in vitro calibration. The specification sheet for each model of scanner should contain this information, but it is not always presented in a standardised manner.

7.3.2 Apparel for All Postures

The environment conditions for scanning include no eyeglasses, watches and jewellery, wearing light form-fitting apparel, tying long hair and wearing a bathing cap to cover the hair. The surface area of clothing and hair can have a direct impact on the measured volume, due to its potential for encapsulating trapped air. As a result, men should wear swimming trunks or single-layer form-fitting shorts without padding. Women should wear a single-layer sports top and form-fitting shorts.

For those using laser scanning, researchers should be aware that the wavelength of the source may restrict the use of dark clothing colours, and so lighter colours are recommended. The burgeoning market in compression sports clothing might appear to fit these requirements; however, if valid measurements of body shape are to be made, clothing should conform to the body contour without compressing it. This may be difficult to achieve in practice, and care must be taken to ensure the clothing surface is smooth and free from creases and also to avoid strong elastic waistbands from altering the uncompressed body shape.

7.3.3 Landmarks

In order to extract traditional anthropometric measurements, the 3D scanner software must be able to identify certain landmarks. There are three common landmarking systems used in 3D anthropometry: (1) automatic landmark recognition (ALR), where the software identifies landmarks from the scan without human intervention; (2) digital landmark placement (DLP), where landmarks are located on a digital image by identifying surface features; and (3) physical-digital landmark location (PDL), where landmarks are placed physically on the body and then located digitally on the scanned image. ALR has proved to be unacceptably inaccurate, while DLP is often difficult on obese or very muscular participants, where underlying bony landmarks are hard to locate. Therefore, we rely heavily on PDL, which has the disadvantage of requiring more time and operator skill. There is no universally accepted protocol for 3D scanning; however, current protocols are being lodged with the J.E. Lindsay Carter Anthropometry Archive (Stewart and Hume 2014).

Physical-digital landmark location landmarking of the body can be undertaken before acquisition of the scan. Landmarks need to be identifiable as a three-dimensional (xyz) point from the rendered scan file and so may be affixed as small triangles, bespoke reflective stickers or some other physical marker such as cod liver oil capsules fixed to the body surface. Bony landmarks require physical palpation to identify and cannot be inferred directly from the scan. This process requires considerable time and technical skill. For example, the acromiale, trochanterion and iliac crest ISAK landmarks (Stewart et al. 2011) might be marked for direct length (or height) measurements or to assist defining the required plane for body segmentation. In addition, the use of scans to measure volumes requires the breathing cycle to be carefully regulated, and this may require extra landmarks. In this respect, the level of the third costal cartilages of the rib cage corresponds to the point of the highest mobility during breathing cycles, which is at the same level as the axilla in most individuals.

7.3.4   Protocols, for Example, Specific Landmarks

The T3 costal landmark is defined as the point on the skin surface corresponding to the midline of the sternum at the level of the third rib costal cartilage (*see* Fig. 7.1). Note that this is superior to the ISAK mesosternale landmark.

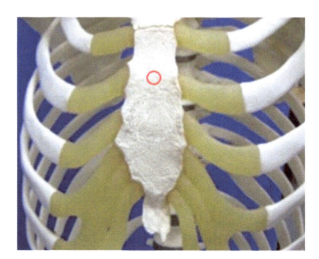

Fig. 7.1 Location of the T3 costal landmark

The T3 posterior landmark is on the dorsal side of the torso, which is defined as the point on the skin surface of posterior median furrow at the corresponding height of the T3 costal landmark.

The lateral deltoid landmarks are defined as the most lateral points on the skin surface overlying the deltoid muscles as observed from the front when the participant is standing erect with feet together and arms against the sides and hands in the mid-prone position (i.e., thumbs pointing forwards) resting on the lateral thighs. These landmarks are described in Stewart and Hume (2014) and are required for bi-deltoid breadth measurement.

7.3.5   Scan Postures

Body posture during scanning is important to ensure accurate measures can be made from the images. Inside the 3D scanning booth, participants are positioned into standard scanning poses (*see* Fig. 7.2) and instructed to hold their breath (at end tidal expiration) for the duration of each scan (~10–12 s).

Generally, the scan position is with arms and legs abducted to permit body segmentation, so enabling calculation of limb segment parameters such as girths, volumes and areas. However, in practice, this posture is not strictly defined in terms of the specifics of positioning, and there is a lack of consensus in terms of arm abduction angle, forearm or elbow angle and hand position and orientation. In addition, a

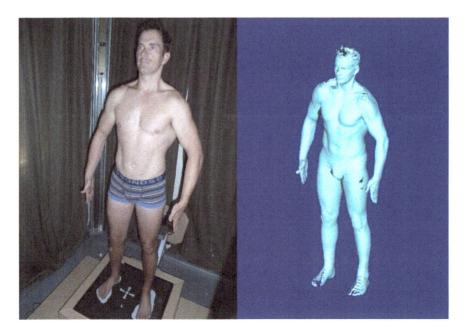

Fig. 7.2 Example scanning pose for 3D scanning and initial 3D image

range of other position definitions may be required to enable standardisation of the breathing cycle and to facilitate range of measurements that compare with conventional anthropometry. For fixed scanners, the acquisition time generally makes it feasible for participants to hold their breath, thereby eliminating the breathing artefact, but depending on the stage of the breathing cycle adopted, there are important consequences for girth and volume measurements.

For optimal results from 3D scanning, a particular posture must be maintained. For example, when scanning with fixed scanners such as the Hamamatsu, the following postures are used: egress position end tidal, egress position inspired, egress position expired and scanner position end tidal. Alternatively, with the portable Artec-L Scanner, scanner position end tidal is used, and participant stability is facilitated with a pair of orthopaedic walking poles.

For the egress position end tidal posture, the participant stands erect with the head facing forwards and the eyes maintained at the horizontal level. Arms are adducted to the lateral aspect of the torso, with forearms extended and in a mid-prone position. Thighs and legs are held together, with feet oriented forwards, to give the entire body an erect posture. The participant adopts shallow breathing to prevent noticeable movements of the thorax, and scanning takes ~8–10 s for the image to be acquired.

For the egress position inspired posture, the participant stands erect in the booth with both feet together in-between two pre-marked foot images on the floor of the scanner. The head is held erect and facing forward, with the eyes maintained at the horizontal level. Arms remain adducted and the forearm extended and in mid-prone position with the palms placed on the lateral aspect of thighs. The thighs and the legs are fully adducted with the feet oriented forward. When alerted by the operator, the participant breathes in maximally and holds the breath. Once again, scanning takes ~8–10 s, whereupon the participant can resume normal breathing. This breath-holding factor is important when quantifying the scan volume (which includes entrapped air within the lungs), which in turn affects body fat predictions using the two-compartment method.

Egress position expired is similar to the egress position inspired posture, except that when alerted by the operator, the participant breathes out maximally leaving the lungs with only the residual gas volume (RGV). In this posture, the rib cage depresses with concomitant reduction of the thoracic volume and increment of the abdominal volume. Care must be taken not to allow the participant to flex forwards out of a vertical position when maximal expiration is undertaken.

The scanner position end tidal posture fixes each of the feet onto the pre-marked foot symbols on the floor of the scanner, thereby causing each leg to be abducted from the midline. The head is oriented forwards with the eyes fixed at the horizontal level. Arms are abducted from the torso, and the forearms flexed at the elbow and in mid-prone position to align the palms parallel to the thighs. The participant maintains shallow breathing throughout the scan to avoid noticeable movements of the rib cage.

When using portable 3D scanners such as the Artec-L scanner, the scanner position end tidal is used. However, postural stability is aided by using a pair of adjust-

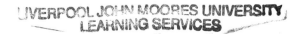

able orthopaedic walking poles since the time for scanning is ~45 s. The use of these poles helps reduce movement artefact caused by the longer scan duration compared to fixed scanners.

There are landmarks and volumetric differences according to breathing cycle in egress positions. In the egress position inspired, there is vertical mobility upwards of all the landmarks and thoracic expansion, and, consequently, there is increase in the body volume. The reverse occurs in the egress position expired where the landmarks undergo vertical mobility downwards, with consequent reduction of thoracic diameters and body volume. The differences in landmark mobility in the two egress positions have been measured up to 25 mm on the mesosternale, and bi-deltoid breadth and chest depth expansion measured up to 4 mm and 10 mm, respectively.

There are also body dimension differences between data extracted from egress position end tidal and scanner position end tidal 3D images (*see* Fig. 7.3). The waist and hip circumference measures vary in the two postures. A participant's waist circumference (812.1 mm) and hip circumference (991.5 mm) in egress position end tidal change to 817.1 mm and 1020.5 mm, respectively, in scanner position end tidal. Abdominal and waist circumferences acquired in the standing position show differences in level, size and shape compared with lying or sitting positions. 3D scan body volume will contain thoracic gas and, therefore, overestimate the true body volume value, which leads to a corresponding inflation of estimated fat content using the two-compartment model. Such breathing directives have led to variation in estimated %fat from 10.3% (expired) to 27.6% (inspired) in a sample of 116 adults (Njoku and Stewart 2016) which underscores the importance of standardising

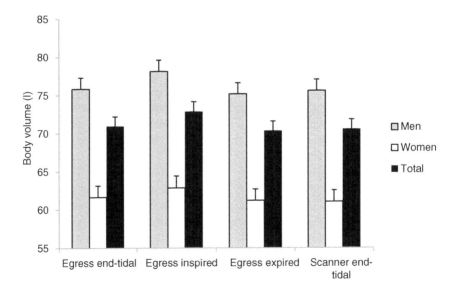

Fig. 7.3 Body volume in 74 male and 39 female healthy adults; all gender differences were significant after Bonferroni adjustment ($p < 0.001$)

breathing. While more in-depth respiratory research could usefully quantify this, such work has yet to be conducted. As a result, it is important that the expiratory reserve volume, plus half of the tidal volume, be subtracted from the scan volume to yield a body composition prediction, when this is required.

The level, shape and size of the abdomen change with different body positions. Waist girth, for example, will generally be largest when sitting, an intermediate value when standing and least when lying. Even within the standing posture, arm position makes a profound difference to the magnitude of the waist (Lennie et al. 2013). It is paradoxical that the health risk imposed by abdominal obesity is almost always predicted by standing anthropometry in field and clinical settings, yet verified by supine medical imaging, without consideration of the influence of positional difference on measurement value. With landmarks on the appropriate level to identify the waist or abdominal girth, the differences can be verified.

This is the background for the development of an "enriched abdominal waist model" by quantifying the waist area using abdominal transverse sections in both standing and lying positions and combining the 3D image of abdominal circumference in different positions with subcutaneous fat measured by ultrasound. Plotting the depth of subcutaneous fat with ultrasound on the abdominal circumference extracted from the standing posture could result in a cascade of errors in the prediction of waist shape, waist area, coronal diameter, sagittal diameter and subcutaneous tissue percentage within the abdominal circumference. However, this error can be corrected by designing a protocol for extracting the abdominal circumference from the 3D scan using a lying posture, since ultrasound measures are performed while the participant lies in prone or supine postures. This technique requires a different protocol and a hand-held scanner.

The supine scan for enriched abdominal waist model requires the alignment of two strong tables of similar height with a gap of 20 cm. Arms are folded across the shoulders in the same way as the ISAK standard waist protocol (Stewart et al. 2011), and the feet are together. The 20 cm gap should correspond with the waist-abdominal region and facilitate access to the torso in almost 360°. Participants should be scanned at the end tidal position, and if a breath is required, the scan should be suspended until the participant has returned to the end tidal position. In a sample of 18 adults, such postural difference between standing and supine has been shown to lead to a mean reduction of 4.9% in abdominal girth and 17.1% in abdominal cross-sectional area (Ng et al. 2016). This is one example of the contribution 3D scanning is making to increasing contemporary understanding of what anthropometric measurements actually mean.

7.4 What Is 3D Scanning Used to Measure?

For measurements to be extracted from traditional fixed scanners, the body scan is modelled by converting point-cloud surface representation to a polygon. Selected body landmarks, such as the vertex (superior aspect of the head), nape of neck, right and left axilla, and crotch are generally required to be located before the scan can be converted into polygon.

When using a portable scanner software such as Artec Studio or similar products, the positioning tool is used to orient the scans in xyz coordinates. Standard practice is for the x axis to point towards the observer, y axis to the right and z axis vertical, when the scanned person is facing the observer. Once in this orientation, successive frames of a particular scan can be aligned together and then registered as a single frame. All the unwanted segments, including the pair of orthopaedic walking poles and the floor, are deleted using the eraser sub-menu. Orienting the scan in xyz space enables planar eraser function which makes a range of processing tasks much more straightforward. Other sub-menu tools include hole filling, applied to re-edit small areas of missing data, while the small object filter removes data sets which are distant from the scanned image. With the edges sub-menu, larger sections of missing data are filled. After this, a solid 3D model is produced using the fusion menu, and measurements can be extracted from it.

Three-dimensional analysis can be extended to calculate segmental and whole-body volumes and, hence, to estimate body fat percentage. If the mass of the participant is known and the volume estimated by 3D scanning, one can calculate the whole-body density. Then, with certain assumptions regarding tissue density made, one may estimate body fat percentage. However, studies examining the accuracy and precision of using 3D scans to predict whole-body density measured against a criterion standard such as dual X-ray absorptiometry or composite models which additionally include bod pod or hydrostatic weighing are needed.

Body changes due to growth, maturation, dietary and training interventions can also be assessed. 3D scanning can be used to visualise and better quantify size and shape changes that occur due to ageing or as a result of exercise or nutrition interventions. Somatotyping using 3D anthropometry has been conducted which moves beyond the traditional triple-view approach in a standard pose and enables interactivity with the image and viewing from any angle (Olds et al. 2013) in addition to other applications to health and exercise science (Olds and Rogers 2004).

7.4.1 Special Challenges for Some Populations

Capturing the body shape of athletes, as compared to the general population, offers some advantages but also some challenges. Firstly, athletes are commonly lean and healthy individuals with positive self-esteem and are generally receptive to being measured, while the population at large (most especially overweight individuals) might have considerable reluctance to be scanned in form-fitting clothing. By contrast, athletes generally are comfortable being scanned in minimum clothing and usually have the type of clothing required, thus avoiding the issue of wearing a size provided by the research lab which may not fit perfectly or indeed alter body shape in a subtle way. Athletes are also used to routine physical measurements and are generally at ease in a laboratory environment, which is in contrast to members of the public who may be much less comfortable. However, athletes may present some difficulties by virtue of their unusual size or proportions; this has also been cited as an issue for other types of measurement (e.g., dual energy X-ray absorptiometry scanning). Extremely tall or large athletes may exceed the detectable scan volume of fixed scanners, either by being too tall (perhaps >195 cm) or too broad.

For 3D scanning, segmentation of the body requires the arms to be separated from the torso and the legs from one another. In stocky individuals, this may not be possible, and the orientation of the head and shoulder girdle in some individuals may be challenging for the default settings on scan software to detect properly, due to extreme development of neck musculature. This also causes a problem when it comes to identifying planes to use when dividing the arms from the torso. Well-developed latissimus dorsi musculature can add to the difficulty in identifying the required plane, underscoring the inadequacy of the default to orthogonal axes in sagittal and transverse planes for the "cut lines" with older scanners, meaning that inevitably some of the arm is included in the torso and vice versa.

7.5 How Do You Report 3D Scanning Data to Athletes and Coaches?

There are currently no standards for reporting 3D scanning to athletes given the recent use of 3D scanning with athletes. Reports are generated by each individual manufacturer's software. There are some company databases that can be used for comparison purposes, usually for a fee.

7.6 Example of a 3D Scanning Protocol for a Large-Scale Survey

The following example 3D scanning protocol was used for a large-scale survey in New Zealand. The survey used a Vitus XXL scanner. The scanner projects non-ionising laser light onto the body with the reflection captured by cameras as a series of points (generally between 700,000 and 1,000,000) with Cartesian coordinates, joined together to create the digital statue. It uses eye-safe class 1 visible red laser light (minimum levels of ionising radiation) and was manufactured and developed in compliance with the regulations of the US Food and Drug Administration (US Department of Health and Human Services) pertaining to laser safety.

7.6.1 Team Personnel

To ensure quality data are collected and participants complete the scanning requirements in as short a time as possible, a team of personnel with specific responsibilities is needed at each survey data collection session:

Team leader

- The survey protocol conduct
- Data sampling site logistics (e.g., liaison and coordination with data collection site manager)
- Overseeing transport, (un)packing, (dis)assembly and calibration of scanner and all equipment
- Recording any incidents on a Serious Events Register
- Timekeeping for workflow
- Ensuring that all data files are backed up regularly
- Assisting other team members when required

Participant receptionist

- Greeting and briefing participants
- Administering informed consent forms and demographic questionnaires
- Collecting and filing all hard copies of paperwork
- Assigning participants an ID number

Anthropometrists

- Locating and placing physical landmarks on participants
- Taking physical measurements
- Recording all measurements
- Observing other anthropometrists to minimise mistakes
- Escorting participants to the scanner technician

Scanner technicians

- Positioning participants in the correct postures for scanning
- Operating the scanner system
- Verifying the scanned images for correct posturing, landmark positioning and checking scan image quality
- Saving the scan

7.6.2 Survey Protocol

The survey protocol consists of five stages with approximately 60 min per participant.

Stage 1: Briefing and informed consent (10 min)

The receptionist greets the individual participants at reception. Prior to their visit, all participants will have been issued with an information sheet (i.e., about the study aims and methods, instructions on level of hydration and food intake, clothing, no prior exercise) and a consent form. At the session they will also be verbally informed of the measurement procedures and their rights as volunteers. After providing written informed consent, participants complete a short demographic questionnaire and are assigned a unique identification number using a four-digit coding convention. The consent form is the only document linking each participant's identification number to their names.

Stage 2: Change to form-fitting clothing (5 min)

Participants are then shown to the private changing area so they can change into light-coloured sports or undergarments (tight-fitting briefs for men and high-rise underpants and stretch midriff tops for women), remove all jewellery and, if necessary, tie their hair up. Participants are able to choose to wear their own underwear, provided it was deemed acceptable for scanning by an anthropometry team member. The apparel must be a light colour and a tight fit. These colours provide minimal reflection during the scanning process. Participants will not wear shoes or socks during the survey.

Participant's personal belongings are stored in a large plastic container for safe-keeping (one container per participant).

Stage 3: Landmarking (8 min) and manual/physical measurements (20 min)

Manual measures from landmarking are required as they are either difficult or impossible to accurately derive automatically from the scan by the Vitus XXL system. Just prior to landmarking, all participants are reminded of the procedures via a poster of photos showing the landmarks and the three postures they are required to assume during landmarking, physical measurement and 3D scanning.

The required landmarks are marked on participants by their trained anthropometrist. Trained personnel must be either a qualified Level 2 anthropometrist or have received suitable training from a qualified Level 3 or 4 anthropometrist. The ideal situation is to have a landmarker and an observer (another anthropometrist from the team). This is to minimise mistakes. Instruction booklets on how to conduct the landmarking are provided for reference. These landmarks are necessary for obtaining measures to be derived post-scan.

To identify each skeletal reference point, each is physically located by palpation on the body surface, marked with a small pen-marked cross, and then raised double-sided adhesive sticker pointing at the landmark is placed on the cross (note: stickers are only placed on participants' bodies after the physical measures have been completed). Once landmarking is complete, anthropometrists check the placement of their landmarks and tick the corresponding box on the datasheet to signify that the landmarks have been located.

Once landmarking is complete, the anthropometric team conducts the manual measurements. This is so participants only get processed by the same two people, in order to protect their privacy. These measures are conducted using ISAK-approved anthropometric kits. Prior to use, the kit contents are calibrated and checked for damage.

An anthropometrist acts as a recorder. Each measure is repeated twice and entered by the recorder onto an Excel spreadsheet, which indicates whether a third measure is needed. Following completion of all of the physical measurements, a review of the datasheet is conducted. Measurements falling outside of normative bounds are rechecked by the anthropometrist, with a third measurement taken if the first and second measurements differed by more than 1.0%.

Stage 4: Scanning (15 min)

After manual measurements, participants proceed to the scanning area. The scanner technician tells participants of the three postures necessary to adopt and what to expect when the scan begins. The scanner technician instructs participants on where to stand, how to stand and when and how to breathe. Scanning will only commence once the operator is happy with how the participant is standing and positioned on the podium. Each scan will last 12 s and will produce a 3D image of the participant. After each scan, participants can relax while the operator visually inspects the image to check whether all the landmarks are clearly visible and that the posture is adopted correctly. The scanner technician takes two scans of each posture, which equals six scans in total. If the scan technician is not happy with the results of any of the scans, then the unacceptable scans are repeated.

Stage 5: Participants get changed back into their regular clothing (5 min)

Following completion of scans, participants are ushered back to the change area where they will change back into their clothes. The anthropometrist will then usher the participant back to reception and return the completed datasheet to either the team leader or the receptionist. The datasheet is checked to confirm whether all physical measurements fall within normative bounds (i.e., the 2.5th–97.5th percentile range). The participant is then released from the data collection process.

7.7   Summary

Three-dimensional body scanning is used to determine surface anthropometry characteristics such as body volume, segment lengths and girths. Body posture during scanning is important to ensure accurate measures can be made from the images. Training is required to ensure successful use of 3D scanning hardware and software.

References

Lennie S, Amofa-Diatuo T, Nevill AM, Stewart AD (2013) Protocol variations in arm position influence the magnitude of waist girth. J Sports Sci 31(12):1353–1358

Ng HY, Njoku CO, Stewart AD (2016) Waist shape, girth and area are affected by posture: insight from 3D scanning. In: Ferreyro Bravo F, Esparza Ros F, Marfell-Jones M (eds) Kinanthropometry XV proceedings of the 15th international society for the advancement of Kinanthropometry conference, Merida, Mexico, pp. 278–279

Njoku CO, Stewart AD (2016) 3D scanning: consequences of the breathing cycle for body composition. In: Ferreyro Bravo F, Esparza Ros F, Marfell-Jones M (eds) Kinanthropometry XV proceedings of the 15th international society for the advancement of Kinanthropometry conference, Merida, Mexico, pp. 267–268

Olds T, Daniell N, Petkov J, David Stewart A (2013) Somatotyping using 3D anthropometry: a cluster analysis. J Sports Sci 31(9):936–944

Olds T, Rogers M (2004) 3D anthropometry–applications to health and exercise science. Sport Health 22:21–23

Ryder JR, Ball SD (2012) Three-dimensional body scanning as a novel technique for body composition assessment: a preliminary investigation. J Exerc Physiol Online 15(1):1–14

Stewart AD, Hume PA (2014) Bideltoid breadth measurement. J.E. Lindsay Carter Kinanthropometry Archive 3D Scanning Protocols, 2. Retrieved from http://jelckca-bodycomp.com

Stewart AD, Marfell-Jones MJ, Olds T, de Ridder JH (2011) International standards for anthropometric assessment. ISAK, Lower Hutt, New Zealand

Chapter 8
Non-imaging Method: Air Displacement Plethysmography (Bod Pod)

Greg Shaw and Ava Kerr

Abstract Air displacement plethysmography is used to measure body volume. The Bod Pod (COSMED USA Inc., Concord, CA) is an easy-to-use, convenient, non-invasive device that can accommodate a large spectrum of athletic physiques, assessing fat and fat-free mass reliably and accurately. Estimates of body density are in close agreement to those using the hydrostatic weighing technique, with Bod Pod now considered the gold standard for assessment of body density in multi-compartment models. It often underestimates fat mass compared to other physique assessment techniques; however, this may be due to poor standardisation practices. When undertaken in a well-controlled standardised manner, Bod Pod has proven to be an accurate and reliable technique for tracking physique changes over time. It is valuable in large athletes who may be more comfortable undertaking physique assessment via Bod Pod compared to other techniques where reliability in this population might be an issue.

Keywords Air displacement plethysmography • Body volume • Bod Pod • Non-invasive • Fat • Fat-free mass • Body density • Multi-compartment models Standardisation practices • Calibration

G. Shaw (✉)
Australian Institute of Sport, Australian Sports Commission,
P.O. Box 176, Canberra, ACT 2616, Australia
e-mail: greg.shaw@ausport.gov.au

A. Kerr
Faculty of Science, Health, Education and Engineering, University of the Sunshine Coast,
Maroochydore DC, QLD 4558, Australia
e-mail: akerr@usc.edu.au

© Springer Nature Singapore Pte Ltd. 2018   87
P.A. Hume et al. (eds.), *Best Practice Protocols for Physique Assessment in Sport*,
https://doi.org/10.1007/978-981-10-5418-1_8

8.1 Introduction

The Bod Pod is used in research and clinical practice and is designed to estimate a person's body composition. The Bod Pod is an air displacement plethysmograph that uses whole-body densitometry to determine body composition (fat vs lean). It is similar in principle to underwater weighing and measures body mass (weight) using a precise scale and volume by sitting inside the Bod Pod. Body density can then be calculated: density = mass/volume. Once the overall density of the body is determined, the relative proportions of body fat and lean mass are calculated via the Siri or Brozek equations.

During a measurement, the Bod Pod produces very small volume changes inside the chamber and measures the pressure response to these small volume changes. For more detailed information, see http://www.cosmed.com/hires/marketing_literature/product_news/Product_News_Air_Displacement_EN_print.pdf.

8.2 Why Measure Physique Using the Air Displacement Plethysmography Technique?

The measurement of physique via densitometric methodologies has been the cornerstone of body composition assessment for the best part of the last century. Utilising the principle that density equals mass/volume, and solving for fat and fat-free compartments (under the assumption that compartments have known and constant densities), has allowed scientists and practitioners to assess body composition in a range of populations. Traditionally, hydrodensitometry (or underwater weighing) has estimated total body volume via Archimedes' principle. Although previous attempts, utilising Boyle's law ($P_1V_1 = P_2V_2$), had demonstrated the principles of air displacement plethysmography, significant errors were reported (Gnaedinger et al. 1963; Dempster and Aitkens 1995). These were associated with the introduction of a human body to the measurement chamber, violating the isothermal requirements of Boyle's law. However, in 1995 Life Measurement Instruments (Concord, CA) designed an air displacement plethysmography device called the Bod Pod (see Fig. 8.1). The device comprises a sealed measuring chamber with a reference chamber linked by a flexible diaphragm which, when perturbed, creates small pressure changes between both chambers. Utilising Poisson's law to correct for errors associated with human addition to the measurement chamber, the device measures the inverse pressure-volume relationship between the two chambers to calculate the volume of the athlete (Dempster and Aitkens 1995). This body volume, corrected for the thoracic gas volume, is divided into the body mass to determine body density. The technique of Bod Pod eliminates the requirement for athletes to be totally submerged underwater to measure body density, instead measuring air displaced from a chamber by the body. This ensures a more comfortable and non-invasive method of body density measurement. Once body density has been calculated, it

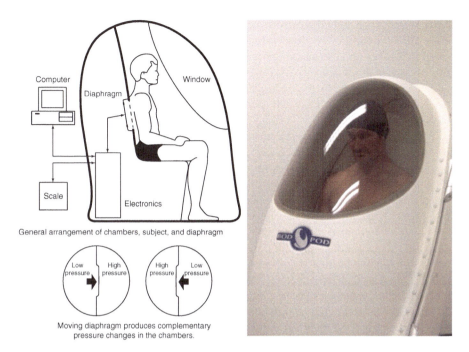

Fig. 8.1 Bod Pod device schematic, including visualisation of diaphragm perturbations utilised to determine body volume of the athlete in the measurement chamber. Schematic from http://www. cosmed.com/hires/marketing_literature/product_news/Product_News_Air_Displacement_EN_ print.pdf

can be converted to a percentage body fat using population-specific equations (Siri 1956; Ortiz et al. 1992). Although population-based equations are available, the increased accuracy available from their use is questionable (Collins et al. 2004), and therefore Siri (Siri 1956) or Brozek (Brožek et al. 1963) equations are sufficient, especially in adult athletic populations.

The current Bod Pod (COSMED USA Inc., Concord, CA) is an easy-to-use, convenient, non-invasive device that can accommodate a large spectrum of athletic physiques, assessing fat and fat-free mass reliably and accurately.

The Bod Pod has been reported to be reliable across a range of body fats, ages and ethnicities (Collins et al. 1999; Collins and McCarthy 2003; Noreen and Lemon 2006; Anderson 2007; Tucker et al. 2014) suggesting a technical error of measurement for percent body fat of between 0.4 and 1.24% (Vescovi et al. 2001; Wells and Fuller 2001) and a coefficient of variation of between 2.0 and 5.3% (Noreen and Lemon 2006; Anderson 2007). As with any device, technical and biological error can influence the reliability and accuracy of the test; therefore strict control of these variables should be implemented to improve the precision of the technique.

Error associated with the volume of air in the lung and the adiabatic air close to the skin requires correction due to assumptions of the technique. Therefore, thoracic gas volume and surface area artefact need to be measured or estimated correctly to ensure an accurate and reliable body volume is measured. Variability in estimates of body surface area and subsequent estimates of surface area artefact are likely to have small influences on estimates of percent body fat (0.1%), potentially increasing as the leanness of the athlete increases (Collins and McCarthy 2003). The measurement of thoracic gas volume by the Bod Pod's inbuilt pulmonary plethysmography device has been shown to be reliable and accurate (Davis et al. 2007). Modest changes in physique may influence measured and predicted lung volume; however, whether this is evident in athletic populations, manipulating physique is yet to be seen. What is evident is that the difference between percent body fat estimates determined using predicted or measured thoracic gas volume is small and likely clinically insignificant (Collins and McCarthy 2003), especially in adult athletic populations. However, when considering individual variability rather than group means, some individuals have shown large differences in percent body fat (as much as 3%) between methods. This may be accounted for by differences in breathing patterns that are significant deviations from a normal breathing pattern (Tegenkamp et al. 2011). This emphasises the requirement that predicted and measured volumes, which ever chosen, should not be used interchangeably (Collins and McCarthy 2003).

Of particular interest to athletes, their coaches and service providers is the ability of the Bod Pod technique to provide a valid measure of two-compartment body composition. The Bod Pod is a useful substitute for underwater weighing showing excellent agreement between devices when estimating body density even across a varying array of percent body fat and ages (Fields et al. 2000). Compared to more potentially accurate composition assessment techniques, Bod Pod has been shown to underestimate fat mass when compared to magnetic resonance imaging (Ludwig et al. 2014), dual-energy X-ray absorptiometry (Collins et al. 1999) and three-compartment (Collins et al. 1999) and four-compartment (Fields et al. 2001; Millard-Stafford et al. 2001) assessment techniques.

In athletic populations when Bod Pod has been compared to percent body fat measures from hydrostatic weighing, dual-energy X-ray absorptiometry and three-compartment and four-compartment models, it has been shown to have good agreement (Utter et al. 2003; Ballard et al. 2004) to underestimate (Collins et al. 2004) or overestimate fat mass (Bentzur et al. 2008). An early study in college footballers showed Bod Pod underestimated fat mass compared to hydrostatic weighing due mostly to a higher measured body density (Collins et al. 1999). Additionally, in the same study when compared to dual-energy X-ray absorptiometry and a three-compartment assessment of composition, Bod Pod consistently underestimated mean percent body fat (Collins et al. 1999). A follow-up study in an ethnically diverse population showed Bod Pod consistently underestimated fat mass across ethnicity and strength training experience (Collins et al. 2004). When female athletes had multiple assessment measures, Bod Pod compared favourably with dual-energy X-ray absorptiometry (Ballard et al. 2004) but also underestimated percent body fat (Bentzur et al. 2008). Although estimations of fat mass may be lower than those of dual-energy X-ray absorptiometry, the measurement of the relative change in fat mass, over time (8 weeks to 16 months), has been shown to have a high measure of agreement between the two techniques (Weyers et al. 2002).

All things considered, Bod Pod when undertaken in a controlled standardised manner can provide accurate and reliable two-compartment measures of physique. It is capable of accurately tracking change in physique whilst being time efficient and non-invasive and requiring minimal technical expertise.

8.3 What Is the Air Displacement Plethysmography Technique and Technology?

Bod Pod is a proprietary air displacement plethysmography system sold and serviced through COSMED USA Inc. (Concord, Ca; www.cosmed.com). The system comes in two configurations: the Pea Pod designed for infants and the Bod Pod Gold Standard, which has an additional paediatric option (2–6 years of age), for the measurement of adolescents and adults. This makes Bod Pod a true cradle-to-grave technology capable of assessing a wide range of physiques and ages (Fields et al. 2015). The device consists of three main components: the measurement POD, a desktop computer and a digital scale (see Fig. 8.1). The pod is separated into two isolated chambers separated by a fibreglass wall moulded to form the seat. The rear reference chamber houses the electronics for pressure analysis and lung volume estimation and is completely sealed from the external environment. The front measurement chamber is accessible via a hinged door with a clear window for athlete comfort. This access point is sealed during measurement by strong electromagnets that prevent the pod being opened and ensuring a sealed chamber of known volume (460 L). The measurement chamber has an athlete capacity of 260 L which is sufficient to accommodate the majority of competitive athletes. The desktop computer runs a Windows-based software package to control the measurement device. A digital calibratable scale is connected to the device for the accurate measurement of body mass.

COSMED recommends the Bod Pod be set up in a well-controlled operating environment to ensure optimal measurement conditions are maintained throughout calibration and testing, ensuring accuracy and precision. The room temperature should be between 21 and 27 °C and relative humidity between 20 and 70% (noncondensing). The Bod Pod should not be placed near a heater, under air conditioning vents or fans, and must be kept out of direct sunlight to avoid temperature fluctuations. A warning sign should be placed on the outside of the door of the Bod Pod room, highlighting that measurement is in process and that no one should enter.

8.3.1 Calibration and Quality Control

The key components of the system are Bod Pod dual chamber capsule, 50 L calibration volume cylinder, Bod Pod PC software, scales and 2 × 10 kg calibration masses.

Due to the mathematics of air displacement plethysmography, assessment of body volume, calibration and quality control activities are essential to ensure valid and reliable results. These must be undertaken prior to any test session.

Quality control functions are in the Bod Pod software. Two failed quality control tests require a system reboot. If problems continue, technical support should be followed up through your local COSMED supplier. The Bod Pod device warm-up processes can be programmed in advance and should finish at least 30 min prior to measurement (commencing 2 h prior to measurement) to allow sufficient time for additional quality control processes (digital scale and measurement system calibration) prior to any measurement.

The most important step is the final calibration of the device with a known volume. Utilising the provided 50 L calibration cylinder, the technician is required to undertake five calibration volume tests. This involves an initial empty Bod Pod test followed by five tests with the calibration cylinder inside the Bod Pod. An average of the five tests is taken with a small tolerance or SD. This is a fundamental step in the measurement process and must be adhered to for accurate measurement of athletes.

Although the Bod Pod software is highly automated with minimal expertise required to operate the system, great care must be taken during quality control procedures. Non-compliance from the outlined quality control and measurement procedures specified by COSMED in their operating manual (COSMED USA 2014) can lead to significant errors in composition assessment. Training on the operation and maintenance of the device is provided by COSMED representatives, and a 3 h orientation course is provided once the instrument has been commissioned. Different university or commercial organisations will have identical quality control procedures, but athlete standardisation protocols may vary. Athletes undertaking Bod Pod assessment for the first time at a new facility should enquire about these requirements and the facilities' quality control/calibration schedule to ensure the assessment completed is reliable and precise.

8.3.2   Equipment

The Bod Pod is available through COSMED USA Inc. (www.cosmed.com) with COSMED regional offices in North America, China and Australia and throughout Europe, with further distributors situated worldwide. The Bod Pod comes in one level of specification suitable for athletic populations—Bod Pod Gold Standard. The 2016 purchase price of the Bod Pod was US$75,000. Traditionally thought of as a research-level technology, due to cost and accessibility, the Bod Pod is now becoming more commercially available in gyms, testing facilities and performance laboratories. This means the Bod Pod is an accessible and affordable technology for body composition analysis with commercial scans in Australia costing in 2016 approximately $A50–100 per scan (sometimes including a subsequent consultation).

8.4   How Do You Use the Air Displacement Plethysmography Technique for Your Athletes?

As with most physique assessment techniques, the Bod Pod requires standardisation of athlete presentation to minimise biological variability. With this in mind, athletes should be given clear guidance prior to presenting for testing to ensure arrival in a suitable state. Hair (Peeters and Claessens 2011), clothing (Fields et al. 2000; Vescovi et al. 2002), prior exercise (Otterstetter et al. 2013), skin temperature (Fields et al. 2004), prior food and fluid intake (Heiss et al. 2009) and extreme breathing or postural movements (Tegenkamp et al. 2011) can significantly impact the reliability and accuracy of the Bod Pod assessment. Therefore, athlete standardisation should be implemented to ensure the accuracy and reliability of results from the Bod Pod are maintained over time. This includes guidance given to athletes in advance of testing regarding no prior exercise or food and fluid intake (see Chap. 5 for more detail). It should also be made clear to athletes utilising Bod Pod for physique assessment and monitoring that any deviation from clothing recommendation can significantly impact their physique assessment. Form-fitting Lycra/spandex-type swimsuit or single-layer compression shorts without padding are recommended for male athletes with the addition of a seam-free sports bra recommended for female athletes. A swim cap (preferably silicon or minimum Lycra) must be worn to compress the hair on the head.

8.4.1   Composition Measurement

Once the quality control processes have been completed, the test can begin, and the technician will be required to complete a single volume calibration, tare the scale and weigh the athlete, all before measuring the athlete's body density. This measurement involves two or three 40 s tests. A third volume measure is dependent on the first two measures being within 150 ml of one another. After a body volume has been measured, the technician will be required to select the density model depending on the population within which the athlete best fits. For consistency once an equation is chosen, it should be utilised with all assessments. Additionally, thoracic gas volume is either measured or the predicted model needs to be reviewed. Thoracic gas volume is measured via a computer-guided procedure with athletes instructed to follow the instructions on the computer screen through the Perspex window. The whole test procedure takes ~10 min per athlete to complete from start to finish (shorter if thoracic gas volume is estimated rather than measured).

8.5   Example of a Bod Pod Standard Operating Procedure

The following example Bod Pod standard operating procedure is to guide a technician to be able to conduct measurement for an athlete.

8.5.1 One Day Prior to Measurement

Set the Bod Pod to automatically start the warm-up for the appropriate time the next morning. Warm-up should be finished at least 30 min before measurement. Select QC > Warmup. Select day and time. Click *Next*.

The scales should be calibrated once a week or whenever moved. Select "Calibrate Scale" and follow the on-screen instructions. You can check when the scales were last calibrated by clicking on Check Scale. Click scale calibration and follow on-screen instructions. Use both 10 kg weights provided. If the test fails, redo the calibration.

The room temperature should be controlled between 21 and 27 °C. Use a timer and oil heater to warm the room sufficiently before the warm-up process. Maintain the room temperature throughout the measurement protocol.

8.5.2 On the Day of Measurement

Perform the following quality control procedures in this order, without interruptions: QC menu > (1) analyse hardware, (2) scale check, (3) autorun and (4) volume—select appropriate cylinder volume—adult/paediatric.

For each procedure, follow the instructions exactly as they are given on the screen. If using the *Measured* option of the thoracic gas volume (TGV), the air tube and filter are required to be fitted prior to calibration. Keep the door of the room closed during these processes to reduce fluctuation in temperature and pressure. If a test fails, repeat. If failures are repeated, contact Bod Pod customer service.

Measure the athlete's height prior to measurement. Ask the athlete to go to the bathroom, get changed and empty their bladder. Clothing should be minimal and tight fitting, for example, Speedo or Lycra-type swimsuit, compression shorts (i.e., no padding) and non-padded sports bra. Ask the subject to wear their own or the specific Bod Pod swim cap. All other articles should be removed, including socks, jewellery, glasses, etc.

Click *Test* > *Body Composition*. Enter subject information: first name/last name; date of birth (DD/MM/YYYY); gender; ID1 (initials and DOB or subject ID); ID2 (measurement number); height, cm; and ethnicity, general population or African/ American. Follow the on-screen instructions or refer to the manual for further assistance.

Choose the density model most appropriate to the population similar to the athlete and thoracic gas volume preference (predicted/measured/entered).

Start calibration process by following instructions on screen. Whilst completing the calibration process, follow on-screen instructions to measure the athlete's mass. This will include taring the scales before and after the measurement of mass. Avoid pressure and temperature changes in the room by avoiding the opening of the room door. Once calibration is complete, remove the calibration cylinder and ask the athlete to sit inside.

Explain the measurement procedure to the athlete. The Bod Pod will take two volume measurements, approximately 20 s in length. A third measurement may be required if the standard deviation between the first two is too great (the operator will be prompted on screen if this is the case). Ask the athlete to relax and breathe normally and stay as still as possible. There will be some clicking noises on the left hand side near the ear. Light changes in pressure may be felt. Should the athlete need to, or wish to, be removed at any time, the light green button on the left hand side (near the knee) can be pressed at any time.

Follow the on-screen instructions. If you need to stop the measurement for any reason, click the *Back* button, and this will allow you to repeat the test. Clicking *Cancel* will cancel the whole procedure.

Explain the thoracic gas volume procedure to the athlete as follows:

This part of the test will use the breathing tube to your left and will measure the amount of air in your lungs. It involves three steps, and you will be in the Bod Pod for about 50 s. (1) After I close the door, please hold the breathing tube in one hand and watch the monitor for the purple and green progress bar telling you when to breathe *IN* and *OUT*. Breathe at the same rate as the progress bar. (2) After about four breaths, a message will appear on the screen that says "Prepare to put tube in mouth and plug up nose". Simply bring the tube close to your mouth. Immediately after, you will see a message that says, "Put tube in mouth". Please put the tube tightly in your mouth creating a seal, plug your nose and continue breathing according to the progress bar. You will hear some pops and clicks inside of the Bod Pod. (3) After a few more breaths, you will see a message on the screen that says "Prepare to Huff". This will alert you that during the next exhalation, the airway connected to the tube will close for 2 s. Immediately after, you will see the final message that says "*huff, huff, huff*". At this point please huff outwards; on the third huff, the measurement is complete.

The results screen for the thoracic gas volume measurement also shows *Merit* and *Airway Pressure*. Merit should be <1 and airway <35. If either of these shows the word *HIGH* next to it, the thoracic gas volume measurement must be repeated by clicking on *Repeat TGV Measurement*. If the merit value is high, ask the subject to make sure their mouth is tightly around the breathing tube. If airway pressure is high, make sure the athlete is not huffing too hard into the breathing tube. Even if merit and airway pressure values are normal, the measured thoracic gas volume may be outside of what is expected in the majority of the population. In this case, a message is displayed, and the thoracic gas volume measurement can be repeated. Thoracic gas volume measurements outside of what is expected in the majority of the population should only be accepted if there is reason to believe the athlete might have an abnormal thoracic gas volume. The thoracic gas volume measurement can be repeated as many times as necessary.

The test is now complete. Ask the athlete to exit the Bod Pod and click *Next* to display results. Select an activity level that best suits the subject in question. Ask the athlete to self-select, if necessary. Click *Next* to choose the printing options. Click *Print* twice, once for the athlete and once for the clinic.

8.6   What Is the Air Displacement Plethysmography Technique Used to Measure?

Bod Pod air displacement plethysmography is the new gold standard for body density measurement. This density value can then be used in a validated equation to provide a two-compartment model of physique assessment. Fat mass and fat-free mass in absolute terms (kg) and a percentage are provided in the subsequent report. Therefore, Bod Pod can be a useful tool for those athletes looking to track whole-body changes in these compartments. Athletes who require high level of precision and validity (e.g., wrestlers determining minimum weight for competition) of physique measures are encouraged to spend significant effort in minimising biological and technical error through standard measurement practices as outlined throughout this and other chapters. Due to the limitations of the air displacement plethysmography technique, segmental composition and more detailed assessment of subsequent fat-free mass compartments are not available from Bod Pod.

Bod Pod can provide a useful alternative to dual-energy X-ray absorptiometry for athletes that need to avoid radiation exposure, for example, females trying to conceive, are pregnant or breastfeeding. Additionally, athletes who are undergoing injury rehabilitation and are being exposed to other radiation sources for diagnostic purposes might choose Bod Pod. Extremely tall and wide athletes, such as NFL players, who are too big for dual-energy X-ray absorptiometry might benefit from more reliable results via Bod Pod compared to utilising correction protocols on dual-energy X-ray absorptiometry.

8.7   How Do You Report the Air Displacement Plethysmography Data to Your Athletes and Coaches?

The Bod Pod has inbuilt reporting templates and an athlete database. Reports (see Fig. 8.2) provide details around measured metrics of the air displacement plethysmography technique with additional reporting capable of charting composition change over time. Reports can be printed with ease at the time of testing and can be modified to the specifications and requirements of the facility. Deviations from standardised procedures cannot be tracked or monitored within the software, and only text-based comments can be added to the end report by the technician allowing for interpretation of results based on changes in standardisation procedures.

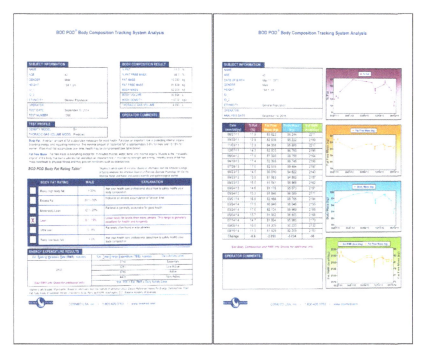

Fig. 8.2 Sample Bod Pod report including change in relative and absolute measures of two-compartment physique

8.8   Summary

The Bod Pod device consists of a measurement pod of two isolated chambers to measure body volume, a calibratable set of scales and a computer attached to each measurement device. Within the measurement pod, a reference chamber houses electronics and technology for estimating lung volume. During measurement the athlete is seated in the measurement chamber, accessible via a hinged, magnetically locking door with a clear window. The Bod Pod can accommodate very large athletes with a volume capacity up to 260 L. The quality control, calibration and measurement processes are guided by software on the attached computer. The Bod Pod software is highly automated and makes the system extremely easy to use with minimal expertise required. However, the quality control and calibration procedures require attention to detail and compliance to the outlined process to ensure significant errors are not introduced.

Composition measurement takes only a few minutes and includes the acquisition of an accurate mass, multiple measures of body volume and either the measurement or estimation of lung gas volume. The measurement process itself is simple with the athlete entering the chamber and sitting quietly, breathing normally and minimising movement. Two measurements of body volume are undertaken with a third required if the first two measures are not within 150 ml. Body volume measurements take approximately 40 s per test, with additional time required if lung volume is measured rather than estimated. The whole measurement process takes approximately 10 min from stepping on the scales to stepping out of the Pod.

Once the body volume has been calculated, the software will quickly provide details of percent body fat and absolute values of fat mass and fat-free mass. This information is displayed on the screen, and a detailed report can be printed off, including information on previous measures and visualisation of this change over time. This information can be used by coaches, athletes and service providers to monitor the effectiveness of physique manipulation interventions or the effect of various training blocks on physique.

References

Anderson DE (2007) Reliability of air displacement plethysmography. J Strength Cond Res 21:169–172

Ballard TP, Fafara L, Vukovich MD (2004) Comparison of bod pod and DXA in female collegiate athlete. Med Sci Sports Exerc 36(4):731–735

Bentzur KM, Kravitz L, Lockner DW (2008) Evaluation of the BOD POD for estimating percent body fat in collegiate track and field female athletes: a comparison of four methods. J Strength Cond Res 22(6):1985–1991

Brožek J, Grande F, Anderson J, Keys A (1963) Densitometric analysis of body composition: revision of some quantitative assumptions. Annals of the New York Academy of Science 110(1):113–140

Collins AL, McCarthy HD (2003) Evaluation of factors determining the precision of body composition measurements by air displacement plethysmography. Eur J Clin Nutr 57(6): 770–776

Collins MA, Millard-Stafford ML, Evans EM, Snow TK, Cureton KJ, Rosskopf LB (2004) Effect of race and musculoskeletal development on the accuracy of air plethysmography. Med Sci Sports Exerc 36(6):1070–1077

Collins MA, Millard-Stafford ML, Sparling PB, Snow TK, Rosskopf LB, Webb SA, Omer J (1999) Evaluation of the bod pod for assessing body fat in collegiate football players. Med Sci Sports Exerc 31(9):1350–1356

COSMED USA (2014) BOD POD gold standard body composition tracking system operators manual–P/N 210–2400, REV-I. Concord, CA

Davis JA, Dorad S, Keays KA, Reigel KA, Valencia KS, Pham PH (2007) Reliability and validity of the lung volume measurement made by the BOD POD body composition system. Clin Physiol Funct Imaging 27(1):42–46

Dempster P, Aitkens S (1995) A new air displacement method for the determination of human body composition. Med Sci Sport Exerc 27(12):1692–1697

Fields DA, Gunatilake R, Kalaitzoglou E (2015) Air displacement plethysmography: cradle to grave. Nutr Clin Pract 30(2):219–226

Fields DA, Higgins PB, Hunter GR (2004) Assessment of body composition by air-displacement plethysmography: influence of body temperature and moisture. Dynamic. Medicine 3(1):3

Fields DA, Hunter GR, Goran MI (2000) Validation of the BOD POD with hydrostatic weighing: influence of body clothing. Int J Obes Relat Metab Disord 24(2):200–205

Fields DA, Wilson GD, Gladden LB, Hunter GR, Pascoe DD, Goran MI (2001) Comparison of the BOD POD with the four-compartment model in adult females. Med Sci Sport Exerc 33(9):1605–1610

Gnaedinger RH, Reineke EP, Pearson AM, Van Huss WD, Wessel JA, Montoye HJ (1963) Determination of body density by air displacement, helium dilution, and underwater weighing. Ann N Y Acad Sci 110(1):96–108

Heiss CJ, Gara N, Novotny D, Heberle H, Morgan L, Stufflebeam J, Fairfield M (2009) Effect of a 1 liter fluid load on body composition measured by air displacement plethysmography and bioelectrical impedance. J Exerc Physiol Online 12(2):1–8

Ludwig UA, Klausman F, Baumann S, Honal M, Hövener JB, König D, Deibert P, Büchert M (2014) Whole-body MRI-based fat quantification: a comparison to air displacement plethysmography. J Magn Reson Imaging 40(6):1437–1444

Millard-Stafford ML, Collins MA, Evans EM, Snow TK, Cureton KJ, Rosskopf LB (2001) Use of air displacement plethysmography for estimating body fat in a four-component model. Med Sci Sports Exerc 33(8):1311–1317

Noreen EE, Lemon PWR (2006) Reliability of air displacement plethysmography in a large, heterogeneous sample. Med Sci Sports Exerc 38(8):1505–1509

Ortiz O, Russell M, Daley TL, Baumgartner R, Waki M, Lichtman S, Wang J, Pierson RNJ, Heymsfield SB (1992) Differences in skeletal muscle and bone mineral mass between black and white females and their relevance to estimates of body composition. Am J Clin Nutr 55(1):8–13

Otterstetter R, Johnson KE, Kiger DL, Agnor SE, Edwards J, Naylor JB, Krone SJ (2013) The effect of acute moderate-intensity exercise on the accuracy of air-displacement plethysmography in young adults. Eur J Clin Nutr 67(10):1092–1094

Peeters MW, Claessens AL (2011) Effect of different swim caps on the assessment of body volume and percentage body fat by air displacement plethysmography. J Sports Sci 29(2):191–196

Siri WE (1956) The gross composition of the body. Adv Biol Med Phys 4:239–280

Tegenkamp MH, Clark RR, Schoeller DA, Landry GL (2011) Effects of covert subject actions on percent body fat by air-displacement plethysmography. J Strength Cond Res 25(7):2010–2017

Tucker LA, Lecheminant J, Bailey BW (2014) Test-retest reliability of the bod pod: the effect of multiple assessments. Percept Mot Skills 118(2):563–570

Utter AC, Goss FL, Swan PD, Harris GS, Robertson RJ, Trone GA (2003) Evaluation of air displacement for assessing body composition of collegiate wrestlers. Medicine Science and Sports Exercise 35(3):500–505

Vescovi JD, Zimmerman SL, Miller WC, Fernhall B (2002) Effects of clothing on accuracy and reliability of air displacement plethysmography. Medicine Science Sport and Exercise 34(2):282–285

Vescovi JD, Zimmerman SL, Miller WC, Hildebrandt L, Hammer RL, Fernhal lB (2001) Evaluation of the BOD POD for estimating percentage body fat in a heterogeneous group of adult humans. Eur J Appl Physiol 85(3-4):326–332

Wells JC, Fuller NJ (2001) Precision of measurement and body size in whole-body air-displacement plethysmography. International Journal of Obesity Related Metabolic Disorders 25(1):1161–1167

Weyers AM, Mazzetti SA, Love DM, Gómez AL, Kraemer WJ, Volek JS (2002) Comparison of methods for assessing body composition changes during weight loss. Med Sci Sports Exerc 34(3):497–502

Chapter 9
Non-imaging Method: Bioelectrical Impedance Analysis

Ava Kerr and Patria A. Hume

Abstract Bioelectrical impedance analysis allows measurement of total body water, which is used to estimate fat-free body mass and, by difference with body mass, body fat. An athlete appointment of 15 min is needed for body mass and standing stature measurement, electrode placement, and then 1 min of data collection. The method is popular due to the procedure being simple and non-invasive, good portability of the equipment and its relatively low cost compared to other methods of body composition analysis. However, precision and validity can be low without a standardised protocol of assessment that includes guidance for subject presentation. Sensitivity to monitor change of physique is low given variation in athlete presentation for testing can affect the results (e.g. levels of hydration). Training is available from equipment suppliers; however, there are no accreditation systems. The techniques to collect the data are easy; however, interpretation of the data is impeded given the black box approach to the data. Studies that compare results from bioelectrical impedance analysis to other body composition techniques are outlined, and example reports to athletes are provided.

Keywords Bioelectrical impedance analysis • Hydration • Calibration • Total body water estimation • Fat-free mass • Fat mass • Body mass • Electrodes • Portable Low cost • Reports

A. Kerr (✉)
University of the Sunshine Coast, Maroochydore DC, QLD, Australia
e-mail: akerr@usc.edu.au

P.A. Hume
Sport Performance Research Institute New Zealand,
Auckland University of Technology, Auckland, New Zealand
e-mail: patria.hume@aut.ac.nz

9.1   Introduction

The International Society for Electrical Bioimpedance (http://www.isebi.org) was founded in 1992 to promote research, development, use and understanding of electrical impedance measurements as a means of assessing normal and abnormal physiological states in medicine and biology. The first international conference on electrical bioimpedance was earlier in 1969 with the 16th conference in 2016. Multi-frequency bioelectrical impedance analysers were first commercially available in the mid-1980s, and their usage has continued to increase from clinical use, commercial fitness centres to sports testing application. Guidelines for clinical bioelectrical impedance analysis have been discussed (Kyle et al. 2004c); however, there are no international standards available. In general, bioelectrical impedance technology may be acceptable for determining body composition of groups and for monitoring changes in body composition within individuals over time. Use of the technology to make single measurements in individual patients, however, is not recommended (Buchholz et al. 2004).

9.2   Why Measure Physique Using This Technique?

Bioelectrical impedance analysis determines the electrical impedance (flow of an electric current through body tissues) which is used to calculate an estimate of total body water. The total body water value is used to estimate fat-free body mass and by difference with body mass, body fat. Although there is risk of inaccurate and unreliable data, other attributes make this a popular field technique for large homogenous groups. These include commercial high availability, low time commitment for data collection, athlete friendly, and low health risk for single or multiple tests. The method is also popular due to the procedure being simple and non-invasive, portability of the equipment and its relatively low cost compared to other methods of body composition analysis. The importance of subject presentation for bioelectrical impedance assessment is a key as it impacts upon results more than any other technique. Furthermore, because of the array of factors that influence results, the actual impact (and direction of change) can be difficult to estimate. If the technician follows a best practice protocol and athletes are given clear guidance regarding presentation for testing, the technique can be a useful and reliable method for estimation of total body water and, consequently, fat-free mass and fat mass.

9.3   What Is This Technique and Technology?

Deuterium dilution is the reference method for laboratory-based total body water measurement but is expensive and time consuming for both testing and analysis (Colley et al. 2007; van Marken Lichtenbelt et al. 1994), whereas bioelectrical impedance analysis has been applied in both athlete and non-athletic populations. It is considered safe, non-invasive and cost-effective with instantaneous total body water results (Kerr et al. 2015b; Moon et al. 2008). Bioelectrical impedance analysis is considered a doubly indirect measurement of body composition utilising algorithms to estimate fat-free mass and fat mass from the total body water assessment. The technique relies on several assumptions including the human body being a series of cylinders that have equal resistivity to an electrical current that passes through water-containing tissue (i.e. fat-free mass). Additionally, the technique is insensitive to water changes in the trunk region, and predictive algorithms assume a relative distribution of water between the limbs and trunk (Ward 2012; Deurenberg et al. 1995).

Bioelectrical impedance analysis measures current, voltage and phase angle throughout human tissue containing water. The premise is that electrical conduction is more pronounced in fat-free tissue due to water and electrolyte content than in fat mass (Lukaski and Bolonchuk 1987). There is a relationship between the impedance of a geometrical system and the conductor length, the cross-sectional area and the signal frequency. The impedance to a flow of current is related to the volume of a conductor assuming the conductor and the signal frequency are constant throughout the system. Typically, this can be expressed as $V = pL2/Z$. This is where Z is impedance ($R = \sqrt{R^2 + Xc^2}$), R is resistance, Xc is reactance, p is volume resistivity, L is conductor length and V is conductor bioelectrical volume (Lukaski and Bolonchuk 1987).

Impedance measurement uses either two or four electrodes. A small current (~1–10 µA) is passed between two electrodes, and the voltage is measured between the same (for a two-electrode configuration) or between the other two electrodes. Electrodes are usually on the wrist to the contralateral ankle. However, commercial devices vary greatly in where electrodes are sited (i.e. hands, feet, foot to hand). The important principle is which path the electrical current is taking in the body. Once the current is measured, the device then calculates its impedance, resistance and reactance. This is then interpreted as total body water, intracellular water and extracellular water in the measurement results. The measurements and calculations can then estimate body composition via fat-free mass, fat mass and fluid distribution by pre-programmed algorithms.

9.3.1 Equipment and Calibration

Single-frequency bioelectrical impedance analysis at 50 kHz measures the sum of extracellular water and intracellular water resistivity. This allows estimates of fat-free mass and total body water. It is however not sensitive enough to determine differences in intracellular water (Kyle et al. 2004a). Therefore, body composition results from athletes with significant hydration variance due to exercise-induced hypohydration, or acute food or fluid intake may not be valid (Saunders et al. 1998). Percent body fat estimates were found to increase due to higher impedance and body mass levels from ingesting fluid 20 min prior to testing (Dixon et al. 2009). Bioelectrical impedance analysis only half predicted the total body water loss after exercise although conditions were standardised across four separate treatments (Koulmann et al. 2000). These studies suggest that bioelectrical impedance analysis is heavily reliant on standardised protocols such as athlete presentation in a euhydrated, rested and fasted state to be reasonably accurate when measuring total body water and subsequent calculation of fat mass and fat-free mass.

Bioelectrical impedance spectroscopy creates frequencies in a range of 1–1300 kHz instead of the solitary 50 kHz from bioelectrical impedance analysis. This system uses the lower spectrum of frequencies to measure extracellular water. At higher frequencies the current can progressively permeate the cell membrane and consequently measure intracellular water and thus enable calculation of total body water (Wagner and Heyward 1999; Cornish et al. 1996). Bioelectrical impedance spectroscopy estimates hydration status more accurately than bioelectrical impedance analysis when compared against the deuterium dilution criterion standard (Martinoli et al. 2003). In contrast, poor accuracy has been reported using bioelectrical impedance spectroscopy in estimating body composition in overweight or obese men compared to a dual-energy X-ray absorptiometry body composition scan. However, dual-energy X-ray absorptiometry assumes body density to be constant and so is less sensitive to variance in hydration status, somewhat explaining the poor levels of agreement between these two methods (Pateyjohns et al. 2006). Bioelectrical impedance spectroscopy has been found to overestimate percentage body fat in lean individuals yet underestimate it in the overweight or obese by significant amounts (Sun et al. 2005). Therefore, interpretation of results of bioelectrical impedance spectroscopy should be made with caution when measuring body composition in overweight or obese individuals.

Although there is information on total body water measurement of athletes using bioelectrical impedance spectroscopy technology (Utter and Lambeth 2010; Svantesson et al. 2008) as well as overweight and obese individuals (Pateyjohns et al. 2006; Moon et al. 2009), there is little research available on the hydration status of athletes with high fat-free mass using bioelectrical impedance spectroscopy. As the fat-free mass contains proportionally most of the total body hydration (Brožek et al. 1963), this parameter is likely to be most responsible for the biological variability in the measurements (Van Loan and Mayclin 1992).

As there are many commercially available bioelectrical impedance analysis devices, we have chosen to describe the use of a device and the associated protocols used at the University of the Sunshine Coast by chapter author Ava Kerr and colleagues. The SFB7 tetra polar bioimpedance spectroscopy device (ImpediMed, Australia) has a single channel that scans 256 discrete frequencies between 4 and 1000 kHz for the estimation of body composition in healthy individuals. The SFB7 utilizes Cole modelling with Hanai mixture theory to determine total body water, extracellular fluid and intracellular fluid from impedance data. Fat-free mass and fat mass are then calculated on the device. Further data analysis can be undertaken in the supporting software. Therefore, no population-specific prediction equations (algorithms) are required for data analysis. The device is portable with a case, electrodes and clips, leads and software, has a touch screen for operation and takes readings in <1 s. Calibration of the device involves connecting each coloured (yellow, red, black, blue) cabled electrode into each colour-matched port in the calibration test unit. Prompts of the device are followed to auto calibrate prior to testing the athlete.

9.3.2 Accuracy of Types Of Devices

One of the main assumptions with bioelectrical impedance analysis technology is that the human body is a series of biological cylinders with standard lengths and cross-sectional areas; however, this is clearly not the case. The limbs are used to measure whole body resistance, yet the trunk, which contains approximately half the total body mass, is only a minor contributor to the conductor resistance. Additionally, the resistance to the electrical current is expected to be constant despite dependence on the type of tissue, hydration status and the concentration of electrolytes (Kushner 1992).

The conductivity of electrical current is related to body water; therefore, acute changes in hydration status due to exercise or food and fluid ingestion will impact upon results. For example, any fluid deficit that results from involuntary hypohydration after exercise is identified as fat mass when assessed via bioelectrical impedance analysis. There is an effect of exercise on body composition estimates with bioelectrical impedance analysis (Rodriguez-Sanchez and Galloway 2015), most likely due to increased cutaneous blood flow and skin electrolyte accumulation which influence electrical conductance and therefore precision of bioelectrical impedance analysis measurement (O'Brien et al. 2002). While this sustained impact on physique assessment using bioelectrical impedance analysis may be resolved via a cold shower (Gatterer et al. 2014), this does not account for body fluid deficits.

Because hydration changes typically involve changes in fluid and electrolyte content, the interpretation of a change in bioimpedance (and thus body composition) can be confounded. Effects of a 1 L fluid load on body composition measured by bioelectrical impedance and air displacement plethysmography have been reported (Heiss et al. 2009). As acute ingestion of fluid can overestimate fat mass by 3.2% (Saunders et al. 1998), it is recommended that athletes arrive early morning after an overnight fast for testing (Kyle et al. 2004b). Even small amounts of fluid intake of 0.59 L increase fat mass estimations (Dixon et al. 2009), so reliability of assessment is heavily dependent on athlete presentation. Acute food and fluid intake can artificially influence body composition estimates, regardless of macronutrient content. An overnight fast is likely sufficient as a pre-assessment dietary control for bioelectrical impedance analysis (Tinsley et al. 2017). Bioelectrical impedance decreased by 4.4% in response to feeding, leading to a 2% increase in total body water and fat-free mass, with individual increases up to 4.5%. Bioelectrical impedance analysis fat mass estimates decreased from 1.4% to 2.4%, with individual decreases of up to 10%.

In agreement, the latest research undertaken by the University of Sunshine Coast group showed a much larger decrease in fat mass from non-standardised presentation (unrestricted food and fluid intake plus exercise) compared to standardised presentation (overnight fasted, euhydrated, rested) after 6 months of self-selected training and diet. Additionally, the small increase in fat-free mass identified via standardised testing (204 g) was increased to 1908 g when presentation was not controlled for. Of interest was the random nature of individual responses to non-standardised presentation with fat-free mass and fat mass determined from bioelectrical impedance spectroscopy ranging from −5.632 kg to 2.223 kg (fat-free mass) and −2.857 kg to 4.909 kg (fat mass). This makes bioelectrical impedance spectroscopy unique regarding its vulnerability to imprecision as the impact can be inconsistent across individuals (Dehghan and Merchant 2008) and prediction of small to moderate changes in physique traits difficult to quantify. Considering these findings, it is recommended that athlete presentation follow previous clinical guidance (Kyle et al. 2004b) before utilising bioelectrical impedance spectroscopy technology for monitoring changes in physique.

Bioelectrical impedance consumer devices for measurement of body composition have been shown to be inaccurate in comparison to whole body magnetic resonance imaging and dual-energy X-ray absorptiometry (Bosy-Westphal et al. 2008). Accuracy of seven consumer grade bioelectrical impedance analysis devices (finger to finger, hand to hand and leg to leg) has been compared to air displacement plethysmography and seven-site skinfold-derived estimated body fat in 82 females (Peterson et al. 2011). There were no systematic differences in percent body fat estimates between skinfold and seven bioelectrical impedance analyses. However, skinfold measures were the most reliable method of estimating body composition.

9.4 How Do You Use the Selected Technique for Your Athlete?

Precision and accuracy, validity and sensitivity to monitor change of physique are potential issues with bioelectrical impedance analysers. Research studies have shown that bioelectrical impedance analysis is variable and does not provide an accurate measure of body composition. Segmental bioelectrical impedance analysis has been developed to overcome inconsistencies between resistance and body mass of the trunk. Although the instruments are straightforward to use, careful attention to the method of use as described by the manufacturer is needed.

9.4.1 Athlete Presentation for Testing

In order to minimise biological variability, it is important to adhere to a standardised protocol and maintain a consistent presentation for assessment each time. With this mind, athletes must be given clear guidance beforehand in order to present for testing in a standardised manner:

- Increase fluid intake with meals and snacks the previous day to ensure good hydration on the morning of assessment
- Avoid any heavy intense training late in the evening prior to the day of assessment or any exercise on the morning of the assessment

- Overnight fast with no food or fluid intake
- Wear comfortable clothing that allows easy access to wrists and ankles
- Void bowel and bladder prior to testing

9.4.2 Athlete Preparation Procedure During Assessment

To conduct the athlete assessment:

- Record body mass in minimal clothing on a calibrated scale
- Measure stretch stature using a calibrated stadiometer
- Enter athlete demographic data into device including age, ethnicity and gender
- Direct athlete to lie on a flat, even surface, e.g. examination table or yoga mat on floor
- Extend the athlete's arms by their sides, palms down, abducted 30° from the trunk
- Abduct the athlete's legs to 45° and maintain this position for a minimum of 10 min prior to assessment to stabilise body water shifts between limb compartments
- Shave electrode sites if necessary to gain good skin contact and clean all sites with alcohol swabs and allow to dry prior to electrode application

9.4.3 Electrode Placement

Electrodes are placed on the hand and foot in the correct position as outlined by the manufacturer's procedure. Each dual tab electrode adhesive is applied to the skin with the tab facing outwards from the body. One electrode is placed central on the dorsal side of the wrist in alignment with the ulnar head. The yellow sense lead alligator clip attaches here. The other end of the electrode is placed on the dorsal surface of the hand 1 cm proximal to the third metacarpophalangeal joint. The red current source lead alligator clip attaches here. One electrode is placed central on the dorsal surface of the ankle between the lateral and medial malleoli. The blue sense lead alligator clip attaches here. The other end of the electrode is placed on the dorsal surface of the foot 1 cm proximal to the second metatarsophalangeal joint. The black current sink lead alligator clip is attached here (see Fig. 9.1).

Tracking results over time requires precision of impedance output. Standardisation of measurement practice is key to this precision. ImpediMed's dual tab electrodes are designed to improve standardisation of measurement technique and data collection. The sense and drive signal leads are separated by a fixed distance of 5 cm, controlling the electrical field effects that can induce variability in results. The green placement line allows reproducible placement at consistent anatomical markers. The dual tab arrangement limits the number of placements and opportunities for variability in placement, especially between operators.

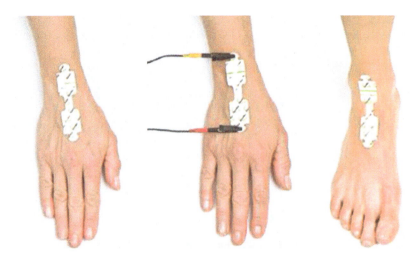

Fig. 9.1 ImpediMed's dual tab electrodes are designed to improve standardisation of measurement technique and data collection

Once the athlete is in the supine position, the electrodes are attached and the leads are plugged into the device (see Fig. 9.2). *Measurement* setup is selected on the device menu, the athlete details are entered and then the measurement setting is selected. The *Measure* tab on the screen is selected to make a measurement for 1 s. Collected files are uploaded to a personal computer and then analysed using the software provided with the device.

9.5   What Is the Technique Used to Measure?

The assessment appointment takes ~15 min resulting in estimates of total body water, extracellular fluid, intracellular fluid, fat-free mass, fat mass and body mass index (see Fig. 9.3 for an example of the bioelectrical impedance analysis results screen from the ImpediMed device).

9.6   How Do You Report the Data to Your Athlete and Coach?

Assessment results should be reported to the athlete, explaining the limitations of a one-off assessment, or providing measurements over several points in time to track changes (see Fig. 9.4 for individual test results from SFB7 bioelectrical impedance spectroscopy focusing on body composition outputs).

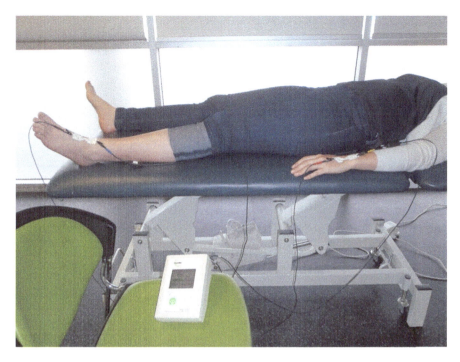

Fig. 9.2 Once the participant is in the supine position, the electrodes are attached and the leads are plugged into the device

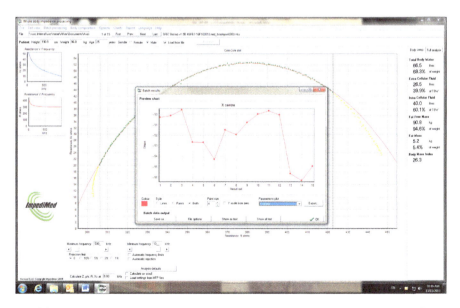

Fig. 9.3 Example of bioelectrical impedance analysis results screen from the ImpediMed device showing 1 of 15 tests processed

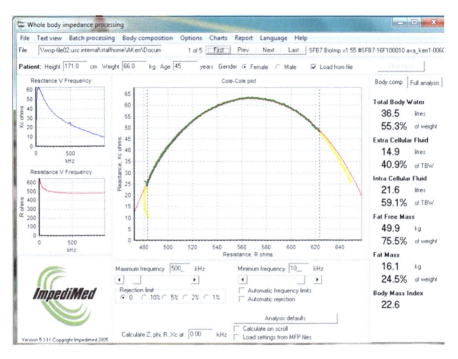

Fig. 9.4 Example of bioelectrical impedance spectroscopy results screen from ImpediMed device of a single test

9.6.1 Example Reports Comparing Techniques

The variance in individual total body water significantly changes estimates of fat mass and fat-free mass especially in large resistance trained males who have high levels of lean mass. A study (Kerr et al. 2015) was conducted to determine the validity of a bioelectrical impedance spectroscopy device against the doubly labelled water reference method for total body water. Data were collected on 29 individuals who also undertook a Bod Pod measurement to measure body density and estimates of fat mass and fat-free mass. The total body water estimations were incorporated with the body density values from the Bod Pod to create 3-compartment models using the Siri equation (Withers et al. 1998). The 3-compartment model using bioelectrical impedance spectroscopy for total body water estimation was more accurate than the simple 2-compartment model from the Bod Pod. The difference was due to the actual total body water measurement from the bioelectrical impedance spectroscopy device or the doubly labelled water being used in the 3-compartment model whereas the Bod Pod assumes a total body water of 73.7% in everyone. A sample report for a participant in the study is shown in Fig. 9.5. Explanation for the difference in results for the participant included:

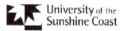

Name: DS   Date: 4/08/2012

Body Mass: 98.7 kg   BMI: 29

Height: 184.9 cm

This report provides a summary of your total body water (TBW) values as measured by the deuterium oxide tracer and the multi-frequency Bioelectrical Impedance Spectroscopy unit (MF-BIS).

	Your TBW (L)	Your TBW (%)
Deuterium oxide	61.7	62.5
MF-BIS	55.64	56.37

	TBW Trained men (%)	TBW Sedentary men (%)
Withers et al 1998 Deuterium oxide	63.7	56.02

Your BOD POD body density value allows us to create a 2-Compartment model of body composition which partitions the body into fat mass (FM) and fat free mass (FFM) (Schematic 2-C).

A 3-Compartment model includes your TBW value in addition to your body density (BD) so the three compartments are FM, TBW and fat free dry mass (FFDM) see Schematic 3-C.

Models of Body Composition

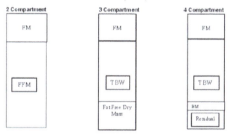

FM, fat mass; FFM, fat free mass; TBW, total body water; BM, bone mass; Residual, everything else.
(Withers et al. Critical Appraisal of the Estimation of Body Composition via 2-, 3- and 4-Compartment Models 1999)

We use the Siri Equation to create the 2-Compartment model of fat mass and fat free mass. This is identical to your BOD POD body composition report so it should look the same.

Your 2-Compartment Model of Body Composition:

1/BD = FM/FM density + FFM/FFM density

FM% = 497.1/BD − 451.9

FM% = 497.1 / 1.0579 − 451.9

FM% = 17.99

We have added your TBW value from the deuterium oxide results in the equation below to create a 3-C model. This is more accurate than the 2-C model which uses a reference value of 72% TBW in the calculation. Therefore, the 3-C model is a more accurate reflection of your body composition. Remember, a measurement is always better than an assumed constant. The 4-C model will improve upon this further by adding your bone mineral density value instead of an assumed constant.

Your 3-Compartment Model of Body Composition:

1/BD = FM/FM density + TBW/H20 density + FFDM/FFDM density

FM% = 211.5/BD − 78.0 (TBW/body mass) − 134.8

FM% = 211.5/1.0579 − 78.0 (61.7/98.7) − 134.8

FM% = 16.36

If you have any questions at all about your results please contact me on Phone 07 5459 4605 or Email aker@usc.edu.au

Thank you so much for participating in my study. Remember that my next study will create a 4-Compartment model of body composition building on the measurements so far. So get busy training so you can improve your results from this study!

Fig. 9.5 Example of a report for a participant in a study that used bioelectrical impedance spectroscopy, doubly labelled water and Bod Pod to calculate 2-compartment and 3-compartment models for fat mass and fat-free mass and total body water

- Deuterium dilution is the reference method for total body water measurement but still has a resolution of $800 \times g$—it is not 100% perfect.
- Bioelectrical impedance spectroscopy has a resolution of 2.4–2.6 kg, so when the total body water estimations are incorporated into the 3-compartment models, the consequent percentage body fat results from both calculations will be different.
- The Bod Pod assumes total body water is a constant 73.7% and the densities of fat mass and fat-free mass are 1.1000 g cm³ and 0.9007 g cm³, respectively. The problem is that these data were collected from only 3–5 elderly male cadavers who are nothing like you and the other subjects in this study. Your Bod Pod results are likely to be less accurate than the reference 3-compartment model as seen in your report.

There are demonstrated effects of food and fluid intake plus exercise on all of the most commonly used methods of body composition assessment used by athletes (Meyer et al. 2013). An additional study (Kerr et al. 2017) showed large variance in fat mass and fat-free mass under non-standardised presentation or post meal conditions. Thirty-two large muscular males were tested five times in 27 h across the most common laboratory and field methods of physique assessment with components used to create 3-compartment and 4-compartment models. The standardised presentation conditions (overnight fasted, rested, euhydrated) were compared against non-standardised presentation conditions (self-selected food and fluid intake plus exercise) and after either a specified 500 g meal or a 500 g meal plus 1000 mL of water. A sample report for a participant in the study is shown in Fig. 9.6. Explanation for the results for the participant included:

- The reason for the difference in results (even though they are from the same standardised presentation testing) for you is because all methods contain some built-in assumptions.
- Bod Pod assumes a constant total body water and fat mass and fat-free mass densities, whereas we know this is not the case in many individuals.
- The dual-energy X-ray absorptiometry scanner does not measure total body water directly; it assumes a constant total body water density. It also has to extrapolate or 'guess' that the tissue overlying the bone is the same as the tissue just outside of the bone, and this may not necessarily be the case especially in the trunk region.
- Bioelectrical impedance spectroscopy measures the impedance to a current and assumes the body is a set of cylinders of constant dimension. The 3-compartment and 4-compartment models, although considered reference methods, are influenced by the bioelectrical impedance spectroscopy values included in their calculations.
- Although skinfold data are the most reliable of all the techniques when incorporated into a body fat percentage, body mass is included which is impacted by prior food and fluid intake or hydration status. You would know this by weighing yourself before and after a big meal (hyper-hydrated) or after a night on the town (dehydrated).

University **of the**
University of the
Sunshine Coast
Queensland, Australia

Test Administrator: Ava Kerr MSc
Contact Phone: 07 5459 4605
Email: akerr@usc.edu.au

Body Composition Reliability Study Athlete Results

| Name: | MC | | Age: | 29 | Test Date: | 5/10/2013 |
| BMI: | 36 | | Height: | 1.76 | Return Date: | 5/04/2014 |

This report provides a summary of your fat mass and fat free mass in kg and percent as measured by the DXA, BOD POD and also when calculated into 3 and 4-Compartment models. The first row is your result and the next is the average of the group.

		Fat Mass %	Fat mass kg	Fat Free Mass %	Fat Free Mass kg
BOD POD					
You		16.80	18.87	83.20	93.66
Average		18.13	16.83	81.88	74.76
DXA					
You		12.85	14.52	83.81	94.70
Average		18.32	17.07	77.48	70.87
3-C Model					
You		12.67	14.26	87.33	98.27
Average		16.26	15.17	83.74	76.42
4-C Model					
You		11.24	12.65	88.76	99.88
Average		15.39	14.35	84.61	77.23
Skinfolds %					
You		7.1			
Average		9.39			

Test results inevitably vary slightly between body composition techniques. This is because, when used in isolation, they all make assumptions...
DXA - Assumes a constant level of hydration

BOD POD - Assumes a constant density of fat mass and fat free mass

Skinfolds Assumes an association between subcutaneous fat (under the skin) and whole body fat

Unlike the above techniques (all 2 compartment models as they break the body up into fat mass and fat free mass), the **3 and 4 compartment models** use a combination of data from all of the measures you had undertaken. Because of this, the **3 and 4 compartment models** are considered the reference method and offer the most precise measure of your TRUE body composition, with all assumptions removed.

Fig. 9.6 Example of a report for a participant in a study that used Bod Pod and dual-energy X-ray absorptiometry to calculate 3-compartment and 4-compartment models for fat mass and fat-free mass. Surface anthropometry was used to calculate skinfold percentage

- Underpinning all this information is not the technique itself but rather the conditions under which is collected. Your testing was undertaken under 'pristine' standardised presentation conditions so you can be sure that despite the slight variance in results per methods, the results are accurate.

9.7   Summary

Bioelectrical impedance analysis can be considered to be low in accuracy and reliability. Regional body assessment is possible but is invalid. Bioelectrical impedance analysis assessment devices are readily available, and assessment is quick compared to other methods. The method is athlete friendly as it is non-invasive and there is low health risk. Athlete preparation for measurement is important given the effect of hydration on results. Training of the technician is preferred to ensure correct preparation of the skin and reliable placement of electrodes.

References

Bosy-Westphal A, Later W, Hitze B, Sato T, Kossel E, Giüer CC, Heller M, Müller MJ (2008) Accuracy of bioelectrical impedance consumer devices for measurement of body composition in comparison to whole body magnetic resonance imaging and dual x-ray absorptiometry. Obes Facts 1(6):6

Brožek J, Grande F, Anderson JT, Keys A (1963) Densitometric analysis of body composition: revision of some qantitative assumptions. Ann N Y Acad Sci 110(1):113–140

Buchholz AC, Bartok C, Schoeller DA (2004) The validity of bioelectrical impedance models in clinical populations. Nutr Clin Pract 19(5):433–446

Colley RC, Byrne NM, Hills AP (2007) Implications of the variability in time to isotopic equilibrium in the deuterium dilution technique. Eur J Clin Nutr 61(11):1250–1255

Cornish BH, Ward LC, Thomas BJ, Jebb SA, Elia M (1996) Evaluation of multiple frequency bioelectrical impedance and Cole-Cole analysis for the assessment of body water volumes in healthy humans. Eur J Clin Nutr 50(3):159–164

Dehghan M, Merchant AT (2008) Is bioelectrical impedance accurate for use in large epidemiological studies? Nutr J 7(1):26

Deurenberg P, Tagliabue A, Schouten FJ (1995) Multi-frequency impedance for the prediction of extracellular water and total body water. Br J Nutr 73(03):349–358

Dixon CB, Ramos L, Fitzgerald E, Reppert D, Andreacci JL (2009) The effect of acute fluid consumption on measures of impedance and percent body fat estimated using segmental bioelectrical impedance analysis. Eur J Clin Nutr 63(9):1115–1122

Gatterer H, Schenk K, Laninschegg L, Schlemmer P, Lukaski H, Burtscher M (2014) Bioimpedance identifies body fluid loss after exercise in the heat: a pilot study with body cooling. PLoS One 9(10):e109729

Heiss CJ, Gara N, Novotny D et al (2009) Effect of a 1 liter fluid load on body composition measured by air displacement plethysmography and bioelectrical impedance. J Exerc Physiol Online 12(2):1–8

Kerr A, Slater G, Byrne N, Chaseling J (2015) Validation of bioelectrical impedance spectroscopy to measure total body water in resistance -trained males. Int J Sport Nutr Exerc Metab 25(5):494–503

Kerr A, Slater GJ, Byrne N (2017) Impact of food and fluid intake on technical and biological measurement error in body composition assessment methods in athletes. Br J Nutr 117(4): 591–601

Koulmann N, Jimenez C, Regal D, Bolliet P, Launay J-C, Savourey G, Melin B (2000) Use of bioelectrical impedance analysis to estimate body fluid compartments after acute variations of the body hydration level. Med Sci Sports Exerc 32(4):857–864

Kushner RF (1992) Bioelectrical impedance analysis: a review of principles and applications. J Am Coll Nutr 11(2):199–209

Kyle UG, Bosaeus I, De Lorenzo AD, Deurenberg P, Elia M, Gómez JM, Heitmann BL, Kent-Smith L, Melchior J-C, Pirlich M, Scharfetter H, Schols AMWJ, Pichard C (2004a) Bioelectrical impedance analysis—Part I: Review of principles and methods. Clin Nutr 23(5):1226–1243

Kyle UG, Bosaeus I, De Lorenzo AD, Deurenberg P, Elia M, Manuel Gómez J, Lilienthal Heitmann B, Kent-Smith L, Melchior J-C, Pirlich M, Scharfetter H, Schols AMWJ, Pichard C (2004b) Bioelectrical impedance analysis—Part II: Utilization in clinical practice. Clin Nutr 23(6):1430–1453

Kyle UG, Bosaeus I, De Lorenzo AD, Deurenberg P, Elia M, Manuel Gomez J, Pichard C (2004c) Bioelectrical impedance analysis-part II: utilization in clinical practice. Clin Nutr 23(6):1430–1453

Lukaski HC, Bolonchuk WW (1987) Theory and validation of the tetrapolar bioelectrical impedance method to assess human body composition. In: Ellis KJ, Yasumura S, Morgan WD (eds) In vivo body composition studies, brookhaven national laboratory. The Institute of Physical Sciences in Medicine, New York, NY

Martinoli R, Mohamed EI, Maiolo C, Cianci R, Denoth F, Salvadori S, Iacopino L (2003) Total body water estimation using bioelectrical impedance: a meta-analysis of the data available in the literature. Acta Diabetol 40(0):s203–s206

Meyer NL, Sundgot-Borgen J, Lohman TG, Ackland TR, Stewart AD, Maughan RJ, Smith S, Müller W (2013) Body composition for health and performance: a survey of body composition assessment practice carried out by the Ad Hoc Research Working Group on Body Composition, Health and Performance under the auspices of the IOC Medical Commission. Br J Sports Med 47(16):1044–1053

Moon J, Tobkin S, Roberts M, Dalbo V, Kerksick C, Bemben M, Cramer J, Stout J (2008) Total body water estimations in healthy men and women using bioimpedance spectroscopy: a deuterium oxide comparison. Nutr Metab 5(1):7

Moon JR, Smith AE, Tobkin SE, Lockwood CM, Kendall KL, Graef JL, Roberts MD, Dalbo VJ, Kerksick CM, Cramer JT, Beck TW, Stout JR (2009) Total body water changes after an exercise intervention tracked using bioimpedance spectroscopy: a deuterium oxide comparison. Clin Nutr 28(5):516–525

O'Brien C, Young AJ, Sawka MN, Koulmann N, Jimenez C, Regal D, Bolliet P, Launay JC, Savourey G, Melin B (2002) Bioelectrical impedance to estimate changes in hydration status. Int J Sports Med 23(5):361–366

Pateyjohns IR, Brinkworth GD, Buckley JD, Noakes M, Clifton PM (2006) Comparison of three bioelectrical impedance methods with DXA in overweight and obese men. Obesity 14(11):2064–2070

Peterson JT, Repovich WES, Parascand CR (2011) Accuracy of consumer grade bioelectrical impedance analysis devices compared to air displacement plethysmography. Int J Exerc Sci 4(3):176–184

Rodriguez-Sanchez N, Galloway SD (2015) Errors in dual energy x-ray absorptiometry estimation of body composition induced by hypohydration. Int J Sport Nutr Exerc Metab 25(1):60–68

Saunders MJ, Blevins JE, Broeder CE (1998) Effects of hydration changes on bioelectrical impedance in endurance trained individuals. Med Sci Sports Exerc 30(6):885–892

Sun G, French CR, Martin GR, Younghusband B, Green RC, Xie Y-g, Mathews M, Barron JR, Fitzpatrick DG, Gulliver W, Zhang H (2005) Comparison of multifrequency bioelectrical impedance analysis with dual energy X-ray absorptiometry for assessment of percentage body fat in a large, healthy population. Am J Clin Nutr 81(1):74–78

Svantesson U, Zander M, Klingberg S, Slinde F (2008) Body composition in male elite athletes, comparison of bioelectrical impedance spectroscopy with dual energy X-ray absorptiometry. J Negat Results Biomed 7(1):1

Tinsley GM, Morales E, Forsse JS, Grandjean PW (2017) Impact of acute dietary manipulations on DXA and BIA body composition estimates. Med Sci Sports Exerc 49(4):823–832

Utter AC, Lambeth PG (2010) Evaluation of multifrequency bioelectrical impedance analysis in assessing body composition of wrestlers. Med Sci Sports Exerc 42(2):361–367

Van Loan MD, Mayclin PL (1992) Use of multi-frequency bioelectrical impedance analysis for the estimation of extracellular fluid. Eur J Clin Nutr 46(2):117–124

van Marken Lichtenbelt W, Westerterp K, Wouters L (1994) Deuterium dilution as a method for determining total body water: effect of test protocol and sampling time. Br J Nutr 72(4):491–497

Wagner DR, Heyward VH (1999) Techniques of body composition assessment: a review of laboratory and field methods. Res Q Exerc Sport 70(2):135–149

Ward LC (2012) Segmental bioelectrical impedance analysis: an update. Curr Opin Clin Nutr Metab Care 15(5):424–429

Withers RT, LaForgia J, Pillans RK, Shipp NJ, Chatterton BE, Schultz CG, Leaney F (1998) Comparisons of two-, three-, and four-compartment models of body composition analysis in men and women. J Appl Physiol 85(1):238–245

Chapter 10
Non-imaging Method: Doubly Labelled Water

Elaine C. Rush

Abstract In athletes the doubly labelled water technique is a non-invasive way of measuring the rate of carbon dioxide production over a period of 7–14 days. It allows the determination of total body water and total energy expenditure. The technique requires an athlete to consume a stable isotope water known as doubly labelled water and then provide urine samples at several days post the initial ingestion. The most sensitive means of measuring the isotopes of deuterium and oxygen-18 in the samples is by isotope ratio mass spectroscopy.

Keywords Body composition • Total body water • Fat mass • Fat-free mass • Total body mass • Energy • Expenditure • Nutritional status • Input • Output • Cadaver Molecules • Deuterium • Oxygen-18

10.1 Why Do You Want to Conduct the Doubly Labelled Water Technique?

The accurate measurement of body composition and energy expenditure is a way of assessing nutritional status. Nutritional status is associated with performance, with physical and cognitive function and with body composition. A simplistic view of the control of body weight is that energy input should equal energy output; if not, then overall weight will change. In its simplest and most common form, body composition can be regarded as fat mass and fat-free mass, and when added together, they are the total body mass. By definition, and measurement on cadavers, the fat mass

E.C. Rush
Faculty of Health and Environmental Sciences, Auckland University of Technology, Private Bag 92006, Auckland 1142, New Zealand
e-mail: elaine.rush@aut.ac.nz

© Springer Nature Singapore Pte Ltd. 2018   117
P.A. Hume et al. (eds.), *Best Practice Protocols for Physique Assessment in Sport*,
https://doi.org/10.1007/978-981-10-5418-1_10

is all the molecules of the body that will dissolve in ether (i.e., fat mass contains no water). In adults and most animals, fat-free mass is 73.2% water—a universal constant (Ritz 2000); however, although this is the accepted constant, this may not be the case in athletes or obesity. If the total body water is known, fat-free mass can be calculated and the fat mass derived by subtraction.

10.1.1   Measuring Body Composition and Energy Expenditure in Athletes

The doubly labelled water technique is considered the "gold standard" for determining total body water and total energy expenditure. The main strength is that it can be used to determine energy requirements in the free-living, healthy state. Other measurement techniques such as heart rate monitoring, accelerometry, activity diaries and records and food intake measures are often compared to the doubly labelled water measures for validation. Detailed descriptions of the doubly labelled water technique and calculation may be found on the International Atomic Energy Agency website (https://humanhealth.iaea.org).

Total energy expenditure (the total energy expended each day) is composed of three main components: resting energy expenditure; the energy associated with the ingestion, digestion and assimilation of food (i.e., the thermic effect of food); and activity energy expenditure. The doubly labelled water technique does not allow measurement of the thermic effect of food and the resting energy expenditure.

10.1.1.1   Accuracy and Precision of the Doubly Labelled Water Technique

The accuracy of the doubly labelled water technique has been examined in a number of validation studies using whole body indirect calorimeters (Schoeller 1988; Schoeller et al. 1986b). A wide range of participants and conditions were represented in these studies. Included participants in these studies ranged from 43 adults to four premature infants and from 39 healthy individuals eating oral diets to five clinical populations receiving parenteral nutrition. The level of energy expenditure in two adult participants was over 35 MJ.day^{-1}. Percent error between the two methods was calculated relative to the reference value and in the two healthy adults did not exceed −2.5% ± 4.9% SD. The greatest range of error was in a study of five adults with a percentage error of 1.5% ± 7.6%.

Given the small sizes of these validation studies, the error is small and judged by Schoeller (1988) as generally valid. A consensus report (Prentice 1990) considered cross-validation data available in 1990. Eight more infants with a changing diet and 16 soldiers were added to the studies reviewed by Schoeller (ibid). Percent error was −8.7 ± 12.9 for the infants and +5.3 (SD not reported) for the soldiers. These two studies both had changing sources of water during the isotope elimination period. The consensus from these experts was that accuracy is in the order of 1–3% and precision 2–8%, with the Coward model using multi-point regression analysis of isotope elimination rates seeming to offer 2–3% better precision than the two-point method (Cole and Coward 1992). The major contribution of this report was that technical recommendations for the use of the doubly labelled water method in humans were made generally available.

Whilst analytical and sampling errors may be reduced, the variation due to physiological changes over a period of time cannot be assessed. Michael Goran's group (Goran et al. 1993; Goran et al. 1994) estimated that the experimental variability of the technique under controlled conditions was ±8.5% with a wide range of variability between participants. Over three separate 14-day assessments, this group also showed an intra-individual variation of ±10%, due to fluctuations in physical activity levels.

Perhaps the best test of the reliability of the analyses for the doubly labelled water technique was a double-blind study (Roberts et al. 1995) that looked at variation amongst 18 laboratories given the same samples to analyse from two participants. Continuous direct calorimetry measurements were performed over the same 10 days as the doubly labelled water sample collection. This study confirmed that the doubly labelled water technique can be accurate in comparison with calorimetry, but the between-laboratory coefficient of variation was 10.3%. If there is high analytical error, the multi-point method is less robust compared to the two-point method for the calculation of the dilution spaces.

10.2 What Is the Doubly Labelled Water Technique?

The doubly labelled water technique is a non-invasive way of measuring the rate of carbon dioxide production in free-living participants over a period of 7–14 days. The term doubly labelled water refers to water that contains higher concentrations of both deuterium and oxygen-18, which are stable isotopes (i.e., not radioactive). These isotopes of hydrogen and oxygen are naturally found in the human body and in water and other molecules that contain hydrogen and oxygen at very low concentrations. Enriched (higher than background concentration) doubly labelled water is consumed by drinking, and timed samples of body fluid (urine, blood or saliva) are taken both before and after consumption.

10.2.1 Isotopes

Isotopes of an element always contain the same number of protons, but the number of neutrons may vary. For example, oxygen-16 contains eight protons and eight neutrons, but the heavier isotope oxygen-18 contains eight protons and ten neutrons. The number of neutrons and protons added together gives the atomic weight of the atom—so there are ^{18}O, ^{17}O and ^{16}O. Similarly, an atom of hydrogen usually has no neutrons and just one proton (^1H), with an atomic weight of 1. However, an atom of deuterium has one proton and one neutron (^2H). There is an isotope of hydrogen, tritium (^3H), that contains two neutrons, but this atom is unstable (i.e., will break down releasing energy). Unstable isotopes are radioactive but are not involved in any way with the doubly labelled water technique. Other stable isotopes such as molecules labelled with carbon-13 or nitrogen-15 can be used as biological tracers and biomarkers of metabolism. The body is composed of many different elements, the most abundant are oxygen (O), carbon (C), nitrogen (N) and hydrogen (H), and smaller quantities of their stable isotopes (*see* Fig. 10.1).

10.2.2 Doubly Labelled Water

The doubly labelled water biomarker consists of a higher-than-normal concentration of the stable isotopes deuterium (^2H_2O) and oxygen-18 ($H_2{}^{18}O$) in the molecules of water. In nature, 15 in 100,000 atoms of hydrogen are deuterium (0.015%), and

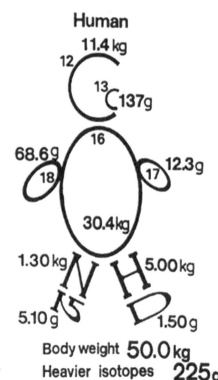

Fig. 10.1 Schematic of the isotopic composition of a 50 kg human. Sourced with permission from https://www.ncbi.nlm.nih.gov/pmc/articles/PMC3524304/ (Wada 2009)

2 in 1000 atoms of oxygen are oxygen-18 (0.20%). As a general guide, the dose for one measurement using doubly labelled water would be around 1 g/kg body weight of a mix of 10% oxygen-18 and 10% deuterium (i.e., ~70 g/person = 70 mL). This represents a relatively small but expensive quantity costing between $US10 and $US20 per gram.

10.2.3 Carbon Dioxide Production

The rate of carbon dioxide production is related to the total quantity of energy expended by the human body as work is done (i.e., energy present in the macronutrients carbohydrate, protein, fat and alcohol is used to pump ions across cell membranes, to propagate nervous impulses, to move actin over myosin and to synthesise [anabolism] new molecules from smaller ones). This change of energy from one form to another is eventually lost from the body as heat. The rate of energy transfer, or work, is also called total energy expenditure and has the units MJ or kcal/day.

10.2.4 Total Energy Expenditure and Subcomponents

When combined with a measurement of resting metabolic rate (e.g., by indirect calorimetry), the total energy expenditure/resting metabolic rate ratio can be calculated as a measure of the daily physical activity level. At perfect rest all day, the value would be 1.0 and, in extreme energy expenditure sports, may exceed a value of 2.0. The total volume of water in the body is also gained, as both the deuterium space and the oxygen-18 space are derived. If the hydration of the fat-free mass (~73.2% water in adults) is known, then fat-free mass may be calculated. In the two-compartment model of body composition, the balance of total body mass is fat mass, which by definition contains no water, so fat mass percent can be derived. In addition, the doubly labelled water technique provides a measure of water turnover measured in L/day.

10.2.5 Safety, Ethical and Cost Considerations

There are no health risks associated with stable isotopes. At the doses used for assessment of total energy expenditure and body composition, there is no evidence related to any long- or short-term effects of deuterium or oxygen-18 consumption in humans (Guo et al. 2000; Klein and Klein 1986; Jones and Leatherdale 1991; Katz 1960).

The production of water containing higher-than-normal concentrations of ^{2}H and ^{18}O may be by prolonged distillation, electrolysis or chemical exchange (Klein and Klein 1986). Water containing ^{18}O is used in biomedical research and diagnostic medicine including positron emission tomography, and since 1991, the price of labelled water has increased and remains relatively high.

The cost of analysis of body fluid samples for the concentrations of ^{2}H and ^{18}O must be considered. Analysis requires an isotope ratio mass spectrometer and expert technicians to operate. As a result, relatively few centres around the world have these facilities. If embarking on a doubly labelled water assessment, it is wise to first cost both the quantity of water for dosing and the number of analyses required as the total can be hundreds of dollars for each resulting sample.

10.3   How Do You Use the Doubly Labelled Water Technique for Athletes?

It is important to understand the principles, athlete presentations and procedural considerations when using doubly labelled water. The doubly labelled water method and standards are overseen by the International Atomic Energy Agency which undertakes training and sends experts to countries to assist and advise new operators.

10.3.1   Principles

The first principle of isotope dilution allows measurement of an unknown volume. If an unknown quantity of water has a known amount of a marker (a dose) introduced (e.g., dye, distinct molecules or stable isotopes) and the two are allowed to mix thoroughly, then the amount of water can be calculated as:

- Amount of marker in known volume $= N_D \times V_D = N_U \times V_U$ (i.e., $V_u = N_D \times V_D / N_U$), where N_D is the amount of the marker, V_D is the volume of the dose and N_U is the amount of the marker in the unknown volume V_U.

The resultant concentration can be measured ($N_U \times V_U$) from a sample of body fluid such as urine. An analogy would be to give a dose of 70 mg of a dye in a 1 mL volume. As body water in an adult may be between 15 and 50 L, this 1 mL is a very small fraction and does not need to be factored in. If the resultant concentration after equilibration was 2 mg/L, $V_u = 50$ mg/2 mg/L. Therefore, the unknown volume (V_u) = 25 L. Assuming that the hydration of fat-free mass is ~73.2%, fat-free mass is therefore 34.2 kg. If the body weight is 60.0 kg, then fat mass is 25.8 kg (60.0 minus 34.2), and fat percentage is 43%. This result is not typical for an athlete but a value commonly found in women.

However, the human body is not a water-tight vessel, and fluid is gained and lost all the time, transcutaneously via food and drink, through inhalation and exhalation and within urine, sweat and faeces. Overall, the volume of fluid in the body stays the same, but the total amount and concentration of biomarker will decrease as it leaves the body. Around 2 L of fluid is exchanged each day, but the amount of remaining biomarker changes. This rate of loss (k) is, for example, with deuterium, denoted as k_2 (*see* Fig. 10.2).

The second principle is the rate of isotope loss in relation to carbon dioxide production. The rate at which the isotopes of hydrogen and oxygen leave the body is related to the rate of production of carbon dioxide. This can be converted to a measure of the number of calories consumed over 14 days.

10.3.2   Measurement of the Isotopes in Body Fluid

The measurement of any biomarker requires that the amount of biomarker added is able to be detected with adequate precision so as to detect small changes. The most sensitive means of measuring the isotopes of deuterium and oxygen-18 is by isotope ratio mass spectroscopy. The use of this measurement technique reduces the amount of dose required but is expensive in terms of the equipment, sample processing and time for an expert to measure the samples. The isotope ratio mass spectroscopy instrumentation determines the ratio of numbers of heavy to light isotopes of a gaseous element. The sample must be processed first so that a gas is formed and then, when accelerated through an energy field, the isotopes will behave differently according to mass, which allows the ratio to be determined. Fourier transform infrared spectroscopy can be used to measure deuterium in saliva and plasma but requires much larger doses as it relies on the properties of the spectrum of infrared light

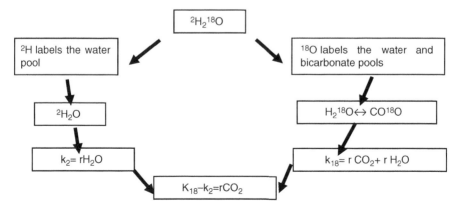

Fig. 10.2 The metabolic pathway of the doubly labelled water isotopes, ^2H deuterium and ^{18}O oxygen-18, in the water and bicarbonate spaces of the body. k rate of loss of isotope and r rate of loss of molecules of water and carbon dioxide

relative to a standard. Relatively few laboratories are able to undertake these analyses with the required precision and reliability; therefore, it is prudent to get quotes for both the labelled isotopes and the analysis, as well as information about the laboratory's quality control measures before undertaking or proposing a doubly labelled water study.

10.3.3 Procedural Considerations for a Doubly Labelled Water Study

The measurements necessary for calculation of total energy expenditure are shown in Table 10.1. A number of procedural questions need to be considered as part of the assessment:

- How much of the isotope is needed to dose each athlete?
- Whether to allow athletes to eat and drink before and after the isotope dose, the body mass of the athlete should be taken with their bladder empty.
- How to sample and time the collection of the urine sample.
- Multi-point or two-point sampling of urine for the exponential decay of the isotopes.
- The use of deuterium or oxygen-18 dilution spaces for the determination of total body water and fatness. The concentrations of deuterium and oxygen-18 in the dose diluted ~500× accurately (i.e., weighed or pipetted) in water. The water used to dilute the dose needs to be analysed for deuterium and oxygen-18. Ideally

Table 10.1 Measurements necessary for calculation of total energy expenditure

Measurement	Unit	Deuterium δ	Oxygen 18 δ
Athlete body mass[a]	70.4 kg		
Mass of dose given[a]	71.1347 g		
Mass of dose diluted[a]	0.1576 g		
Amount of tap water used to dilute dose[a]	55.299 g	−37.0	−8.82
Diluted dose[a]		1444.0	146.23
Baseline urine[a]	δ	−11.0	−3.29
Days			
Time of each sample	0.154	882.6	95.56
Either 5 h or 1 day[a]	0.189	883.0	92.18
	2.033	796.1	76.39
	4.954	692.3	61.41
	6.960	608.7	50.51
End of period of interest[a]	14.049	385.0	25.52
Food quotient	Ratio, e.g., 0.82		

Example values and precision of measurement required are in italics
[a]Measurements required if only two-point determination to be made

only one large mixture of deuterium and oxygen-18 is prepared, and therefore this diluted dose is to be measured only once and the values used for all athletes.

- The reliability of the doubly labelled water technique.

10.3.4 Dosing

A pre-dose body fluid sample must be collected for baseline measurements. The dose given is determined by the body size, the size of the pool of body water (73.2% of fat-free mass), the level of physical activity and the duration in days of the measurement. It is important to have a sufficient dose so that, on the final day of sampling, the enrichment of the isotopes in body fluid can be measured precisely and is sufficiently greater than the baseline value. As a guide, 0.12 g.kg^{-1} body water of 99 atom% deuterium-labelled water and 1.8 g.kg^{-1} body water of 10 atom% oxygen-18 water are the standard dose consumed. A subsample of the dose which is accurately diluted 500 times with water is then stored with the urine samples in the same type of container. All samples must be stored in tightly sealed containers. They do not need to be frozen, but if they are, ensure that there is sufficient head space so that as the frozen sample expands, the container is not ruptured.

The dose is weighed (in gram to four decimal places) with a high precision balance. Then the athlete washes the dose down with two 50 mL aliquots of tap water in the same cup which had contained the weighed isotope dose. If any dose is lost, this must be accounted for and should be collected on tissues and placed in a sealed container. Storage of the dose in a capped and sealed glass bottle and provision of a straw for drinking are recommended to reduce loss of the dose by evaporation or spillage. If a straw is used, this must not be removed from the bottle until the entire dose plus rinses are consumed.

Elite athletes are likely to have higher water content (due to less fat mass) and to have higher water turnover due to sweating and increased energy expenditure than less active athletes. Therefore, the dose for total energy expenditure should be determined carefully to ensure that at the end of the measurement period, the enrichment in body fluids is above the background/baseline values. Sampling at more points may be necessary to ensure the slope of the line is valid. If athletes change location during the measurement period, background isotope concentration may change—it is best to undertake tests within the same environment.

It is worthwhile to collect more samples of urine that will be analysed to protect against sample loss. After ingestion of the dose, two or three bladder evacuations may be required over a period of up to 6 h before a timed urine sample that is equilibrated with all the body water may be obtained. Labelling of all sample pots with athlete name, date and time of voiding is essential.

10.3.5   Eating and Drinking Before and After the Isotope Dose

The technical recommendations for use of doubly labelled water in humans (Prentice 1990) require that participants should be fasted at least 4 h before administration of the dose. The recommendations state that whilst earlier protocols insisted that the participant remains fasted during the 3–6 h equilibration period, recent studies have often permitted moderate food and fluid intake. This question has been examined in a number of studies (Calazel et al. 1993; Schoeller et al. 1986a; Streat et al. 1985) which have shown that withholding of parenteral nutrition or prolonged fasting and feeding before and after the isotope dosing is not necessary in doubly labelled water studies. In rats the measurement of total body water using isotopic dilution (tritium) is independent of the flux of water through the rat (Brigant et al. 1993). Albeit that tritium is not present in the drinking water, whilst the stable isotopes of deuterium and oxygen-18 are, the withholding of fluid and food partially negates the free-living advantage of the technique. As the calculation of the isotope spaces in the multi-point method is affected by the other sampling points, not just the equilibration phase, it seems sensible that at all samples are obtained under the same conditions (i.e., in the normal fed and hydrated state).

Another important consideration to gain the cooperation of athletes is not to induce discomfort by fasting any longer than necessary. Therefore, the baseline sample can be collected before the athlete comes into the laboratory, which could be the first urination of the day. At this time a larger sample (more than 100 mL) could be collected, and then there is not the need to pass a urine sample before the dose can be consumed.

10.3.6   Collection and Timing of Urine Samples Including Baseline/Background Isotope Concentrations

Urine is usually chosen as the physiological fluid to be sampled because of its relative ease of collection compared with saliva and plasma. Any uncertainty around the cost and time commitment for analysis of samples means that an initial decision whether to use the two-point or multi-point method of analysis may be deferred and samples collected to fit both sampling regimes. Equilibration of the dose with total body water and urine samples has been shown to take between 4 and 5 h (Matthews and Gilker 1995), though this can be longer in the elderly (Blanc et al. 2002). For the two-point method, a partial correction for dose lost before equilibration involves measuring the concentration and volume of the dose in urine formed before equilibration. For this reason, samples may be collected at 2 and 3 h after dosing, so that the loss can be calculated, and then two further samples at 4 and 5 h can be collected to measure the plateau/equilibrium concentration. Further samples of urine can be collected on days 2, 5, 7 and 14.

Second void urine, rather than a 24 h composite of the whole day's urine, gives the lowest variation in the determination of total energy expenditure (Seale et al. 1989). This indicates that samples close to isotopic equilibrium, with the entire body water pool at the time of collection, offer the best results. Therefore, the time for each sample could be calculated as the midpoint of the time between the first emptying of the bladder in the morning and the time of the second emptying of the bladder for the day when the urine sample was collected. Always store duplicates of samples in glass bottles sealed securely with lined caps—they may be frozen, but be sure there is plenty of headspace as if bungs are used, they may dislodge during defrosting.

Whilst stable isotopes do not change if they change physical phase (i.e., as liquid to gas or solid to liquid), the concentration of the isotopes in each phase will be different. This is particularly important when storing the biomarker or samples to be analysed. If the container is not sealed, then the lighter isotopes will evaporate more quickly, and the liquid left will have a higher concentration than that needed to be measured.

10.3.7   How Many Sampling Points for Calculation of Energy Expenditure?

Combined precision and accuracy of the multi-point method has been demonstrated to be better than the two-point method when compared to whole body calorimetry. The coefficient of variation of the multi-point method has been shown to be 3.6% compared with 5.4% for the two-point method (Cole and Coward 1992). The two-point method is cheaper as it requires less sample collection, handling and mass spectrometric analysis, but it is less robust to random error in isotope enrichments. However, the multi-point method is more robust to random errors and does allow an individual estimate of precision. But it does involve more sample collection and analysis and may be affected by systematic variations that produce curvature in the exponential decay lines. If the washout of the isotope from the body is not a logarithm-transformed straight line, the dilution space estimated may be incorrect.

10.3.8   Differences in Dilution Spaces: Fractionation

A further consideration related to fractionation is that the heavier isotopes, as part of biological molecules, may react differently in the metabolic pathways, and an unequal transfer between molecules can occur. In other words, when a molecule undergoes a change of physical state, medium or chemical reaction, the heavier isotopic molecules will tend to remain in the state of lower energy. This phenomenon needs to be taken into account when determining the flux rates of water and carbon dioxide.

The measurement of total body water with oxygen-18 gives smaller values than the deuterium dilution volume. The greater deuterium space is because there is an exchange of the deuterium with the labile hydrogen of protein and other body molecules (Schoeller et al. 1980). The assumption that the oxygen-18 space is 1.01 times greater than total body water is generally accepted and applied in the literature. Technically, oxygen-18 may be measured with more precision and accuracy than deuterium, particularly if the zinc method is used to measure deuterium (Ritz et al. 1994). This means that the use of the oxygen-18 space to calculate body composition could be a better choice. The calculated ratio of the dilution spaces is a procedural check as part of the calculation of the carbon dioxide output—the ratio should be between 1.03 and 1.07.

10.4 How Do You Report the Doubly Labelled Water Technique Data to Athletes and Coaches?

The values for total body water, fat-free mass and fat mass are calculated and can be reported back to the athlete and coach.

10.5 Summary

The use of doubly labelled water (commonly known as deuterium dilution) amongst athletic populations is uncommon due to the technical nature, cost and lack of availability of the assessment. The reliability of the technique is high. Regional body assessment is not possible, rather total body water, fat-free mass and fat mass are calculated. The time commitment for the athletes is approximately 6 h given the repeat samples required.

References

Blanc S, Colligan AS, Trabulsi J, Harris T, Everhart JE, Bauer D, Schoeller DA (2002) Influence of delayed isotopic equilibration in urine on the accuracy of the (2)H(2)(18)O method in the elderly. J Appl Physiol (1985) 92(3):1036–1044

Brigant L, Rozen R, Apfelbaum M (1993) Tritium dilution space measurement is not modified by a doubling in fluid intake. J Appl Physiol 75:412–415

Calazel CM, Young VR, Evans WJ, Roberts SB (1993) Effect of fasting and feeding on measurement of carbon dioxide production using doubly labeled water. J Appl Physiol 74(4):1824–1829

Cole TJ, Coward WA (1992) Precision and accuracy of doubly labeled water energy expenditure by multipoint and two point methods. Am J Physiol 263:E965–E973

Goran MI, Beer WH, Wolfe RR, Poehlman ET, Young VR (1993) Variation in total energy expenditure in young healthy free-living men. Metabolism 42(4):487–496

Goran MI, Poehlman ET, Danforth E (1994) Experimental reliability of the doubly labeled water technique. Am J Physiol 266(3 Pt 1):E510–E515

Guo ZK, Cella LK, Baum C, Ravussin E, Schoeller DA (2000) De novo lipogenesis in adipose tissue of lean and obese women: application of deuterated water and isotope ratio mass spectrometry. Int J Obes Relat Metab Disord 24(7):932–937

Jones PJ, Leatherdale ST (1991) Stable isotopes in clinical research: safety reaffirmed. Clin Sci 80(4):277–280

Katz JJ (1960) The biology of heavy water. What happens to experimental organisms that have been raised on water in which the hydrogen is not the common isotope of mass one but the heavy isotope of mass two? Sci Am 203:106–116

Klein PD, Klein ER (1986) Stable isotopes: origins and safety. J Clin Pharmacol 26(6):378–382

Matthews DE, Gilker CD (1995) Impact of 2H and 18O pool size determinations on the calculation of total energy expenditure. Obes Res 3(Suppl 1):21–29

Prentice AM (ed) (1990) International Dietary Energy Consultancy Group. The doubly-labeled water method for measuring energy expenditure: Technical recommendations for use in humans. (A consensus report by the IDECG working group). 1990 edn. Nutritional and Health-Related Environmental Studies International Atomic Energy Agency, Vienna, Austria

Ritz P (2000) Body water spaces and cellular hydration during healthy aging. Ann N Y Acad Sci 904:474–483

Ritz P, Johnson PG, Coward WA (1994) Measurements of 2H and 18O in body water: analytical considerations and physiological implications. Br J Nutr 72:3–12

Roberts SB, Dietz W, Sharp T, Dallal GE, Hill JO (1995) Multiple laboratory comparison of the doubly labelled water technique. Obes Res 3(Suppl1):3–13

Schoeller DA (1988) Measurement of energy expenditure in free-living humans by using doubly labeled water. J Nutr 118:1278–1289

Schoeller DA, Leitch CA, Brown C (1986a) Doubly labelled water method: in vivo oxygen and hydrogen isotope fractionation. Am J Physiol 251(20):R1137–R1143

Schoeller DA, Ravussin E, Schutz Y, Acheson KJ, Baertschi P, Jequier E (1986b) Energy expenditure by doubly labeled water: validation in humans and proposed calculation. Am J Physiol 250(19):R823–R830

Schoeller DA, van Santen E, Peterson DW, Dietz W, Jaspan J, Klein PD (1980) Total body water measurement in humans with 18O and 2H labeled water. Am J Clin Nutr 33:2686–2693

Seale J, Miles C, Bodwell CE (1989) Sensitivity of methods for calculating energy expenditure by use of doubly labeled water. J Appl Physiol 66(2):644–653

Streat SJ, Beddoe AH, Hill GL (1985) Measurement of total body water in intensive care patients with fluid overload. Metabolism 34(7):688–694

Wada E (2009) Stable δ15N and δ13C isotope ratios in aquatic ecosystems. Proc Jpn Acad Ser B Phys Biol Sci 85(3):98–107

Chapter 11
Imaging Method: Ultrasound

Timothy R. Ackland and Wolfram Müller

Abstract The ultrasound technique for measurement of subcutaneous adipose tissue and embedded fibrous structures employs image capture from any standard brightness mode ultrasound machine followed by an image analysis procedure. The technique avoids compression of the tissues and movement that occurs when using skinfold calipers. The ultrasound method only samples the subcutaneous adipose tissue and does not measure the fat stored in deeper depots.

Keywords Ultrasound • Subcutaneous • Adipose • Tissue • Fibrous structures Image capture • Brightness mode • Image analysis • Compression • Tissue • Standard locations

11.1 Why Measure Physique Using This Technique?

Subcutaneous adipose tissue (SAT) measurement using skinfolds has a long tradition, but the accuracy obtained using this technique is limited because skin and subcutaneous adipose tissue are measured together in a compressed state without considering the compressibility and viscous-elastic behaviour at the individual measurement sites (Ackland et al. 2012; Müller et al. 2013a, 2016). In the past 3 years, a novel ultrasound technique for measurement of subcutaneous adipose tissue and

T.R. Ackland (✉)
School of Sport Science, Exercise and Health, The University of Western Australia,
Crawley, WA 6009, Australia
e-mail: tim.ackland@uwa.edu.au

W. Müller
Institute of Biophysics, Medical University of Graz, Harrachgasse 21, A-8010 Graz, Austria
e-mail: wolfram.mueller@medunigraz.at

© Springer Nature Singapore Pte Ltd. 2018   131
P.A. Hume et al. (eds.), *Best Practice Protocols for Physique Assessment in Sport*,
https://doi.org/10.1007/978-981-10-5418-1_11

embedded fibrous structures has been introduced (Müller et al. 2013a, 2013b). This technique employs image capture from any standard B-mode (brightness mode) ultrasound machine followed by an image analysis procedure and avoids compression of the tissues and movement that occurs when using skinfold calipers. The method has little participant involvement, does not require ionising radiation and can be applied to children, adolescents and adults of varying size and levels of body composition (Störchle et al. 2016). With the advent of portable ultrasound devices, this technique can be used in field and laboratory environments.

Several manufacturers distribute A-mode US equipment that employ unknown algorithms for estimating subcutaneous adipose tissue. Many assumptions must be adopted and serious errors can be made using A-mode US models because fibrous structures are embedded in the subcutaneous adipose tissue and the resulting complex image structures cannot be interpreted correctly by an automatic processing algorithm.

B-mode images are generated by sequences of US beams that are sent into the tissue to create an image in which the brightness of the screen corresponds to the echo intensity in the plane of the scan. The differences in acoustic impedance are quite large between skin and subcutaneous adipose tissue and between subcutaneous adipose tissue and muscle fascia; therefore, the transition from subcutaneous adipose tissue to adjacent tissues can usually be seen clearly when US imaging parameters are chosen properly. The captured image is then analysed via proprietary software (Fat Analysis Tool FAT 3.3, Rotosport, Graz, Austria; http://rotosport.com) to provide mean (±SD) subcutaneous adipose tissue thickness for the ultrasound beams contained within the specified region of interest (ROI).

Ultrasound measurements of subcutaneous adipose tissue in excised pig tissue have been compared with direct vernier caliper measurements (Horn and Müller 2010). For this comparison, a linear probe (7.5 MHz) was positioned with its centre at a marked position on the skin of the excised tissue, and US measurement of subcutaneous adipose tissue thickness was made without compression, due to a thick layer of gel. Subcutaneous adipose tissue thickness was evaluated in the vicinity of the centre of the US image. The authors reported the standard error of estimate (SEE) was 0.21 mm, and the slope of the regression line was 0.98 when conventional sound speed of $c = 1540$ ms^{-1} was used. Using a lower speed of sound propagation in subcutaneous adipose tissue (1510 ms^{-1}) for the distance calculation resulted in the best fit for these data (slope of 1.00).

Inter-tester reliability data for a sample of 19 female athletes measured by three observers has been reported (Müller et al. 2013b). The observers applied diagnostic B-mode US combined with the evaluation software for subcutaneous adipose tissue measurements at eight ISAK skinfold sites. Subcutaneous adipose tissue thickness sums at eight sites measured with fibrous structures included (D_{INCL}) resulted in a SEE = 0.60 mm, $R^2 = 0.98$ ($p < 0.001$), limit of agreement LOA = 1.18, ICC = 0.968 [0.957−0.977]. Similar values were found when fibrous structures were excluded (D_{EXCL}): SEE = 0.68 mm, $R^2 = 0.97$ ($p < 0.001$).

In subsequent research it was found that several ISAK sites are not suited for US measurements because of complex structures surrounding the subcutaneous adipose tissue and because of thickness changes of the subcutaneous adipose tissue layer in the vicinity of the centre of the site. Therefore, a new set of sites that are well suited for B-mode ultrasound measurements of subcutaneous adipose tissue patterning had to be developed, and both landmarking and ultrasound measurement procedures required standardising in order to obtain maximum accuracy and reliability. The eight standard sites were chosen to represent trunk (three sites), arms (two) and legs (three) for subcutaneous adipose tissue patterning studies. This standardised approach is described in a recent publication (Müller et al., 2016) which also contains interobserver results (three observers measured 12 athletes; for D_{INCL}, SEE = 0.55, R^2 = 0.998 ($p < 0.01$), ICC = 0.998; for D_{EXCL}, SEE = 0.66, R^2 = 0.997 ($p < 0.01$), ICC = 0.996).

Intra-tester measurements (three measurement series in each person) performed in 38 untrained, normal weight, overweight, and obese persons (body mass indices ranged from 18.5 to 40.3 kgm^{-2}; 19 men and 19 women) resulted in SEE = 1.1 mm for thickness sums D_{INCL}, 95% of measurement sums were within ±2.2 mm and Spearman's rank correlation coefficient ρ was 0.999 ($p < 0.01$). For D_{EXCL}, SEE was 1.5 mm, 95% of measurement sums were within ±3.2 mm and ρ was 0.997 ($p < 0.01$). In the normal weight subgroup, 95% of D_{INCL} deviations were below 1.4 mm, and 95% of D_{EXCL} deviations were below 1.6 mm. In the overweight/obese subgroup, 95% of D_{INCL} deviations were below 2.9 mm and below 3.8 mm for D_{EXCL}. Relative deviations (in percent of the subcutaneous adipose tissue thickness) were smaller in the overweight/obese group (where D ranged from 53 to 245 mm; median deviation of the subcutaneous adipose tissue thickness sum was 0.5% for D_{INCL} and 0.9% for D_{EXCL}) when compared to the normal weight group (where D ranged from 12 to 77 mm; median deviation was 1.1% for both D_{INCL} and D_{EXCL}). This is not surprising because the biologically given tissue border detection errors (Müller et al. 2016) play a larger role for relative errors in lean persons where the sum of fat thicknesses is small.

This body composition method samples the subcutaneous adipose tissue depots of the body with measurement sites at eight standard locations on the right side of the body. These standard sites are approached from distinct anatomical structures, then located relative to stature of the individual and finally marked with precision. Additional sites can be measured for any specific purpose; however, the standard eight sites should be measured as a minimum to account for interindividual variation in subcutaneous adipose tissue deposition. With appropriate training and experience, the US technique is very accurate, reliable and time-efficient. Individual participants can be marked, images captured and data analysed by a single operator within 20 min.

11.2   What Is This Technique and Technology?

The FAT software will adapt to any good-quality B-mode US image obtained with a linear transducer (probe). In slim people, high frequencies ranging from about 10 to 20 MHz should be used to maximise the accuracy of tissue border detection, and in overweight or obese groups, lower frequencies ranging from about 5 to 10 MHz will be necessary to penetrate the thick subcutaneous adipose tissue layers. Scan parameters (depth, frequency, focus, gain and the depth-gain compensation setting) should be adjusted to optimise all relevant tissue boundaries within the image. With a thick (3–5 mm) layer of gel applied, the centre of the probe is held perpendicular to the skin surface, directly over the marked site and without compressing the skin.

It is strongly recommended to participate in a training program to reach the high accuracy and reliability level obtainable with this standardised US technique. Details of training courses (generally 2–3 days) and costs can be found at http://rotosport.com or on the homepage of the International Association for Sciences in Medicine and Sports (www.iasms.org).

11.3   How Do You Use the Selected Technique for Your Athlete?

All participants must be marked prior to measurement. The measurement sites, marked on the right side with the participant either standing or sitting according to the standard protocol, are shown in Fig. 11.1. An abbreviated description of these site locations is given below, whereas the full description is provided in Müller et al. (2016):

- Upper abdomen (UA)—0.02 h (2% of height) superior and lateral to the centre of the umbilicus
- Lower abdomen (LA)—0.02 h inferior and lateral to the centre of the umbilicus
- Erector spinae (ES)—0.14 h superior to the surface of a table on which the participant is seated and 0.02 h lateral to the most adjacent lumbar spinous process
- Distal triceps (DT)—0.05 h superior to a supporting surface with the participant's forearm (mid-prone position) resting on that surface and on the most posterior aspect of the arm
- Brachioradialis (BR)—0.02 h distally from the biceps brachii tendon with the forearm in the mid-prone position and flexed to 90° and on the most superior aspect of the tensed brachioradialis muscle
- Lateral thigh (LT)—the midpoint of the sagittal thigh diameter at the level of the gluteal fold
- Front thigh (FT)—0.14 h proximally from the most anterior aspect of the patella with the foot placed on an anthropometry box, the thigh horizontal and the patella touching a wall in front. Mark the most anterior aspect of the thigh at this level
- Medial calf (MC)—0.18 h superior to an anthropometry box with the thigh horizontal, leg vertical and right foot positioned on the box. Mark the most medial aspect of the calf at this level. In individuals or ethnic groups with exceptionally long legs, 0.20 h should be used to keep the site at the muscle (and not below it)

These sites were finalised after 2 years of testing, beginning with the ISAK skinfold sites and then moving to more appropriate positions. The final eight sites can

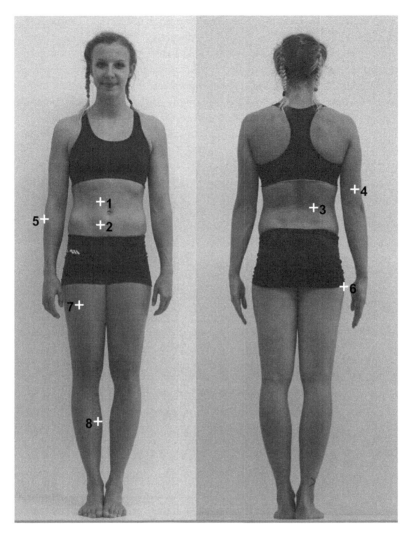

Fig. 11.1 The eight standard ultrasound measurement sites. 1, upper abdomen (UA); 2, lower abdomen (LA); 3, erector spinae (ES); 4, distal triceps (DT); 5, brachioradialis (BR); 6, lateral thigh (LT); 7, front thigh (FT); 8, medial calf (MC)

be located easily and reproducibly, with only a minimum knowledge of human anatomy, and allow for clear images of the important tissues in almost all cases. Importantly, these measurement sites generally have simple underlying anatomy structures that are relatively easy to interpret and a subcutaneous adipose tissue layer that does not vary greatly in thickness within the image.

With the room light dimmed and with the participant lying on a plinth (in supine, prone or side-lying depending on the site being imaged), the operator places the centre of the linear probe over the marked site to capture an US image. The probe is held perpendicular to the skin surface in a manner that does not compress the skin; the thick layer of gel helps to achieve this important criterion and should be visible as a dark black layer above the dermis. This image must include a scale and the following identifiable layers: gel, dermis, subcutaneous adipose tissue, fascia and part of the muscle. The subcutaneous adipose tissue borders should be clear to the investigator—appearing dark in the image compared to the brighter skin above and the muscle fascia below the subcutaneous adipose tissue. The image should be dark within the subcutaneous adipose tissue layer except for any embedded fibrous structures (see Fig. 11.2).

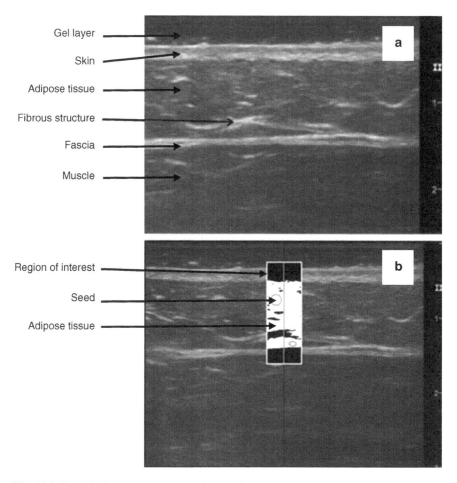

Fig. 11.2 Typical ultrasound image showing the important layers to be identified for analysis (panel **a**) and the region of interest overlaying this image during the analysis process (panel **b**). The light section of the region of interest indicates the subcutaneous adipose tissue region excluding fibrous structures and two seeds to define the subcutaneous adipose tissue

With experience, the operator will be able to manipulate the ultrasound machine parameters to accommodate participants of varying size and body composition. For example, lean athletes have thin subcutaneous adipose tissue layers, so the image depth should be adjusted to maximise the important structures within the image, the frequency increased for better clarity, focal depths arranged to advantage and the gain set to provide optimal contrast.

Image analysis should also be performed in a dimmed room. Once the image scale has been calibrated, the operator creates a region of interest around the centre (i.e., over the landmarked site) which incorporates some of the gel layer down into the muscle layer. Placement of seeds to identify the subcutaneous adipose tissue enables the software to distinguish adipose tissue from other structures. Note in Fig. 11.2 (panel b), two seeds have been placed in the subcutaneous adipose tissue (which is displaying white in the region of interest), while the fibrous structures within the subcutaneous adipose tissue plus all other layers are coloured black.

11.4   What Is the Technique Used to Measure?

The semiautomated analysis software (Fat Analysis Tool FAT 3.3, Rotosport, Graz, Austria) outputs a mean (±SD) subcutaneous adipose tissue thickness value for each measurement site, with embedded tissue structures both included and excluded from the score. It remains the prerogative of the coach or sport scientist as to which value to use or monitor depending on the fundamental research question or practical application.

With practice, and using the full functionality of the FAT 3.3 software, a set of eight images can be measured and analysed in 10–15 min. Once completed, a standardised report is then generated for the participant which includes the ultrasound images, the evaluated images, and all resulting data, including a basic set of anthropometric values and indices.

11.5   How Do You Report the Data to Your Athlete and Coach?

As with the ISAK approach to reporting skinfold values, we favour reporting of a sum of eight subcutaneous adipose tissue values for general monitoring purposes. This approach helps to accommodate interindividual variability in fat deposition. Since this technique has only been in existence for a short time, one of the challenges is to publish normative data for comparison purposes. However, this can also be seen as an advantage, since the normative data (based on currently available data) displayed in Table 11.1 has been gathered using a single,

Table 11.1 Preliminary normative data for the subcutaneous adipose tissue sum of eight sites

Sum of SAT (mm)	Valuation	Comment
Competitive athletes: Female		
Below 25	Extremely low	Medical surveillance recommended
25–35	Very low	Surveillance recommended
35–50	Low	Desirable range
50–70		Noticeable ballast weight
Above 70		Considerable ballast weight
Competitive athletes: Male		
Below 12	Extremely low	Medical surveillance recommended
12–20	Very low	Surveillance recommended
20–30	Low	Desirable range
30–50		Noticeable ballast weight
Above 50		Considerable ballast weight
General public: Female		
Below 25	Extremely low	Medical surveillance strongly recommended
25–35	Very low	Medical surveillance recommended
35–80	Low	Desirable range
80–110		Noticeable ballast weight
110–140		Considerable ballast weight
140–180	High	Medical surveillance recommended
Above 180	Very high	Medical surveillance strongly recommended
General public: Male		
Below 12	Extremely low	Medical surveillance strongly recommended
12–20	Very low	Medical surveillance recommended
20–60	Low	Desirable range
60–100		Noticeable ballast weight
100–130		Considerable ballast weight
130–180	High	Medical surveillance recommended
Above 180	Very high	Medical surveillance strongly recommended

SAT subcutaneous adipose tissue

standardised measurement protocol—this cannot be said for the mass of published data on skinfolds.

Serial monitoring of subcutaneous adipose tissue patterning may also be important in certain applications. To facilitate this, the FAT software reports, in graphic form, the individual site thicknesses (see Fig. 11.3). In this example of a female swimmer (height 1.830 m, mass 67.0 kg, BMI 20.0 kgm^{-2}), the sum of subcutaneous adipose tissue thicknesses D_{INCL} was 60.6 mm, and D_{EXCL} was 54.2 mm. Sites: UA, upper abdomen; LA, lower abdomen; ES, erector spinae; DT, distal triceps; BR, brachioradialis; LT, lateral thigh; FT, front thigh; MC, medial calf.

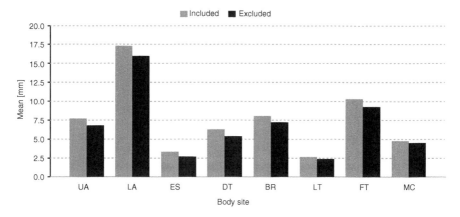

Fig. 11.3 The pattern of subcutaneous adipose tissue thickness across eight sites, with embedded structures both excluded and included

11.6   Limitations

This methodology has some inherent limitations. As with skinfolds, the ultrasound method only samples the subcutaneous adipose tissue and does not measure the fat stored in deeper depots. There are some equipment costs, but these are substantially less than for other imaging devices (like magnetic resonance imaging or computed tomography) or other methods to determine body fat (like dual energy X-ray absorptiometry or Bod Pod). Since this is a novel measurement technique, it will take some time to build a comprehensive pool of normative data.

11.7   Examples of Ultrasound Measurement of Subcutaneous Adipose Tissue

The advantages of using a semiautomated analysis tool can be illustrated with the following examples. Depending on the quality of, and anatomical structures contained within, the captured US image, operators may be called upon to vary the assessment parameters so as to minimise analysis errors.

The existence of Camper's fascia is common within the subcutaneous adipose tissue at the abdominal sites (see Fig. 11.4, panel a). When present, this thick band of fascia can occur in any part of the subcutaneous adipose tissue and can extend across the full width of the US image. Interrogation of the tissue below this fascia layer by an experienced operator reveals it to be part of adipose tissue rather than muscle. The muscle fascia and muscle tissue beneath can be clearly identified at the bottom of this image, and the region of interest for analysis extends into this muscle layer. Such intermediate fibrous structures can also occur at other sites, particularly at the front thigh, where there is quite often an intermediate structure (which may be the reason for problems taking skinfolds there).

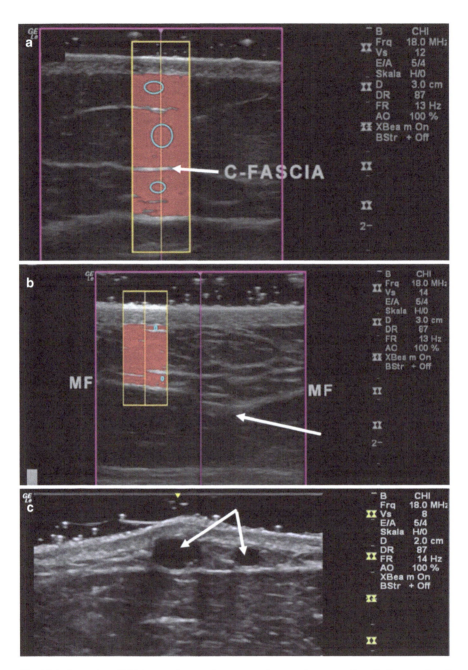

Fig. 11.4 Examples of US images that require operator intervention to avoid analysis errors Panel **a**, embedded structure (Camper's fascia); panel **b**, tendinous inscription of the rectus abdominis; panel **c**, blood vessels located within the SAT

Figure 11.4 (panel b) shows an image taken at the upper abdomen site. The muscle layer is that of rectus abdominis, and there is a tendinous inscription (or intersection) in the central portion of the image which narrows the muscle fibres and, consequently, increases the adipose tissue thickness at that specific location. The region of interest for analysis has been moved to the left of the image so as to avoid this central location in this particular case (that can occur at the upper abdomen site only).

The example of a thin subcutaneous adipose tissue layer shown in Fig. 11.4 (panel c) contains two peripheral blood vessels. Such blood vessels can sometimes be seen at the brachioradialis site. Clearly, these anatomical structures must be avoided during analysis, so the operator would either move the region of interest to one side of the image or capture another US image slightly away from the marked site.

11.8 Summary

The ultrasound technique for measurement of subcutaneous adipose tissue and embedded fibrous structures employs image capture from any standard brightness mode ultrasound machine followed by a semi-automatic image analysis procedure. No other measurement method is capable of measuring subcutaneous adipose tissue at the accuracy and reliability levels obtainable with this standardised ultrasound technique. An international certification for training is available.

References

Ackland TR, Lohman TG, Sundgot-Borgen J, Maughan RJ, Meyer NL, Stewart AD, Müller W (2012) Current status of body composition assessment in sport. Sports Med 42(3):227–240

Horn M, Müller W (2010) Towards an accurate determination of subcutaneous adipose tissue by means of ultrasound. In: 6th World Congress of Biomechanics, Singapore. pp. abstract WCB-A01448–02611

Müller W, Horn M, Fürhapter-Rieger A, Kainz P, Kröpfl J, Ahammer H (2013a) Body composition in sport: a comparison of a novel ultrasound imaging technique to measure subcutaneous fat tissue compared with skinfold measurement. Br J Sports Med 47:1028–1035

Müller W, Horn M, Fürhapter-Rieger A, Kröpfl J, Ackland T, Lohman T, Maughan R, Meyer N, Sundgot-Borgen J, Stewart A, Kainz P, Ahammer H (2013b) Body composition in sport: inter-observer reliability of a novel ultrasound measure of subcutaneous fat. Br J Sports Med 47:1036–1043

Müller W, Lohman TG, Stewart AD, Maughan RJ, Meyer NL, Sardinha LB, Kirihennedige N, Reguant-Closa A, Risoul-Salas V, Sundgot-Borgen J, Ahammer H, Anderhuber F, Fürhapter-Rieger A, Kainz P, Materna W, Pilsl U, Pirstinger W, Ackland TR (2016) Subcutaneous fat patterning in athletes: selection of appropriate sites and standardisation of a novel ultrasound measurement technique: ad hoc working group on body composition, health and performance, under the auspices of the IOC medical commission. Br J Sports Med 50:45–54

Störchle P, Müller W, Sengeis M, Ahammer H, Fürhapter-Rieger A, Bachl N, Lackner S, Mörkl S, Wallner-Liebmann S (2016) Standardised ultrasound measurement of subcutaneous fat patterning: high reliability and accuracy in groups ranging from lean to obese. Ultrasound Med Biol 43(2):427–438. https://doi.org/10.1016/j.ultrasmedbio.2016.09.014

Chapter 12
Imaging Method: Computed Tomography and Magnetic Resonance Imaging

Kristen L. MacKenzie-Shalders

Abstract Magnetic resonance imaging and computed tomography are imaging techniques that provide a highly accurate measure of human body composition at the tissue-organ level. Computed tomography works through measuring the attenuation of X-rays through body tissues, whereas magnetic resonance imaging uses a strong magnetic field to align positively charged protons in the body's tissues which are digitised to provide a greyscale image. Magnetic resonance imaging is emerging as a safe method of choice over computed tomography as it does not expose participants to radiation. Due to constraints in cost and availability, the techniques are generally only used for athletes as part of a research project or for clinical purposes.

Keywords Magnetic resonance imaging • Computed tomography • Imaging techniques • Accurate • Body composition organ • X-rays • Body tissues • Magnetic field • Radiation • Clinical

12.1 Introduction

Human body composition at the tissue-organ level can be assessed via magnetic resonance imaging and computed tomography imaging techniques. Computed tomography works through measuring the attenuation of X-rays through body tissues, whereas magnetic resonance imaging uses a strong magnetic field to align positively charged protons in the body's tissues which are digitised to provide a

K.L. MacKenzie-Shalders
Faculty of Health Sciences and Medicine, Bond Institute of Health and Sport,
Bond University, Robina, QLD 4226, Australia
e-mail: kmackenz@bond.edu.au

© Springer Nature Singapore Pte Ltd. 2018   143
P.A. Hume et al. (eds.), *Best Practice Protocols for Physique Assessment in Sport*,
https://doi.org/10.1007/978-981-10-5418-1_12

greyscale image. Full body composition assessment by magnetic resonance imaging or computed tomography can take ~30 min in total depending on which machine and technique are used (Ross et al. 2000). Single or multiple scans which take ~25 s have been trialled to estimate total body composition (Shen et al. 2004a, b); however, this does not permit assessment of regional differences in athletes. Analysis can be fast and automated or take up to 3 h depending on the information that is required. A new technique (quantitative magnetic resonance or QMR) has been developed in an attempt to address some of these limitations but is subject to more validation work in humans. For all techniques, controls such as participant preparation, positioning and measures to minimise motion artefact are important, and there are several contraindications to scanning that should be screened by trained personnel.

There are multiple machine manufacturers that support the installation, training, calibration and quality assurance related to their machines. However, they are costly to purchase and maintain, and in many cases, body composition assessment and analyses with magnetic resonance imaging or computed tomography will be outsourced. The techniques often require radiographers or radiologists for operation and analysis, but there are situations where other health professionals are trained to undertake specific roles in their application.

Common application of magnetic resonance imaging and computed tomography for athlete body composition assessment outside of clinical or research settings is premature. In these cases, the information provided and how it is interpreted will be highly dependent on the purpose of the research or clinical assessment. While there has to be strong ethical justification of the use of computed tomography for body composition assessment, magnetic resonance imaging and computed tomography may be used opportunistically when assessments are undertaken for other purposes. As the techniques become further refined and increasingly sensitive, they can provide high-quality information on body composition during development, growth and injury and can have a range of applications in high performance sport. However, it is important that they are not applied without consideration of the athlete's situation and performance level.

12.2   Why Measure Physique Using Computed Tomography or Magnetic Resonance Imaging?

Magnetic resonance imaging and computed tomography are imaging techniques that provide a highly accurate measure of human body composition at the tissue-organ level (Wang et al. 1992; Heymsfield et al. 1997; Shen et al. 2003). The techniques provide high image resolution of body tissues including the adipose tissue, connective tissue, vessels, skeletal muscle and organs in the sagittal, coronal and axial anatomic planes (Heymsfield et al. 1997). Both techniques are considered reference methods for body composition assessment due to their high precision and validity in cadaver and live human models (Heymsfield et al. 1997, 1979; Mitsiopoulos et al. 1998; Abate et al. 1994; Rossner et al. 1990). Magnetic resonance imaging is emerging as a safe method of choice over computed tomography as it does not require radiation (Brenner and Hall 2007; Orchard et al. 2005) and due to its ability to measure regional and tissue-specific changes in body tissues with more detail than other body composition assessment methods (Kullberg et al. 2009a).

The coefficient of variation (precision) of magnetic resonance imaging and computed tomography measurements has been shown to be <15%; however, this is highly dependent on the method and participant positioning, algorithms used, number of scans and the extent of interpolation required for whole-body analysis (Silver et al. 2010). Since the widespread proliferation and development of magnetic resonance imaging and computed tomography for body composition assessment in the 1970s and 1980s, there have been several developments for the measurement of body composition in both computed tomography and magnetic resonance imaging techniques. A technique to measure whole-body composition with computed tomography using 22 or more cross-sectional images at well-defined anatomical locations was published in 1986 (Kvist et al. 1986). In the early 1990s, a similar method was posed for magnetic resonance imaging using 28–41 images to measure adipose and lean tissue at a system level (Fowler et al. 1991; Ross et al. 1992). More recently, a method was devised to automate the assessment of whole-body adipose tissue using a developed algorithm using magnetic resonance imaging (Kullberg et al. 2009b). As well as further validation and refinement of the technique, studies in nonathlete populations have successfully used magnetic resonance imaging or computed tomography imaging methods as a method to effectively monitor body composition changes (LeBlanc et al. 2000; Manini et al. 2014).

Magnetic resonance imaging is increasingly being applied in sports medicine by kinanthropometrists and biomechanists to diagnose and make structural and functional measurements in a variety of clinical and experimental contexts including building and validating computational models. Recent developments have allowed the use of magnetic resonance imaging to measure skeletal muscle distribution (Janssen and Ross 1999) and muscular concentration of fat or water through hydrogen ion shifts (Tsubahara et al. 1995). In addition, magnetic resonance imaging is being used for biomechanical assessment, including quantitative measurements of fluid flows, measurements of tissue mechanical properties and joint and muscle kinematics.

Computed tomography and to a lesser extent magnetic resonance imaging are relatively common in nations with well-established healthcare systems and may be paid for by the government or private health companies. However, funding support for their use for non-diagnostic purposes is often not available, and therefore both techniques are costly for body composition assessment (~US $300) and generally limited to research or other specialised settings. In addition, the techniques require specialised skills for machine operation, analysis and effective interpretation and application. It is common for athletes to have several magnetic resonance imaging or computed tomography scans throughout their athletic career for medical, biomechanical or diagnostic purposes. However, with the widespread availability of kinanthropometry and recently increased use of dual-energy X-ray absorptiometry for imaging purposes (see additional chapters on these topics), there are several considerations before magnetic resonance imaging and computed tomography can be justified for athlete body composition assessment.

Computed tomography has an effective radiation dose of 5000–15,000 μSv—a dose that the US Food and Drug Administration estimates may carry a 1-in-2000 lifetime risk of inducing fatal cancer (United States Food and Drug Administration 2017). Comparatively, a whole-body dual-energy X-ray absorptiometry scan has an effective dose of ~0.2 μSv (Albanese et al. 2003). Ethically, computed tomography is not supported for individual or repeat body composition assessments which are arguably more important for athletes and sports performance. In contrast, magnetic resonance imaging provides no radiation dose as it uses magnetic pulses for image generation. The advantages and disadvantages of magnetic resonance imaging and computed tomography for assessing body composition of athletes are summarised in Table 12.1.

Table 12.1 Advantages and disadvantages of magnetic resonance imaging and computed tomography for assessing body composition of athletes

	Magnetic resonance imaging	Computed tomography
Advantages	• Quick and painless • Clear compartmental tissue data including the bone, subcutaneous, regional and visceral adipose tissue, connective tissue, vessels, skeletal muscle and organs • High image resolution • High validity and repeatability • Safe method using magnetic fields	• Quick and painless • Clear compartmental tissue data including the bone, subcutaneous, regional and visceral adipose tissue, connective tissue, vessels, skeletal muscle and organs • High image resolution • High validity and repeatability
Disadvantages	• More expensive than computed tomography, dual-energy X-ray absorptiometry and kinanthropometry • Restricted availability • Highly trained personnel required to operate and analyse • Cannot accommodate large body size (e.g., >body mass index 40) • Slight movement can impact measurement and require remeasurement • No clear documented reference ranges for body composition assessment	• High radiation exposure • Not supported for individual or repeated measurements without clear justification due to radiation dose • High cost and access • Cannot accommodate large body size (e.g., >body mass index 40) • No clear documented reference ranges for body composition assessment

Cited from (Lee and Gallagher 2008)

12.3 What Is Computed Tomography or Magnetic Resonance Imaging?

There are several major medical supply companies that produce computed tomography or magnetic resonance imaging technologies including Toshiba, Phillips, Siemens and GE Healthcare. Further details on the machines, their inclusions and details of purchase are available through the manufacturers' websites (Toshiba Medical (International) n.d.; Philips Healthcare (Country Selector) n.d.; GE Healthcare Global (Country Selector) n.d.; Siemens Healthineers n.d.). Additional costs, including staffing, maintenance, quality assurance and overheads need to be considered. Computed tomography and magnetic resonance imaging machines can look quite similar and usually feature a moveable bed/platform and either a stationary or moveable arm or compartment. They feature an X-ray or magnetic scanner which can rotate 360° around the individual as part of the scanning process. Magnetic resonance imaging machines can range in the strength of the magnetic fields which influences the speed of the measurement, while computed tomography scanners can have multiple X-ray beams which can influence scanning speed and radiation dose.

In clinical practice, magnetic resonance imaging and computed tomography scans are generally undertaken by radiographers (radiologic technologists, diagnostic radiographers or medical radiation technologists) that undergo extensive training and accreditation processes. Radiologists (specialist medical doctors) are trained to analyse the generated images for clinical diagnostic purposes. However, other health professionals including sport scientists and biomechanists may be trained to use certain magnetic resonance imaging machines or analyse scans for specialised interpretation. Machines that use radiation require operator and site accreditation and ongoing manufacturer servicing support. Magnetic resonance imaging and computed tomography scanners will have manufacturer-prescribed calibration and quality assurance processes. Site personnel responsible for the machines will undergo training related to ongoing care, service and software updates.

While mechanistically alike and similarly named, it is important to note that quantitative magnetic resonance (QMR) is a distinctly different method to traditional magnetic resonance imaging. The QMR system from EchoMRI (Echo Medical Systems, Houston, Texas, USA) has been used to measure animal body composition. An assessment model for humans is now specifically designed for universities and research institutions. Each scan requires less operator training and minimal participant preparation, takes 3–5 min and is easily installed (EchoMRI n.d.). QMR has been shown to accurately measure growth in pigs to 50 kg (Andres et al. 2010); however, when validated against a four-compartment model in adults, QMR underestimated fat mass (Swe Myint et al. 2010). There are validation studies, mostly in animals, reported on the EchoMRI website http://www.echomri.com/.

12.4 How Do You Use Computed Tomography or Magnetic Resonance Imaging for Athletes?

In most cases, body composition assessment and analyses with magnetic resonance imaging or computed tomography will be outsourced. However, it is important to understand the basics of the techniques as this will provide detail on the suitability of the measurement for its intended purpose and key considerations for the interpretation of results.

Computed tomography machines measure the attenuation of X-rays through body tissues to create an image. The cross-sectional images are represented by a 2D map of pixels and given a numerical value called a Hounsfield unit (HU) related to electron density (Kvist et al. 1986). Body tissues including the skeletal muscle, bone, visceral organs and brain are identified due to their known HU ranges and are represented by different shades from white (most dense, water) to black (least dense, air) (Kvist et al. 1986). The tissue area is assessed by multiplying the pixels of known depth and number by the width of the cross-sectional image to create a 3D image where required. For further information there are several resources that review the methods in more depth (Heymsfield et al. 1997; Silver et al. 2010; Prado and Heymsfield 2014). Once computed tomography data are collected, the software automatically analyses the tissue type based on HUs and provides summary information.

Magnetic resonance imaging uses a strong magnetic field 15,000–30,000 times stronger than the Earth's natural magnetic field (1.5–3.0 T) to align positively charged protons in the body's tissues. A radio-frequency wave activates the protons, and they actively absorb this wave until the pulse ceases, at which time they release energy. Different tissues contain varying amounts of hydrogen depending on their water content. The alignment, relaxation time and density of protons in different body tissues are detected and digitised, and a greyscale image quantifying the different body tissues is generated for analysis.

For computed tomography, a whole-body protocol using 28 slices has been used (Chowdhury et al. 1994), but this may be impractical since the measurement may take ~30 min and require approximately ~3 h to analyse. Using current technologies, each cross-sectional image for magnetic resonance imaging takes ~25 s to generate and requires the individual to hold their breath to eliminate motion artefact (Ross 1996). For magnetic resonance imaging assessment, the full complement of cross-sectional images required for body composition assessment can take ~30 min depending on which machine and technique are used (Ross et al. 2000). A technique has also been trialled with a single slice at L4–L5 to estimate total body skeletal muscle mass and adipose tissue volumes (Shen et al. 2004a, b). The application of this technique will be problematic in athletes due to the regional variation in body composition and the importance of measuring regionality for most applications. QMR can take from 0.5 to 3.0 min for a full body composition assessment in humans.

For both techniques, the radiographer or technician will ensure that clothing is suitable and not obstructive, or they may provide a gown if needed. No metal is permitted on or in the body for the computed tomography scan, and small metal fragments or pacemakers are contraindicated for magnetic resonance imaging. During the measurement, participants will usually lie supine with arms by their side or above the head and be instructed to keep still for the duration of the measurement. Individuals may also be instructed to hold their breath at intermittent times during the scan. On some occasions, participants may be requested to consume a contrast material to assist with identifying individual tissues. Computed tomography scans are unsafe for use during pregnancy.

12.5 What Is Computed Tomography or Magnetic Resonance Imaging Used to Measure?

Magnetic resonance imaging and computed tomography assessment for athlete body composition is not common outside of clinical or research settings. In these cases, the information provided and how it is interpreted will be highly dependent on the purpose of the research or clinical assessment. While there has to be convincing justification for the ethical use of computed tomography for body composition assessment, some example applications of magnetic resonance imaging include:

- Assessment of skeletal muscle mass or muscle cross-sectional area in athletes with disabilities
- Monitoring of skeletal muscle mass or muscle cross-sectional area/wasting following injury or immobilisation
- Monitoring growth and development of body tissues and organs in athletes with higher risk of developmental delays due to low energy availability (e.g., aesthetic sports)
- Abnormalities in bones, muscles, joints, ligaments and cartilage in development or pre and post-surgery
- Assessment of organ mass and its impact on RMR in comparison to skeletal muscle mass
- Assessments of sodium content of body tissues
- Specific assessments of visceral fat where clinically relevant (e.g., steatosis, type II diabetes)
- Assessment of biomechanical advantages in sports where body composition assessment may result in performance benefits (e.g., weight lifting, lightweight rowing)
- Determining regional, tissue-specific, differences in body composition in response to an intervention (e.g., training, medication, dietary)
- Determining inter-athlete comparisons in body composition characteristics that require specific quantitation of body tissues (e.g., by gender, ethnicity, position, age)
- As a criterion method for comparing other body composition methods (e.g., subcutaneous fat via magnetic resonance imaging assessment in comparison to ultrasound analysis, determining visceral fat mass in comparison to dual-energy X-ray absorptiometry compartmental analyses)

Magnetic resonance imaging and computed tomography may be used opportunistically when assessments are done for other reasons. For example, if an athlete has magnetic resonance imaging monitoring for an injury and are going through an immobilisation period, the same scan can also be assessed for muscular and fat cross-sectional area and quality. Other common uses for magnetic resonance imaging or computed tomography in athlete populations include trauma, abdominal injury, fracture detection and evaluation, cardiac function and the detection of foreign bodies. With appropriate permissions and ethical considerations, this approach can be used effectively when there is close communication between support services staff, the athlete and the athlete's medical practitioner.

12.6   How Do You Report Computed Tomography or Magnetic Resonance Imaging Data to Athletes and Coaches?

In many cases, the information will require expert interpretation or may need repeat measurements to be meaningful. Depending on how the information is interpreted, there may be appropriate reference ranges. Phantom comparison may be useful for determining absolute lipid concentration of tissues by using a regression equation to compare to materials of known composition (Ross et al. 2000).

As these techniques become further refined and increasingly sensitive, it is important that they are not applied without consideration of the athlete's situation (e.g., age, skill ability). "Defects" or trends that aren't considered beneficial for health or sport-specific performance are not a problem if the athlete is asymptomatic and if the results do not directly influence the individual. In addition, magnetic resonance imaging used for body composition assessment will plausibly detect a range of medical defects or physiological states (e.g., pregnancy and cancer) which raises a range of ethical issues in the conduct, analysis, application and communication of magnetic resonance imaging results to athletes from well-intentioned sports personnel (Orchard et al. 2005).

12.7   Summary

Magnetic resonance imaging and computed tomography are imaging techniques that provide a highly accurate measure of human body composition at the tissue-organ level. Both techniques are considered reference methods for body composition assessment due to their high precision and validity. Due to constraints in cost and availability, the techniques are generally only used for athletes as part of a research project or for clinical purposes.

References

Abate N, Burns D, Peshock RM, Garg A, Grundy SM (1994) Estimation of adipose tissue mass by magnetic resonance imaging: validation against dissection in human cadavers. J Lipid Res 35(8):1490–1496

Albanese CV, Diessel E, Genant HK (2003) Clinical applications of body composition measurements using DXA. J Clin Densitom 6(2):75–85

Andres A, Mitchell AD, Badger TM (2010) QMR: validation of an infant and children body composition instrument using piglets against chemical analysis. Int J Obes 34(4):775–780

Brenner DJ, Hall EJ (2007) Computed tomography–an increasing source of radiation exposure. N Engl J Med 357(22):2277–2284

Chowdhury B, Sjostrom L, Alpsten M, Kostanty J, Kvist H, Lofgren R (1994) A multicompartment body composition technique based on computerized tomography. Int J Obes Relat Metab Disord 18(4):219–234

EchoMRI (n.d.) http://www.echomri.com/. Accessed 21 Oct 2016

Fowler PA, Fuller MF, Glasbey CA, Foster MA, Cameron GG, McNeill G, Maughan RJ (1991) Total and subcutaneous adipose tissue in women: the measurement of distribution and accurate prediction of quantity by using magnetic resonance imaging. Am J Clin Nutr 54(1):18–25

GE Healthcare Global (Country Selector) (n.d.). http://www3.gehealthcare.com/en/global_gateway. Accessed 21 Oct 2016

Heymsfield SB, Fulenwider T, Nordlinger B, Barlow R, Sones P, Kutner M (1979) Accurate measurement of liver, kidney, and spleen volume and mass by computerized axial tomography. Ann Intern Med 90(2):185–187

Heymsfield SB, Wang Z, Baumgartner RN, Ross R (1997) Human body composition: advances in models and methods. Annu Rev Nutr 17:527–558

Janssen I, Ross R (1999) Effects of sex on the change in visceral, subcutaneous adipose tissue and skeletal muscle in response to weight loss. Int J Obes Relat Metab Disord 23(10):1035–1046

Kullberg J, J Brandberg J, Angelhed JE, Frimmel H, Bergelin E, Strid L, Ahlström H, Johansson L, Lönn L (2009a) Whole-body adipose tissue analysis: comparison of MRI, CT and dual energy X-ray absorptiometry. Br J Radiol 82(974):123–130

Kullberg J, Johansson L, Ahlstrom H, Courivaud F, Koken P, Eggers H, Bornert P (2009b) Automated assessment of whole-body adipose tissue depots from continuously moving bed MRI: a feasibility study. J Magn Reson Imaging 30(1):185–193

Kvist H, Sjostrom L, Tylen U (1986) Adipose tissue volume determinations in women by computed tomography: technical considerations. Int J Obes 10(1):53–67

LeBlanc A, Lin C, Shackelford L, Sinitsyn V, Evans H, Belichenko O, Schenkman B, Kozlovskaya I, Oganov V, Bakulin A, Hedrick T, Feeback D (2000) Muscle volume, MRI relaxation times (T2), and body composition after spaceflight. J Appl Physiol 89(6):2158–2164

Lee SY, Gallagher D (2008) Assessment methods in human body composition. Curr Opin Clin Nutr Metab Care 11(5):566–572

Manini TM, Buford TW, Lott DJ, Vandenborne K, Daniels MJ, Knaggs JD, Patel H, Pahor M, Perri MG, Anton SD (2014) Effect of dietary restriction and exercise on lower extremity tissue compartments in obese, older women: a pilot study. J Gerontol A Biol Sci Med Sci 69(1):101–108

Mitsiopoulos N, Baumgartner RN, Heymsfield SB, Lyons W, Gallagher D, Ross R (1998) Cadaver validation of skeletal muscle measurement by magnetic resonance imaging and computerized tomography. J Appl Physiol 85(1):115–122

Orchard JW, Read JW, Anderson IJ (2005) The use of diagnostic imaging in sports medicine. Med J Aust 183(9):482–486

Philips Healthcare (Country Selector) (n.d.). http://www.usa.philips.com/healthcare/country-selector. Accessed 21 Oct 2016

Prado CM, Heymsfield SB (2014) Lean tissue imaging: a new era for nutritional assessment and intervention. JPEN J Parenter Enteral Nutr 38(8):940–953

Ross R (1996) Magnetic resonance imaging provides new insights into the characterization of adipose and lean tissue distribution. Can J Physiol Pharmacol 74(6):778–785

Ross R, Goodpaster B, Kelley D, Boada F (2000) Magnetic resonance imaging in human body composition research. From quantitative to qualitative tissue measurement. Ann N Y Acad Sci 904:12–17

Ross R, Leger L, Morris D, de Guise J, Guardo R (1992) Quantification of adipose tissue by MRI: relationship with anthropometric variables. J Appl Physiol 72(2):787–795

Rossner S, Bo WJ, Hiltbrandt E, Hinson W, Karstaedt N, Santago P, Sobol WT, Crouse JR (1990) Adipose tissue determinations in cadavers--a comparison between cross-sectional planimetry and computed tomography. Int J Obes 14(10):893–902

Shen W, Punyanitya M, Wang Z, Gallagher D, St-Onge MP, Albu J, Heymsfield SB, Heshka S (2004a) Total body skeletal muscle and adipose tissue volumes: estimation from a single abdominal cross-sectional image. J Appl Physiol 97(6):2333–2338

Shen W, Punyanitya M, Wang Z, Gallagher D, St-Onge MP, Albu J, Heymsfield SB, Heshka S (2004b) Visceral adipose tissue: relations between single-slice areas and total volume. Am J Clin Nutr 80(2):271–278

Shen W, Wang Z, Punyanita M, Lei J, Sinav A, Kral JG, Imielinska C, Ross R, Heymsfield SB (2003) Adipose tissue quantification by imaging methods: a proposed classification. Obes Res 11(1):5–16

Siemens Healthineers (n.d.). https://www.healthcare.siemens.com. Accessed 21 Oct 2016

Silver HJ, Welch EB, Avison MJ, Niswender KD (2010) Imaging body composition in obesity and weight loss: challenges and opportunities. Diabetes Metab Syndr Obes 3:337–347

Swe Myint K, Napolitano A, Miller SR, Murgatroyd PR, Elkhawad M, Nunez DJ, Finer N (2010) Quantitative magnetic resonance (QMR) for longitudinal evaluation of body composition changes with two dietary regimens. Obesity (Silver Spring, Md) 18(2):391–396

Toshiba Medical (International) (n.d.) http://www.toshibamedicalsystems.com/. Accessed 21 Oct 2016

Tsubahara A, Chino N, Akaboshi K, Okajima Y, Takahashi H (1995) Age-related changes of water and fat content in muscles estimated by magnetic resonance (MR) imaging. Disabil Rehabil 17(6):298–304

United States Food and Drug Administration (2017) What are the radiation risks from CT? United States Food and Drug Administration. http://www.fda.gov/Radiation-EmittingProducts/RadiationEmittingProductsandProcedures/MedicalImaging/MedicalX-Rays/ucm115329.htm. Accessed 10 July 2017

Wang ZM, Pierson RN Jr, Heymsfield SB (1992) The five-level model: a new approach to organizing body-composition research. Am J Clin Nutr 56(1):19–28

Chapter 13
Imaging Method: Dual-Energy X-Ray Absorptiometry

Gary Slater, Alisa Nana, and Ava Kerr

Abstract Dual energy X-ray absorptiometry is used for the assessment of physique traits of athletes. Given the use of X-rays and thus exposure to radiation, specific training by a suitably accredited national organisation is required before dual energy X-ray absorptiometry can be operated, and consideration of the cumulative X-ray dose for athletes needs to be considered. Standardisation of subject presentation (euhydrated and glycogen replete, overnight fasted and in minimal clothing) and positioning on the scanning bed (centrally aligned in a standard position using custom-made positioning aids) and manipulation of the automatic segmentation of regional areas of the scan results are necessary. The International Society for Clinical Densitometry has established good clinical practice guidelines relating to the acquisition and analysis of dual energy X-ray absorptiometry data.

Keywords Dual energy X-ray absorptiometry • Physique traits • X-Rays • Radiation Training • Standardisation • Euhydrated • Glycogen replete • Overnight fasted Clothing • Positioning • Scanning bed • Positioning aids • Segmentation • Clinical densitometry • Clinical practice • Guidelines • Acquisition • Analysis

G. Slater (✉) • A. Kerr
University of the Sunshine Coast, Sippy Downs, QLD, Australia
e-mail: gslater@usc.edu.au; akerr@usc.edu.au

A. Nana
Mahidol University, Salaya, Thailand
e-mail: alisa.nan@mahidol.ac.th

© Springer Nature Singapore Pte Ltd. 2018
P.A. Hume et al. (eds.), *Best Practice Protocols for Physique Assessment in Sport*,
https://doi.org/10.1007/978-981-10-5418-1_13

153

13.1   Introduction

Given the wide-ranging data outputs, increasing accessibility and convenience of assessment for both technician and athlete, dual energy X-ray absorptiometry is becoming a more widely used technique for the assessment of physique traits of athletes. When technical and biological factors that influence precision and reliability of dual energy X-ray absorptiometry are accounted for, it is an excellent method for capturing both one-off assessments and tracking longitudinal changes in physique traits of athletes.

Every dual energy X-ray absorptiometry machine contains three essential components: an X-ray energy source, a detector and a computer interface. The dual energy X-ray absorptiometry machine emits two different sources of X-ray energies which pass through the body. The detector then measures the attenuation ratio of these two energies, with the computer converting the ratio of each individual region using the manufacturer's proprietary equations into whole-body output in three different components, i.e. bone mineral content, lean mass and fat mass for the whole body and for regional areas. Given the use of X-rays and thus exposure to radiation, specific training by a suitably accredited national organisation is required before dual energy X-ray absorptiometry can be operated, and consideration of the cumulative X-ray dose for athletes needs to be given. Registration with regional and/or national government-funded radiation health organisations is also required. Hardware and software vary between manufacturers, as do reference databases from which outputs are generated, and these should be standardised when monitoring athletes longitudinally. Quality control calibration procedures are required prior to assessments each day of operation.

Standardisation of subject presentation (euhydrated and glycogen replete, overnight fasted and in minimal clothing) and positioning on the scanning bed (centrally aligned in a standard position using custom-made positioning aids) and manipulation of the automatic segmentation of regional areas of the scan results are necessary. Body composition assessment implemented with such a protocol ensures a high level of precision while still being practical in an athletic setting. While scan duration varies between manufacturers, an assessment can usually be completed within 10 min.

Dual energy X-ray absorptiometry is unique amongst physique assessment techniques given that it provides measures of both whole body, regional fat mass and lean mass, plus indices of bone health including bone area, mineral density and content.

Reports vary based on the manufacturer, but a wide range of automated reports are available presenting information on bone, fat and lean masses, both at a whole-body and regional level, in the form of both tables and insightful figures. Reports can also be constructed so as to allow direct comparison between assessments, making dual energy X-ray absorptiometry particularly valuable when monitoring longitudinal changes in body composition of athletes.

13.2   Why Measure Physique Using Dual Energy X-Ray Absorptiometry?

Dual energy X-ray absorptiometry has historically been used in a clinical setting to assess bone mineral content (BMC) and density (BMD) at specific bone sites to diagnose osteopenia and osteoporosis. It is considered the reference technique for such assessments (Blake and Fogelman 2009; Lewiecki 2005). However, dual energy X-ray absorptiometry is also able to measure soft tissue, rapidly gaining popularity in recent years as one of the most widely used and accepted laboratory-based methods for body composition analysis amongst athletes (Meyer et al. 2013). Dual energy X-ray absorptiometry not only provides a measure of whole-body BMC, fat mass and lean mass, but it also provides information on regional body composition (i.e. arms, legs, trunk, differences between left and right side), making dual energy X-ray absorptiometry technology unique amongst physique assessment tools and particularly appealing amongst healthcare practitioners and sports scientists in understanding and monitoring changes in physique traits. Dual energy X-ray absorptiometry has also been validated to provide a measure of visceral adipose tissue (Neeland et al. 2016) making it useful for the monitoring of health aspects of body fat distribution. Given this, dual energy X-ray absorptiometry technology is making a transition from a laboratory research tool to a servicing tool amongst athletic populations.

Increased access to dual energy X-ray absorptiometry technology through sporting institutes, universities and commercial radiology clinics has generated interest in its potential to provide rapidly generated and detailed information on body composition. A cursory summary of the advantages and disadvantages of the use of dual energy X-ray absorptiometry for physique assessment of athletes is provided in Table 13.1, while the limitations of dual energy X-ray absorptiometry, previously identified in its use for monitoring body composition in the general population, merit specific exploration in relation to athletes.

Table 13.1 Advantages and disadvantages of dual energy X-ray absorptiometry for physique assessment of athletes

Advantages	Disadvantages
• Suitable for most athletes	• Radiation exposure
• Fast (~5 min)	• Expensive equipment
• Provides regional body composition	• Not portable
• Low radiation dose (~0.5 μSv) and safe for sequential measurements	• Scanning bed is smaller than typical physique of many athletes
• Nonintrusive	• Trained technician required
• Valid measure of visceral adipose tissue	• Unable to directly compare results between different dual energy X-ray absorptiometry machines (need specific regression equations)
	• Lack of comprehensive normative data for athletes

The interpretation of body composition measurements via dual energy X-ray absorptiometry requires an appreciation of the validity and reliability of the technique. While studies in general populations have investigated the validity (comparing results of body composition measurement from other indirect techniques) and reliability of dual energy X-ray absorptiometry assessments of physique (Lohman et al. 2000; Toombs et al. 2012), there are fewer studies related to these issues in athletic populations. This is an important consideration if dual energy X-ray absorptiometry is to be used to assess body composition changes in athletic populations, given the anticipated changes throughout the athlete's sporting career or following a nutrition and/or training intervention are likely small compared to those documented following lifestyle or other interventions in obese populations.

Dual energy X-ray absorptiometry has been validated against the four-compartment model, which accounts for variation in the water and mineral fractions and the density of the fat-free mass. While there is some data suggesting good agreement between dual energy X-ray absorptiometry-derived measures of body composition and the four-compartment model in healthy, young males and females (Prior et al. 1997), others have indicated that dual energy X-ray absorptiometry underestimates body fat (Deurenberg-Yap et al. 2001), especially amongst leaner individuals (Van Der Ploeg et al. 2003; Withers et al. 1998). This has been attributed to individual variation in fat-free mass hydration (Deurenberg-Yap et al. 2001) or differences in anterior-posterior tissue thickness (Van Der Ploeg et al. 2003). However, amongst athletes where the primary focus is on monitoring change in body composition, dual energy X-ray absorptiometry appears to offer sufficient sensitivity to identify small changes in body composition (Weyers et al. 2002; Houtkooper et al. 2000), a necessity within athletic populations where small but important changes in physique traits may be evident throughout a season (Lees et al. 2017).

The precision of measurement for dual energy X-ray absorptiometry in sedentary populations has been shown to be superior to hydrodensitometry and surface anthropometry (Pritchard et al. 1993), with a coefficient of variation of less than 1.0 kg for fat mass, fat-free mass and total mass (Mazess et al. 1990; Tothill et al. 1994). Any variability of results achieved by dual energy X-ray absorptiometry can be divided into two categories: technical and biological error. In an effort to enhance precision of measurement, a best practice protocol for assessment of body composition has been established (Nana et al. 2015). Components of this protocol include standardisation of subject presentation and positioning on the scanning bed and manipulation of the automatic segmentation of regional areas of the scan results. Assessments implemented with such a protocol ensure a high level of precision while still being practical in an athletic setting.

Of particular relevance to athletic populations is the impact of variation in hydration status on dual energy X-ray absorptiometry precision, given fat-free soft tissue mass is assumed to be 73% water (Pietrobelli et al. 1998) yet can vary from 67 to 85% (Moore and Boyden 1963), leading to errors in the estimate of lean mass but not fat mass (Lohman et al. 2000). Current recommendations for standardisation of dual energy X-ray absorptiometry scanning protocols recognise the impact of presenting hydration status (Rodriguez-Sanchez and Galloway 2015), plus acute food/

fluid intake (Horber et al. 1992) and/or exercise (Nana et al. 2012a, 2013; Kerr et al. 2017) on estimates of body composition. However, recent research suggests variance in intramuscular solutes, specifically glycogen (Bone et al. 2016; Rouillier et al. 2015), and to a lesser degree, creatine monohydrate (Safdar et al. 2008; Bone et al. 2016) may also need to be considered given their impact on lean mass hydration (Olsson and Saltin 1970).

Recent investigation into the potential use of dual energy X-ray absorptiometry for the estimation of body density and subsequent efficiencies in the creation of an improved four-compartment physique assessment model warrants further exploration (Wilson et al. 2012; Smith-Ryan et al. 2016). Similarly, the use of dual energy X-ray absorptiometry for estimating body segment inertial parameters in the investigation of human motion kinetics highlights the application of this technology to a broad reaching audience (Wicke and Dumas 2008). Taken together, the unique regional and whole-body estimates of body composition, plus bone health and fat distribution obtained via dual energy X-ray absorptiometry, have ensured it has resulted in its widespread use for the monitoring of body composition of athletes (Meyer et al. 2013).

13.3   What Is Dual Energy X-Ray Absorptiometry?

Dual energy X-ray absorptiometry technology is based on the differential attenuation of transmitted photons at two energy levels by bone, fat and lean tissue (Mazess et al. 1990). Attenuation of low-energy photons is then expressed as a ratio to attenuation observed for the high-energy photons, the outcome of which is specific to different molecular components, including fatty acids, protein and bone. In theory, assessment of all three components would require measurement at three different photon energies. The dual energy X-ray absorptiometry system can thus only be used to estimate the fractional masses of two components in any one pixel. That is, in bone-containing pixels, bone mineral and soft tissue can be measured, while in non-bone-containing pixels, fat and bone mineral-free lean can be measured (Pietrobelli et al. 1996). The proportion of fat and bone mineral-free lean in bone-containing pixels is assumed to be the same as the adjacent non-bone-containing pixels (Pietrobelli et al. 1996), with the software subsequently incorporating individual pixel data into whole-body output. This assumed ratio of fat to bone mineral-free lean in soft tissue pixels is applied to upwards of one-third of pixels in a whole-body scan and particularly evident in regions of low bone-free pixels such as thorax, arm or head, ensuring the identification of composition changes in these regions being less reliable (Lands et al. 1996; Roubenoff et al. 1993).

There are primarily two commercial manufacturers of dual energy X-ray absorptiometry machines, GE Lunar Radiation Corp. (Madison, Wisconsin) and Hologic Inc. (Waltham, Massachusetts), with a third manufacturer, Norland (Fort Atkinson, Wisconsin), recently releasing a new machine with extra-large dimensions and weight capabilities. Although each manufacturer uses slightly different technology (see Table 13.2 for specifications on each manufacturer and their dual energy X-ray

Table 13.2 Specifications of dual energy X-ray absorptiometry scanners commercially available from the two primary manufacturers measuring body composition

Brand names	Hologic		Lunar	
Types	Horizon	Discovery	iDXA	Prodigy
Material				
X-ray sources	Alternating voltage of two energies		Constant potential (76 kV)	
Two energies differentiation	–		K-edge filter	
Effective photon energies	100 and 140 kV		38 and 70 kV	
Scanning geometry	Fan beam		Narrow-fan beam	
Characteristic of detector	Not energy-discriminating		Energy discrimination	
Composition of detector	Multi-element detector array		Solid state linear array	
Table dimension (scan area)	66 cm x 195 cm	65 cm x 195 cm	66 cm x 198 cm	60 cm x 198 cm
Weight (scanner)	365 kg	310 kg	360 kg	272 kg
Maximum weight of subject	227 kg	204 kg	204 kg	159 kg
Quality assessment				
Soft tissue calibration	Step phantom of Lucite and aluminium		Plastic polyoxymethylene (40% fat), water (5% fat)	
Bone calibration	Internal rotating drum		Internal hydroxyapatite calibration	
	Hydroxyapatite spine phantom in epoxy resin		Block phantom and spine aluminium phantom	
Total body precision				
Bone mineral density (CV)	<1%	<1%	<1%	<1%
Body composition (CV)	BMC 0.7%, FM 0.8%, LM 0.5%[a]	<1.9%	BMC 0.5%, FM 1%, LM 0.5%[b]	FM 1.9%[c]
Measurement				
Total body effective radiation	0.007 µGy	0.012 µGy	0.3 µGy	0.04 µGy
Scan time	3 min	7 min	7 min	5 min
Data processing	Automatic and manual analysis of vertebral bone, femoral and forearm regions, total body with soft tissue, patient trending, previous scan comparison, T- and Z-scores, reference comparison, visceral fat assessment, FRAX assessment		Automatic and manual analysis of vertebral bone, femoral and forearm regions, total body with soft tissue, patient trending, previous scan comparison, T- and Z-scores, reference comparison, visceral fat assessment, FRAX assessment	

Table 13.2 (continued)

Brand names	Hologic		Lunar	
Types	Horizon	Discovery	iDXA	Prodigy
Reference database				
Default	NHANES III[d]		Combined Geelong/Lunar[e]	
Alternate	Non-NHANES III		Lunar USA/Northern European[f], NHANES III	

[a]Nowitz and Monahan (2017)
[b]Rothney et al. (2009)
[c]Kaminsky et al. (2014)
[d]NHANES III—USA population ($n > 20,000$), male and female, multi-ethnicities and exclusion criteria: under 20 years of age, pregnant females and hip implants
[e]Combined Geelong/Lunar—Geelong-Australian adult females ($n = 1494$) and males ($n = 1540$) aged 20–79 years, random population based. [f]USA/Northern European—ambulatory population ($n > 12,000$), no chronic diseases, male and female, multi-ethnicities and all ages. Modified from (Genton et al. 2002)

absorptiometry models), every dual energy X-ray absorptiometry machine contains three essential components: two sources of X-ray energies, a detector and a computer interface. The dual energy X-ray absorptiometry machine emits two different sources of X-ray energies which pass through different tissues in the body (Mazess et al. 1990). The detector then measures the attenuation ratio of these two energies (commonly referred to R value) in each pixel of the body, with the computer converting the ratio of each individual pixel using the manufacturer's proprietary equations into whole-body output in three different components. In this way, most dual energy X-ray absorptiometry machines are able to provide a measure of bone mineral content, lean mass and fat mass for the whole body and for regional areas (right and left sides of arms, legs and trunk).

The commercial manufacturers of dual energy X-ray absorptiometry machines make use of three different types of beam technologies: pencil-, fan- and narrow-fan beams. The type of beam technology controls the path of the X-ray beam and therefore determines the scanning time, radiation exposure and potentially the accuracy of the estimates. Pencil beam is regarded as more accurate, but the scanning time per one whole-body scan is also relatively long (up to ~17 min) (Toombs et al. 2012; Lohman et al. 2000). On the other hand, fan beam densitometers are considerably faster in scanning time; however, they are known to produce magnification errors or geometric distortions inherited from magnification of scanned structures as the distance from the X-ray source decreases (Tothill et al. 2001; Tothill and Hannan 2000; Griffiths et al. 1997) and exposes subjects to higher radiation compared to pencil beam (Steel et al. 1998). The influence of magnification has been shown to affect measurements of bone mineral content, bone area and parameters of hip geometry (Tothill et al. 2001; Tothill and Hannan 2000; Griffiths et al. 1997). The newer technology, narrow-fan beam (e.g. GE Lunar Prodigy), is the compromise of older technologies where it has the advantage of fast scanning time (~5 min) while potentially producing less magnification errors compared with a fan beam densitometer (Norcross and Van Loan

2004; Oldroyd et al. 2003), with similar accuracy and precision as pencil-beam scanners (Bilsborough et al. 2014). Nevertheless, due to algorithm differences used in tissue imaging, high and low X-ray beam generation and calibration methodology, longitudinal monitoring should be undertaken on the same scanner and administered by the same qualified technician to optimise measurement precision (Genton et al. 2002).

One of the concerns with dual energy X-ray absorptiometry technology is the radiation exposure. Although dual energy X-ray absorptiometry technology exposes subjects and technicians to radiation, the dose is small. A typical dual energy X-ray absorptiometry machine exposes subjects to a radiation dose of approximately 0.5 μSv per one whole-body scan, approximately equivalent to 1/100th of a radiation dose from a typical chest X-ray or a single transcontinental air flight (Toombs et al. 2012). Although radiation exposure from one whole-body dual energy X-ray absorptiometry scan is small, cumulative exposure from serial scanning as part of routine longitudinal tracking over time could be significant for athletes who may be exposed to ionising radiation from other diagnostic imaging techniques (Cross et al. 2003; Orchard et al. 2005) or frequent aeroplane travel. In Australia, legislative requirements limit exposure for the general public to 1 mSv per year and to volunteers in research to 5 mSv per year. The total amount of radiation exposure an athlete would typically receive from routine body composition monitoring by dual energy X-ray absorptiometry up to 6 whole-body scans per year (~3.0 μSv) is well below these guidelines. Nevertheless, the total number of scans undertaken per year should be capped and strictly documented and monitored to prevent unnecessary radiation exposure. Scanning should not be undertaken in athletes who are pregnant. If there is any doubt, then a pregnancy test should be undertaken or the female athlete scanned in the first 10 days of their cycle. The radiation dose associated with a dual energy X-ray absorptiometry scan typically limits assessments to no more frequently than every 2–3 months. When more frequent review of progress is necessary, dual energy X-ray absorptiometry should be complemented with surface anthropometry, a technique with very high precision that affords more frequent assessments, i.e. every 3 or 4 weeks if necessary during periods of rapid body composition change.

13.4 How Do You Dual Energy X-Ray Absorptiometry for Your Athlete?

The International Society for Clinical Densitometry (ISCD) has established good clinical practice guidelines relating to the acquisition and analysis of dual energy X-ray absorptiometry data (Hangartner et al. 2013). These guidelines have been further refined in an attempt to optimise the precision of measurement of body composition using dual energy X-ray absorptiometry (Nana et al. 2015). Components of this most recent protocol include standardisation of subject presentation (subjects euhydrated, glycogen replete, overnight fasted and bladder voided in minimal clothing and free of any metal) and positioning on the scanning bed (centrally aligned in a standard position using custom-made positioning aids) and manipulation of the automatic segmentation of regional areas of the scan results.

Body composition assessment implemented with such a protocol ensures a high level of precision while still being practical in an athletic setting. Example text used in a letter provided by the authors to athletes prior to a scan to enable the athlete prepare for the scan is shown below:

A few things to prepare for your appointment:

- We are required by Queensland Health to have you complete the following informed consent prior to your scan https://www.smartwaiver.com/w/549351e79a7e3/web/.
- For the most accurate scan result, we recommend that you refrain from eating, drinking or exercising the morning of your scan. Research by our group over the last 10 years shows that food and fluid intake in the few hours before a scan impact the interpretation of your body composition. This is also one of the main reasons we only open early in the morning.
- Wear only clothes that do not contain any metal, including zips, bra clips, etc. The best options include leggings (check for a back zipper) and sports bra (no metal clips) for females and shorts (no zips) or Lycra shorts/Speedo's for males.
- Present to your scan in a well-hydrated state. While you can't drink anything prior to your scan, we encourage you to drink one to two glasses of water with each meal/snack the day prior to your scan. This will help to ensure you wake on the day of your scan well hydrated.
- Ensure your muscle glycogen stores are full. It is important to remember that significant changes in muscle energy reserves (glycogen) can impact on our measurement of muscle mass. If you present glycogen depleted (say, e.g. if you have really pulled back on the carbs in recent weeks or had heavy training the day before), then our measure of muscle mass could be lower by upwards of 1–1.5 kg. We do the very best to ensure the technical reliability of the results but entrust in you to present well hydrated and not energy depleted.

Of particular relevance to athletic populations is the defined scanning area available for assessment when using dual energy X-ray absorptiometry, typically within the range of 60–65 cm × 193–198 cm depending on the manufacturer. It is therefore difficult to perform whole-body dual energy X-ray absorptiometry scans on particularly tall or broad and very muscular athletes, physique traits common to some sports such as rowing, basketball, volleyball and rugby union. A solution is to have taller individuals undertake two partial scans with the body divided at the neck resulting in the most accurate estimates of bone and soft tissue composition (Evans et al. 2005). Until recently, very broad individuals were 'mummy wrapped' in a sheet, bringing the arms forward, so as to fit within the scanning area. While this afforded a whole-body scan to be undertaken, the number of bone-containing pixels is significantly increased while also limiting the ability to assess regional body composition. Further guidance on the capture of data on particularly tall and/or broad athletes is available (Nana et al. 2012b). Norland have recently released a new model (Noland Elite) that will accommodate larger individuals, including athletes with extremes in physique traits having an allowance of 283.5 kg, 137 cm wide and 228 cm tall (Shepherd et al. 2017). Newer dual energy X-ray absorptiometry instruments have larger scanning areas and come with software that allows an estimate of whole-body composition from a half body scan (Rothney et al. 2009), a concept validated previously in obese individuals (Tataranni and Ravussin 1995).

13.4.1 Subject Positioning Protocol

The Nana et al. (2015) protocol involves scans undertaken that emphasises a consistent positioning of athletes on the scanning bed of the dual energy X-ray absorptiometry machine. This involves an athlete lying centrally in the scanning area with their head positioned in the Frankfort plain and with their feet placed in custom-made radio-opaque Styrofoam blocks to maintain a constant distance of 15 cm between the feet for each scan. Similarly, the athletes' hands are to be placed in shaped Styrofoam blocks, so they are in a mid-prone position with a consistent gap of 3 cm between the palms and trunk. Two Velcro straps are used to minimise any athlete movement during the scan and to provide a consistent body position for subsequent scans. One strap is secured around the ankles above the foot positioning pad, and the other strap is secured around the trunk at the level of the mid-forearms as shown in Fig. 13.1.

13.5 What Is Dual Energy X-Ray Absorptiometry Used to Measure?

Whole-body scans are rapid (~5 min), non-invasive and associated with very low radiation doses with precise estimates of whole body and regional fat mass and lean mass, making the technology safe for longitudinal monitoring of body composition. This has application in the monitoring of a range of targeted training and/or dietary

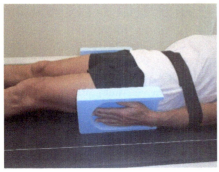
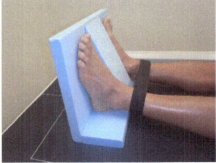

Fig. 13.1 Positioning Styrofoam blocks for dual energy X-ray absorptiometry scanning

interventions amongst athletes, but also other scenarios in which physique traits are likely to change such as the disuse atrophy that often accompanies significant injuries and the subsequent rehabilitation, or when issues of symmetry are of interest. However, due to radiation exposure limits on assessment frequency, dual energy X-ray absorptiometry is often used concurrently with surface anthropometry, a highly precise technique, which affords much more frequent monitoring. Dual energy X-ray absorptiometry has also been accepted by the National Collegiate Athletic Association in their weight certification programme requiring minimum weight via body composition analysis (Clark et al. 2007), with likely wider application to other weight category sports to assist in the identification of an appropriate weight category. Dual energy X-ray absorptiometry has been shown to accurately quantify visceral adipose tissue in both males and females of different ethnicities (Neeland et al. 2016), a potentially important variable to monitor amongst athletes in sports emphasising high absolute mass (Murata et al. 2016). Because of its additional application in the assessment of bone mineral density, dual energy X-ray absorptiometry technology is also becoming increasingly available.

13.6 How Do You Report the Dual Energy X-Ray Absorptiometry Data to Your Athlete and Coach?

There are a selection of reports that can be generated depending on the information required and the dual energy X-ray absorptiometry scanner used. These include bone density, body composition and metabolic and visceral fat. Some dual energy X-ray absorptiometry models afford an opportunity to create reports that populate data from the current assessment with prior scans, creating an excellent medium for interpreting changes in physique traits longitudinally. When interpreting results, an appreciation of test-retest reliability or precision of measurement is necessary. The ISCD advocate recommended minimum performance standards of 2% for percent fat, 3% for fat mass and 2% for lean mass (Hangartner et al. 2013). This should be established across a minimum of 20 volunteers and ideally undertaken on individuals with physique traits that are reflective of the athletic population typically assessed by the dual energy X-ray absorptiometry technician, using the same equipment and protocols. An example report from the Hologic dual energy X-ray absorptiometry scanner is shown in Fig. 13.2.

13.7 Summary

Dual energy X-ray absorptiometry is a widely used technique for the assessment of physique traits of athletes. The dual energy X-ray absorptiometry machine emits sources of X-ray energies which pass through the body enabling determination of bone mineral content, lean mass and fat mass for the whole body and for regional

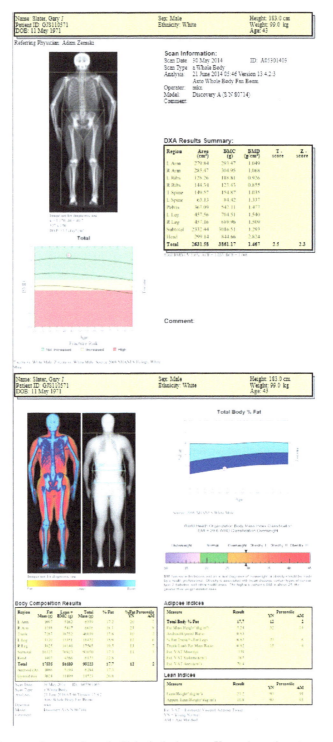

Fig. 13.2 An example report from the Hologic dual energy X-ray absorptiometry scanner

areas. Given the exposure to radiation, specific training by a suitably accredited national organisation is required before dual energy X-ray absorptiometry can be operated. Consideration of the cumulative X-ray dose for athletes needs to be considered. Standardisation of athlete presentation, positioning on the scanning bed and manipulation of the automatic segmentation of regional areas of the scan results are necessary. Body composition assessment implemented with such a protocol ensures a high level of precision while still being practical in an athletic setting. An assessment can usually be completed within 10 min.

References

Bilsborough JC, Greenway K, Opar D, Livingstone S, Cordy J, Coutts AJ (2014) The accuracy and precision of DXA for assessing body composition in team sport athletes. J Sports Sci 32(19):1821–1828

Blake GM, Fogelman I (2009) The clinical role of dual energy X-ray absorptiometry. Eur J Radiol 71(3):406–414

Bone JL, Ross ML, Tomcik KA, Jeacocke NA, Hopkins WG, Burke LM (2016) Manipulation of muscle creatine and glycogen changes DXA estimates of body composition. Med Sci Sports Exerc 49(5):1029–1035

Clark RR, Sullivan JC, Bartok CJ, Carrel AL (2007) DXA provides a valid minimum weight in wrestlers. Med Sci Sports Exerc 39(11):2069–2075

Cross TM, Smart RC, Thomson JE (2003) Exposure to diagnostic ionizing radiation in sports medicine: assessing and monitoring the risk. Clin J Sport Med 13(3):164–170

Deurenberg-Yap M, Schmidt G, van Staveren WA, Hautvast J, Deurenberg P (2001) Body fat measurement among Singaporean Chinese, Malays and Indians: a comparative study using a four-compartment model and different two-compartment models. Br J Nutr 85(4):491–498

Evans EM, Prior BM, Modlesky CM (2005) A mathematical method to estimate body composition in tall individuals using DXA. Med Sci Sports Exerc 37(7):1211–1215

Genton L, Hans D, Kyle UG, Pichard C (2002) Dual-energy X-ray absorptiometry and body composition: differences between devices and comparison with reference methods. Nutrition 18(1):66–70

Griffiths MR, Noakes KA, Pocock NA (1997) Correcting the magnification error of fan beam densitometers. J Bone Miner Res 12(1):119–123

Hangartner TN, Warner S, Braillon P, Jankowski L, Shepherd J (2013) The official positions of the international society for clinical densitometry: acquisition of dual-energy x-ray absorptiometry body composition and considerations regarding analysis and repeatability of measures. J Clin Densitom 16(4):520–536

Horber FF, Thomi F, Casez JP, Fonteille J, Jaeger P (1992) Impact of hydration status on body composition as measured by dual energy X-ray absorptiometry in normal volunteers and patients on haemodialysis. Br J Radiol 65(778):895–900

Houtkooper LB, Going SB, Sproul J, Blew RM, Lohman TG (2000) Comparison of methods for assessing body-composition changes over 1 y in postmenopausal women. Am J Clin Nutr 72(2):401–406

Kerr A, Slater G, Byrne N (2017) Impact of food and fluid intake on technical and biological measurement error in body composition assessment methods in athletes. Br J Nutr 117:591–601

Lands LC, Hornby L, Hohenkerk JM, Glorieux FH (1996) Accuracy of measurements of small changes in soft-tissue mass by dual-energy x-ray absorptiometry. Clin Invest Med 19(4):279–285

Lees MJ, Oldroyd B, Jones B, Brightmore A, O'Hara JP, Barlow MJ, Till K, Hind K (2017) Three-compartment body composition changes in professional rugby union players over one competitive season: a team and individualized approach. J Clin Densitom 20(1):50–57

Lewiecki EM (2005) Clinical applications of bone density testing for osteoporosis. Minerva Med 96(5):317–330

Lohman TG, Harris M, Teixeira PJ, Weiss L (2000) Assessing body composition and changes in body composition. Another look at dual-energy X-ray absorptiometry. Ann N Y Acad Sci 904:45–54

Kaminsky LA, Ozemek C, Williams KL, Byun W, (2014) Precision of total and regional body fat estimates from dualenergy X-ray absorptiometer measurements. J Nutr Health Aging 18(6):591–594

Mazess RB, Barden HS, Bisek JP, Hanson J (1990) Dual-energy x-ray absorptiometry for total-body and regional bone-mineral and soft-tissue composition. Am J Clin Nutr 51(6):1106–1112

Meyer NL, Sundgot-Borgen J, Lohman TG, Ackland TR, Stewart AD, Maughan RJ, Smith S, Muller W (2013) Body composition for health and performance: a survey of body composition assessment practice carried out by the Ad Hoc Research Working Group on Body Composition, Health and Performance under the auspices of the IOC Medical Commission. Br J Sports Med 47(16):1044–1053

Moore FD, Boyden CM (1963) Body cell mass and limits of hydration of the fat-free body: their relation to estimated skeletal weight. Ann N Y Acad Sci 110:62–71

Murata H, Oshima S, Torii S, Taguchi M, Higuchi M (2016) Characteristics of body composition and cardiometabolic risk of Japanese male heavyweight Judo athletes. J Physiol Anthropol 35:10

Nana A, Slater GJ, Hopkins WG, Burke LM (2012a) Effects of daily activities on dual-energy X-ray absorptiometry measurements of body composition in active people. Med Sci Sports Exerc 44(1):180–189

Nana A, Slater GJ, Hopkins WG, Burke LM (2012b) Techniques for undertaking dual-energy X-ray absorptiometry whole-body scans to estimate body composition in tall and/or broad subjects. Int J Sport Nutr Exerc Metab 22(5):313–322

Nana A, Slater GJ, Hopkins WG, Burke LM (2013) Effects of exercise sessions on DXA measurements of body composition in active people. Med Sci Sports Exerc 45(1):178–185

Nana A, Slater GJ, Stewart AD, Burke LM (2015) Methodology review: using dual-energy X-ray absorptiometry (DXA) for the assessment of body composition in athletes and active people. Int J Sport Nutr Exerc Metab 25(2):198–215

Neeland IJ, Grundy SM, Li X, Adams-Huet B, Vega GL (2016) Comparison of visceral fat mass measurement by dual-X-ray absorptiometry and magnetic resonance imaging in a multiethnic cohort: the Dallas Heart Study. Nutr Diabet 6(7):e221

Norcross J, Van Loan MD (2004) Validation of fan beam dual energy x ray absorptiometry for body composition assessment in adults aged 18–45 years. Br J Sports Med 38(4):472–476

Nowitz M, Monahan P (2017) Short term in vivo precision of whole body composition measurements on the Horizon A densitometer. J Med Imaging Radiat Oncol. doi: 10.1111/1754-9485.12646

Oldroyd B, Smith AH, Truscott JG (2003) Cross-calibration of GE/Lunar pencil and fan-beam dual energy densitometers—bone mineral density and body composition studies. Eur J Clin Nutr 57(8):977–987

Olsson KE, Saltin B (1970) Variation in total body water with muscle glycogen changes in man. Acta Physiol Scand 80(1):11–18. d

Orchard JW, Read JW, Anderson IJ (2005) The use of diagnostic imaging in sports medicine. Med J Aust 183(9):482–486

Pietrobelli A, Formica C, Wang Z, Heymsfield SB (1996) Dual-energy X-ray absorptiometry body composition model: review of physical concepts. Am J Phys 271(6 Pt 1):E941–E951

Pietrobelli A, Wang Z, Formica C, Heymsfield SB (1998) Dual-energy X-ray absorptiometry: fat estimation errors due to variation in soft tissue hydration. Am J Phys 274(5 Pt 1):E808–E816

Prior BM, Cureton KJ, Modlesky CM, Evans EM, Sloniger MA, Saunders M, Lewis RD (1997) In vivo validation of whole body composition estimates from dual-energy X-ray absorptiometry. J Appl Physiol 83(2):623–630

Pritchard JE, Nowson CA, Strauss BJ, Carlson JS, Kaymakci B, Wark JD (1993) Evaluation of dual energy X-ray absorpiometry as a method of measurement of body-fat. Eur J Clin Nutr 47(3):216–228

Rodriguez-Sanchez N, Galloway SD (2015) Errors in dual energy x-ray absorptiometry estimation of body composition induced by hypohydration. Int J Sport Nutr Exerc Metab 25(1):60–68

Rothney MP, Brychta RJ, Schaefer EV, Chen KY, Skarulis MC (2009) Body composition measured by dual-energy X-ray absorptiometry half-body scans in obese adults. Obesity (Silver Spring) 17(6):1281–1286

Roubenoff R, Kehayias JJ, Dawson-Hughes B, Heymsfield SB (1993) Use of dual-energy x-ray absorptiometry in body-composition studies: not yet a "gold standard". Am J Clin Nutr 58(5):589–591

Rouillier MA, David-Riel S, Brazeau AS, St-Pierre DH, Karelis AD (2015) Effect of an acute high carbohydrate diet on body composition using DXA in young men. Ann Nutr Metab 66(4):233–236

Safdar A, Yardley NJ, Snow R, Melov S, Tarnopolsky MA (2008) Global and targeted gene expression and protein content in skeletal muscle of young men following short-term creatine monohydrate supplementation. Physiol Genomics 32(2):219–228

Shepherd JA, Ng BK, Sommer MJ, Heymsfield SB (2017) Body composition by DXA. Bone. https://doi.org/10.1016/j.bone.2017.06.010

Smith-Ryan AE, Mock MG, Ryan ED, Gerstner GR, Trexler ET, Hirsch KR (2016) Validity and reliability of a 4-compartment body composition model using dual energy x-ray absorptiometry-derived body volume. Clin Nutr 36:825–830

Steel SA, Baker AJ, Saunderson JR (1998) An assessment of the radiation dose to patients and staff from a Lunar Expert-XL fan beam densitometer. Physiol Meas 19(1):17–26

Tataranni PA, Ravussin E (1995) Use of dual-energy X-ray absorptiometry in obese individuals. Am J Clin Nutr 62(4):730–734

Toombs RJ, Ducher G, Shepherd JA, De Souza MJ (2012) The impact of recent technological advances on the trueness and precision of DXA to assess body composition. Obesity (Silver Spring) 20(1):30–39

Tothill P, Hannan WJ (2000) Comparisons between hologic QDR 1000W, QDR 4500A, and lunar expert dual-energy X-ray absorptiometry scanners used for measuring total body bone and soft tissue. Ann N Y Acad Sci 904:63–71

Tothill P, Avenell A, Love J, Reid DM (1994) Comparisons between hologic, lunar and Norland dual-energy X-ray absorptiometers and other techniques used for whole-body soft-tissue measurements. Eur J Clin Nutr 48(11):781–794

Tothill P, Hannan WJ, Wilkinson S (2001) Comparisons between a pencil beam and two fan beam dual energy X-ray absorptiometers used for measuring total body bone and soft tissue. Br J Radiol 74(878):166–176

Van Der Ploeg GE, Withers RT, Laforgia J (2003) Percent body fat via DEXA: comparison with a four-compartment model. J Appl Physiol 94(2):499–506

Weyers AM, Mazzetti SA, Love DM, Gomez AL, Kraemer WJ, Volek JS (2002) Comparison of methods for assessing body composition changes during weight loss. Med Sci Sports Exerc 34(3):497–502

Wicke J, Dumas GA (2008) Estimating segment inertial parameters using fan-beam DXA. J Appl Biomech 24(2):180–184

Wilson JP, Mulligan K, Fan B, Sherman JL, Murphy EJ, Tai VW, Powers CL, Marquez L, Ruiz-Barros V, Shepherd JA (2012) Dual-energy X-ray absorptiometry-based body volume measurement for 4-compartment body composition. Am J Clin Nutr 95(1):25–31

Withers RT, LaForgia J, Pillans RK, Shipp NJ, Chatterton BE, Schultz CG, Leaney F (1998) Comparisons of two-, three-, and four-compartment models of body composition analysis in men and women. J Appl Physiol 85(1):238–245

Chapter 14
Imaging Method: Technological and Computing Innovations

Jacqueline A. Alderson

Abstract Technological and computing innovations are rapidly transforming the tools we employ for recording, measuring, collating and interpreting body dimension and composition assessments. Three-dimensional body scanning systems integrated with other imaging modalities to create multi-faceted digital human profiles, and artificial intelligence techniques such as deep learning and artificial neural networks, are set to revolutionise the physique assessment landscape over the coming decade. Dual-energy X-ray absorptiometry is regarded as the current gold standard for determining body fat percentage and lean mass. Leveraging computer vision techniques, it is now possible to register an individual's dual-energy X-ray absorptiometry-derived body composition with the mesh exported by the same individual's three-dimensional body scan.

Keywords Technological • Computing • Three dimensional • Imaging modalities • Digital human • Artificial intelligence • Deep learning • Neural networks • Dual-energy X-ray absorptiometry • Computer vision • Body scan

14.1 Introduction

Technological and computing innovations are rapidly transforming the tools we employ for recording, measuring, collating and interpreting body dimension and composition assessments. We are witnessing historically unprecedented rates of advancement in technology and data analytic techniques that will fundamentally transform scientists', health practitioners' and the residential consumers' approach to physique assessment. Three-dimensional body scanning systems integrated with other imaging modalities to create multi-faceted digital human profiles, and artificial intelligence techniques such as deep learning and artificial neural networks, are set to revolutionise the physique assessment landscape over the coming decade.

J.A. Alderson
University of Western Australia, Crawley, WA, Australia
e-mail: Jacqueline.Alderson@uwa.edu.au

© Springer Nature Singapore Pte Ltd. 2018
P.A. Hume et al. (eds.), *Best Practice Protocols for Physique Assessment in Sport*,
https://doi.org/10.1007/978-981-10-5418-1_14

Three-dimensional body scanning is now more widely accessible, user-friendly and less cost prohibitive than ever before. Yet, digitally derived three-dimensional body hull reconstructions have not been shown to be more reliable than manual forms of anthropometric measurement (Kuehnapfel et al. 2017). However, three-dimensional scanning is faster than manual measurement, does not require extensive training to operate and provides substantially greater levels (higher granularity) of information. Considered in isolation, three-dimensional body scanning is not new or novel, but when integrated with other participant-specific imaging modalities, the creation of multi-dimensional human body models may be realised.

Dual-energy X-ray absorptiometry is regarded as the gold standard for determining body fat percentage and lean mass (Lands et al. 1996). Using computer vision techniques, it is now possible to register an individual's dual-energy X-ray absorptiometry-derived body composition with a 3D mesh exported using the same individual's body scan (El-Sallam Abd et al. 2013). The two-dimensional transverse plane dual-energy X-ray absorptiometry pixel areal density information can be internally distributed across the segment volume of a 3D hull to provide an informed representation of segmental mass distribution (Rossi et al. 2016). This 3D hull/dual-energy X-ray absorptiometry image registration process occurs automatically in custom software and requires no manual user input, or specific calibration routine other than that undertaken at the hardware level (i.e. scanner and dual-energy X-ray absorptiometry manufacturer specifications). Further, the automatic image scaling procedures allow for the two images to be scaled to one another using key features from both images.

This technique allows for the estimation of subject-specific body dimension and body segment inertial parameter values. These are ideal for biomechanical modelling purposes and are required for athletic populations where anatomically based regression equations based on normative populations are often not valid (Rossi et al. 2013). Importantly, from a physique assessment perspective, the approach can provide data on body composition changes relative to body shape, valuable in situations where no discernible shape change is identifiable but where the underlying composition has altered.

14.2 Why Measure Physique Using a 3D Scan with an Integrated Dual-Energy X-Ray Absorptiometry Image?

Athlete physical characteristics, especially those required by biomechanists for neuromusculoskeletal modelling purposes such as segment, length, mass location and mass distribution, can vary considerably from those in traditional regression tables based upon normal population samples. Similarly, the science of quantifying human phenotype with respect to dimension and gross composition has shifted in recent years towards a subject-specific approach that aims to establish a 'full-body digital profile' of an athlete. This involves obtaining direct measures of size, shape and function and fitting this information to pre-existing generic models. Research shows that the outputs resulting from a subject-specific approach improve validity by way of modelling error/discrepancy when compared with using normative data assumptions (Winby et al. 2008).

14.3   What Is the Technology Behind the 3D Scan/Dual-Energy X-Ray Absorptiometry Merge Pipeline?

The developed technique requires two scans: (1) a 3D full-body scan (see Fig. 14.1a) and (2) a dual-energy X-ray absorptiometry scan (see Fig. 14.1b). An Artec video scanner was used to record the three-dimensional body scan in the present example, but as discussed later in this section, a range of low-cost, accurate scanners will soon enter the market which will put three-dimensional scanning opportunities in the reach of the average consumer.

In overview, computer vision techniques are used to register the dual-energy X-ray absorptiometry and 3D body scan. This involves deforming the three-dimensional scan silhouette to obtain a best fit (local minima) within the dual-energy X-ray absorptiometry silhouette (see Fig. 14.2a). Once this deformation is achieved, the dual-energy X-ray absorptiometry mass information, determined by proprietary techniques using a Lunar Prodigy dual-energy X-ray absorptiometry machine (GE Healthcare, Buckinghamshire, UK), is distributed over the scanning surface represented by a matrix of squared (0.20 × 0.20 cm) elements (Rossi et al. 2013). Estimation of the mass distribution within the mesh volume is performed by creating a volumetric template (Pataky et al. 2003) which assumes the body as a collection of parallelepipeds (one for each squared element) of uniform density

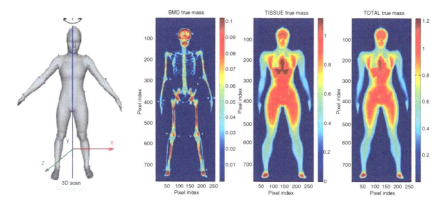

Fig. 14.1 (**a**) 3D body scan, (**b**) dual-energy X-ray absorptiometry scan. Adapted with permission (El-Sallam Abd et al. 2013)

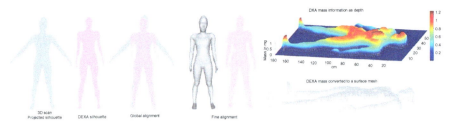

Fig. 14.2 (**a**) Three-dimensional and dual-energy X-ray absorptiometry scan alignment, (**b**) dual-energy X-ray absorptiometry mass information. Reprinted with permission (El-Sallam Abd et al. 2013)

($\rho = 1$ g/cm^3), whose height is computed as shown in Fig. 14.2b. The inertia tensor of the subject is then computed by combining the mass, centre of mass and principal moments of inertia from a sum of each parallelepiped. Importantly, this approach is agnostic to hardware type, and as such, any three-dimensional and dual-energy X-ray absorptiometry scanner can be used to implement the approach.

Humans have been attempting to record and replicate the human form for millennia. Since its introduction in the early 1960s, three-dimensional body scanning technology has materialised vast applications ranging from computer games and animation to virtual fitting and design applications. Methods employed to record and reconstruct the three-dimensional body scan most commonly fall into three broad categories: displacement (e.g. single-point laser), profile (e.g. projected laser) and snapshot (e.g. structured light, photogrammetry). The adoption of three-dimensional body scans over manual anthropometry measurement removes any likelihood of tester bias, allows for large quantities of scans to be recorded and interpreted in a short period of time and, importantly, requires limited operator training (relative to manual method training and accreditation which is time-consuming and labour intensive). Historical constraints associated with three-dimensional body scanning have primarily centred upon the cost of the hardware. However, new technologies are now opening up this avenue for kinanthropometrists and general consumers alike. One pertinent example is that of Microsoft's Kinect—a motion sensor add-on distributed with the Xbox 360 gaming console. Kinect V2 has replaced the Kinect V1 laser scanner/projector in combination with a time-of-flight sensor. Research reports that both sensors demonstrate high accuracy (<2 mm) and precision (mean point to plane error <2 mm) at an average resolution of at least 390 points per cm^2 (Pöhlmann et al. 2016).

Also emerging in this space are turnkey three-dimensional scanning systems that will soon proliferate the consumer market. Examples include a home three-dimensional scanner embedded in a mirror with weight sensor by https://naked.fit/ and a similar Kinect-based home turntable system by http://www.styku.com/. While both commercial examples have yet to be fully released at the time of writing and therefore have not undergone independent validity and reliability testing, manufacturer claims of 2.54 mm depth map accuracy and ±2.5% body fat calculation accuracy in the case of Naked, and Styku claims of 76% more precise measurements than most skilled hand-measuring experts, are impressive results for home-based scanning systems.

What is likely to have the greatest impact on this sector looking forward will be the leveraging of artificial intelligence techniques on the existing body shape and composition databases that already exist. A prime use case is the prediction of three-dimensional avatars from two-dimensional images by https://www.bodylabs.com/ who utilise machine learning deep neural networks to accurately compute the pose and shape of people from a single two-dimensional image or video. Products are based upon the work from leading computer vision research groups worldwide, and a large research portal can be found on the site https://www.bodylabs.com/resources/read/. The companies listed here are just a few examples of many who are currently invested in revolutionising the physique assessment landscape.

14.4   How Do You Use the Selected Technique for Your Athlete?

The merged three-dimensional/dual-energy X-ray absorptiometry scan technique outlined above requires the athlete to be present for dual scan time of 30–40 min. For three-dimensional scanning, the athlete should stand in an A-pose (palms facing the side of the body) such that adequate under arm and between legs coverage is obtained (see Fig. 14.3). During the dual-energy X-ray absorptiometry scan, the operator should position the athlete's arms as close towards an A-pose as possible while remaining within the scanning table. Ideally, the posture during the three-dimensional and dual-energy X-ray absorptiometry scans should be as close as possible to minimise the error associated with deforming the three-dimensional scan during the registration process. The scan dual registration in custom Matlab code requires <5 min of run time, and all desired subject-specific outputs are auto-generated upon completion.

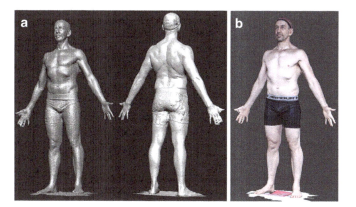

Fig. 14.3 (**a**) Multiview of an initial 3D stereophotogrammetric scan using Logemas Pty Ltd CapJaq scanner. (**b**) Resulting 3D scan with final colour and course textures added

14.5   What Is the Technique Used to Measure?

In addition to subject-specific total body mass and centre of mass location, segment girth (entire segment length), segment length, segment mass and segment centre of mass location can be obtained using the three-dimensional/dual-energy X-ray absorptiometry scan technique.

14.6   How Do You Report the Data to Your Athlete and Coach?

Relevant data is transferred into musculoskeletal modelling pipelines with any physique variables requested by the athlete or coach passed to them privately.

14.7   Summary

Three-dimensional body scanning systems integrated with other imaging modalities to create multi-faceted digital human profiles, and artificial intelligence techniques such as deep learning and artificial neural networks, are set to revolutionise the physique assessment landscape over the coming decade. Using computer vision techniques, it is now possible to register an individual's dual-energy X-ray absorptiometry-derived body composition with the mesh exported by the same individual's three-dimensional body scan.

References

El-Sallam Abd A, Bennamoun M, Sohel F, Alderson JA, Lyttle AD, Rossi M (2013) A low cost 3D markerless system for the reconstruction of athletic techniques. Paper presented at the IEEE Workshop on Applications of Computer Vision (WACV), USA

Kuehnapfel A, Ahnert P, Loeffler M, Scholz M (2017) Body surface assessment with 3D laser-based anthropometry: reliability, validation, and improvement of empirical surface formulae. Eur J Appl Physiol 117(2):371–380

Lands LC, Hornby L, Hohenkerk JM, Glorieux FH (1996) Accuracy of measurements of small changes in soft-tissue mass by dual-energy x-ray absorptiometry. Clin Invest Med 19(4):279–285

Pataky TC, Zatsiorsky VM, Challis JH (2003) A simple method to determine body segment masses in vivo: reliability, accuracy and sensitivity analysis. Clin Biomech 18(4):364–368

Pöhlmann S, Harkness E, Taylor C, Astley S (2016) Journal of Medical and Biological Engineering. valuation of Kinect 3D Sensor for Healthcare. Imaging 36:857

Rossi M, Lyttle A, El-Sallam A, Benjanuvatra N, Blanksby B (2013) Body segment inertial parameters of elite swimmers using DXA and indirect methods. J Sports Sci Med 12(4):761–775

Rossi MM, Alderson J, El-Sallam A, Dowling J, Reinbolt J, Donnelly CJ (2016) A new validation technique for estimations of body segment inertia tensors: principal axes of inertia do matter. J Biomech 49(16):4119–4123

Winby CR, Lloyd DG, Kirk TB (2008) Evaluation of different analytical methods for subject-specific scaling of musculotendon parameters. J Biomech 41(8):1682–1688

Part III

Application of Physique Assessment in Athletes

Is a body type more suitable to a particular sport? How can you predict whether a child might be good at a sport based on their physique? What normative data are there to compare results of your collected data? Does assessment of physique cause anxiety in athletes? How can you gain training and accreditation in body physique techniques? These are some of the many questions raised by practitioners and the reason why part III of the book focuses on applications of physique assessment in athletes. Chapters provide information on physique assessment in practice, large-scale sampling of athletes, body image for athletes, anthropometry profiles for types of sport, and training and accreditation systems.

Chapter 15
Physique Assessment in Practice

Kagan J. Ducker, Deborah A. Kerr, and Patria A. Hume

Abstract Physique assessment provides valuable information to the athlete and coach. However, taken in isolation physique assessment can easily be misinterpreted or misused. Additional information, such as the dietary intake and training load, and input from exercise and health professionals are required to fully interpret the findings and make recommendations. Strengths and limitations of methods of physique assessment are outlined, along with best practice approaches to collection and reporting of data.

Keywords Physique • Assessment • Best practice • Interpretation • Dietary intake Training load • Longitudinal data

15.1   Introduction

Physique assessment provides valuable information to the athlete and coach. However, taken in isolation physique assessment can easily be misinterpreted or misused. Additional information, such as the dietary intake and training load, and input from exercise and health professionals are required to fully interpret the findings and

K.J. Ducker (✉)
Curtin University, Perth, Australia
e-mail: kagan.ducker@curtin.edu.au

D.A. Kerr
School of Public Health, Curtin University, Perth, West Australia, Australia
e-mail: D.Kerr@curtin.edu.au

P.A. Hume
Sport Performance Research Institute New Zealand,
Auckland University of Technology, Auckland, New Zealand
e-mail: patria.hume@aut.ac.nz

© Springer Nature Singapore Pte Ltd. 2018   179
P.A. Hume et al. (eds.), *Best Practice Protocols for Physique Assessment in Sport*,
https://doi.org/10.1007/978-981-10-5418-1_15

to make recommendations. Other health professionals that may need to be consulted to provide further information include the coach, sports physician, sports dietitian, sports physiologist, sports psychologist and strength and conditioning coach.

Physique status will be influenced by factors including genetics, diet, training load and physique requirements for the sport or event that the athlete is competing in. It's important to remember that physique assessment provides information on one aspect of athlete performance, and ideally interpretation should be based on longitudinal data rather than one single measurement. As there is considerable individual variation in physique, cross-sectional comparisons between athletes are not recommended. By having their physique assessed, the individual will have an accurate assessment and objective measure of their current physique status. If the individual is wanting to change their physique, this may provide the necessary motivation for the person.

This chapter will focus on the interpretation of physique assessment in the individual athlete and additional information required to fully interpret the data. It will also include the strengths and limitations of each of these methods.

15.2   Why Measure Physique Status in Relation to Performance, Health Status and Diet?

Prior to conducting physique assessment, the health professional needs to identify the reason for assessing physique in the first place. Too often data are collected without a real understanding of the reason why it is being collected or how to interpret the findings. More importantly, without a clear rationale for undertaking physique assessment, methods may be overused or incorrectly interpreted. This has important cost and resource implications for all concerned. The main goals of physique assessment are to:

- Provide an objective measure of physique status in relation to performance, health status and diet.
- Identify athletes who require additional support to restore or maintain physique status (e.g. at-risk athletes who have lost or gained weight rapidly).
- Monitor the progress of athletes in meeting their physique goals (e.g. strength and conditioning goals to increase muscle mass).
- Monitor the growth of young athletes.

15.3   Optimising Physique for Sporting Performance

Knowledge of the sport and event that the athlete is competing in is important as some sports or events have greater tolerance to physique differences than others. It's important to remember that physique is only one aspect of performance. Whilst in some sports there is a distinct competitive advantage to lower levels of body fat (e.g.

aesthetic, weight bearing and weight class sports), how the athlete achieves this needs to be considered. This is particularly of concern as an energy deficit that could result from maintaining a low fat mass or altering body composition could lead to increased prevalence of relative energy deficiency in sport (RED-S), particularly in females. Relative energy deficiency in sport can have widespread effects on metabolic rate, protein synthesis, menstrual function, bone health, immunity and cardiovascular health (Mountjoy et al. 2014). It is often noted by health practitioners that athletes will start to have a higher incidence of flu-like symptoms, general fatigue and reduced exercise performance when they are aiming to lean down to extremes. It is important to identify the individuals' response so that this optimal body composition is maintained and not surpassed.

15.4 Factors to Consider When Choosing a Physique Assessment Technique

There is no perfect method for assessing physique, and it is critical to consider how the method is going to be applied. All methods have their own advantages and disadvantages as has been outlined in the previous chapters (see Table 15.1 for a summary). It is important to have a clear rationale for why physique is being assessed. The selection of a suitable method for research purposes may be quite different to the method used for individual monitoring by a health professional. Some methods are more portable and suitable for use in the field, such as anthropometry, whilst other more accurate methods such as dual-energy X-ray absorptiometry (DXA) are laboratory based but may not be suitable for some individuals. For example, DXA has a radiation dose associated with it, and although this dose is considered small, this method cannot be used in women that may be or are pregnant.

Being clear on the question will guide the technique chosen, for example, if the purpose is purely to assess body size and shape, techniques such as anthropometry or three-dimensional photonic scanning may be sufficient, whereas if the purpose is to assess or monitor changes in body composition (adipose tissue, muscle mass), there may be more choices of techniques to use.

One of the key considerations will be what options for physique assessment are available, as, practically speaking, this will often be a constraining factor in the decision. Whilst it may be tempting to find the latest and often most expensive technique, for regular monitoring there is usually not enough benefit to offset the costs for using these tools. In an applied sport setting, consider the ability of the technique to measure the variables wanted, with the precision required to detect meaningful change. In practice, a laboratory method (e.g. DXA, air displacement plethysmography—Bod Pod) could be considered as a relatively accurate assessment of body composition to be used occasionally (i.e. annually). Concurrent anthropometric assessment by a certified (i.e. ISAK accredited) anthropometrist will provide a benchmark to allow tracking of changes in body composition more regularly

Table 15.1 Summary of factors to consider when choosing a physique assessment technique

Technique	Advantages	Disadvantages	Best used for
Surface anthropometry	• Portable and robust • Relatively cheap equipment and training • Can easily compare to normative data	• Requires a skilled and certified (ISAK) anthropometrist • Prediction equations are often inaccurate—typically better to have multiple measures over time to assess change rather than absolute values	• Tracking change in physique over time • Assessing body size and shape
Air displacement plethysmography (Bod Pod)	• Accurate and quick assessment of body volume and density • Similar technique to underwater weighing but less downsides	• Relies on suitable room to house unit • Sensitive to participant attire, body hair and moisture on the skin • Often under predicts body fat in an athletic population	• Assessing body density and volume
3D scanning	• Quick scan times • Can assess surface area • Can potentially assess segment lengths	• Sensitive to participant attire and body hair	• Assessing body shape, surface area and volume • Ergonomics and textiles • Assessing large sample sizes
Bioelectrical impedance	• Cheap, quick and widely available	• Relies on participant preparation, e.g. standard hydration status • Body composition often estimated based on unknown regression equations	• Assessing body composition where low cost, easy access and low operator skill are the priorities
Dual-energy X-ray absorptiometry (DXA)	• Allows for the assessment of bone health • Allows for assessment of regional composition • Fast and easy for participant	• Small dose of radiation—can cause access issues • Often small bed sizes • Cannot be used on women who are or may be pregnant	• Assessing bone health • Whole and regional body composition
Ultrasound	• Similar to surface anthropometry but with more objective measures • Can assess greater skin and subcutaneous tissue thickness than anthropometry	• Relatively new and not yet fully validated • Requires significant operator training	• Assessing subcutaneous fat • Tracking change over time

(continued)

Table 15.1 (continued)

Technique	Advantages	Disadvantages	Best used for
Computed tomography and magnetic resonance imaging	• Very accurate • Magnetic resonance imaging has no radiation • Ability to assess visceral composition	• Cost and access is limited • Computed tomography has a relatively large radiation dose • Relatively long scan times	• Research where high accuracy and the ability to assess visceral composition are the priorities

between the laboratory assessments. Anthropometry has the advantage of being a relatively cheap, safe, non-invasive, portable and accurate method of tracking changes in physique in athletes.

A factor that can influence the choice of method is the availability of suitable normative data, particularly if this will be the first assessment of an athlete. Considerable anthropometric normative data is available on elite-level athletes for some sports (Carter and Ackland 1994; Ackland et al. 2003; Ong et al. 2005; Keogh et al. 2007; Kerr et al. 2007; Ridge et al. 2007; Makhter et al. 2008). There is limited normative data on athletes for laboratory methods, and the values obtained (e.g. % fat) are not directly comparable between methods. If the purpose is to monitor changes over time, then the lack of normative data may be less of an issue for data interpretation.

15.5 Best Practice Approaches to Data Collection

When collecting any data, best practice to standardise procedures should be followed, such as following a standard protocol. These approaches have been outlined in other chapters.

Preparing the athlete for physique assessment should follow the guidelines as outlined in Chap. 5 (Athlete Considerations for Physique Measurement) and includes factors such as considering if fasting is required and standardising hydration status. The purpose of physique assessment and the potential benefits to exercise performance should also be discussed with the athlete prior to the measurements. Athletes, particularly those in weight-sensitive sports, may not be completely comfortable with having their physique assessed (Sundgot-Borgen et al. 2013). This can be related to body image issues, eating disorders or pressure to meet unrealistic body composition goals. The paper by Sundgot-Borgen et al. (2013) provides a comprehensive discussion on the complex issues with weight-sensitive sports. It is important that health professionals undertaking the physique assessment are sensitive to these issues and respond appropriately to potential issues when measuring athletes. If there is concern that physique assessment is stressful for the athlete, then a review of the need to undertake physique assessment and the frequency of measurements should be considered.

15.5.1   Consent and Confidentiality

Practitioners should ensure that the requirements of the assessments planned are explained, including why they are being completed, the benefits and risks of the procedures and who will have access to the data, prior to obtaining verbal or preferably written consent from each athlete. Ideally this would occur on each testing occasion; however, a more practical solution may be to obtain an ongoing consent for the tests that are commonly completed, with a regular review process. This consent should include details about who has access to the results. Even if written or verbal consent has been obtained previously, it is considered good practice to always request verbal consent from the athlete prior to starting any physique assessments, particularly if the measures require you to touch them in any way. When working with underage athletes, the consent of their parents and considerations for having a chaperone with the athlete should also be considered.

To assist with maintaining confidentiality, the assessment area should be private. This can be difficult in a team environment where there are often a lot of athletes to be measured in a short space of time. This scenario is not ideal as it becomes more difficult to maintain confidentiality. Athletes are by nature competitive, so this can put extra pressure on an athlete when their data is not kept confidential. Ideally you should put protocols in place that will ensure the data is kept confidential and body composition assessment takes place in a separate room from general club or organisation duties where possible.

15.5.2   Cultural, Gender and Para-Sport Issues

Cultural and gender issues that may be encountered whilst assessing physique should be considered. All athletes should have the option to access a similar sex anthropometrist and a private area where possible. Thought should be given to cultural issues with exposing, touching or marking parts of the body. For example, the Maori people of New Zealand regard their head as sacred, and so the measurer should avoid touching their head unless invited to do so. People of the Muslim faith may require someone of the same gender to assess them, and when landmarking for anthropometric assessment, they will likely object to having a cross drawn on them for religious reasons. Instead a dot with a circle around can be used to mark a skinfold site.

Working with para-sport athletes can present some unique challenges to assessing physique, and little information has been published in this sector. The interindividual differences in body shape and function should be considered when deciding what, if any, techniques are appropriate. For example, when working with amputee athletes, they may not have limbs on the right side of their body to conduct anthropometric assessments. In this situation the left side could be utilised for ongoing tracking in that athlete, or any measurements on that limb could be excluded from their test battery. In most cases it would be prudent to only use a para-athlete's results to track progress longitudinally as opposed to making comparisons to other athletes. Considering issues such as these will ensure that athletes feel safe and comfortable when having their physique assessed.

15.6 Best Practice Approaches to Reporting Results

Basic interpretation of results uses comparison with normative data. Typically for an athlete, this will mean comparing them to averages reported in other athletes from the same sport and age category or by benchmarking them against mean data from the most elite athletes in that sport. You can refer to results from large-scale athlete surveys that occur occasionally to determine if your sport has been surveyed (Carter and Ackland 1994; Ackland et al. 2003; Ong et al. 2005; Keogh et al. 2007; Kerr et al. 2007; Ridge et al. 2007; Makhter et al. 2008), or you could refer to the current literature where the physique of similar athletes has been assessed as part of the study protocols. Some textbooks contain sections on physique, which often contain data sets that are amalgamated from multiple sources to provide quality normative data based on years of data collection (Ackland et al. 2009; Slater et al. 2013).

Comparing athletes' physiques is not recommended for reasons already outlined. However, if comparisons are made between athletes' results, the concept of proportionality should be considered. Many physique assessment techniques are absolute in their nature; however, we need to consider how a variable measured on one athlete compares to that same measurement on another athlete. Consider the situation of determining which rower has a proportionally larger flexed arm girth. There are several different ways to assess proportionality, but one of the simplest methods is by scaling variables, usually by using a standard height (typically 170.18 cm). By considering proportionality, you are evening the playing field between your athletes so that you are better able to make comparisons. For example, we can calculate corrected flexed arm girths for two rowers to assess proportionality:

- Athlete 1 is 195 cm tall and has a flexed arm girth of 36.5 cm; therefore, the corrected flexed arm girth is 36.5 × (170.18/195) = 31.9 cm.
- Athlete 2 is 185 cm tall and has a flexed arm girth of 35 cm; therefore, the corrected flexed arm girth is 35 × (170.18/185) = 32.2 cm.

The first time an athlete is measured, comparisons to normative data will likely be the only comparisons that can be made to interpret your data. However, regular ongoing data collection will provide insights into what is the optimal physique for each athlete, and their results can be tracked over time rather than simply interpreting absolute values. This allows for individual variability in physique and rates of adaptation or change to be taken into account.

Reporting back to athletes should happen as soon as it is appropriate. Importantly, the report should be completed in such a way that athletes and support staff can understand the results and how they may affect training and competition performance. Using easy to understand metrics, such as comparisons to normative data, somatotypes and ratios, may help an athlete to understand their results. The inclusion of a brief explanation about the meaningfulness of the results in the context of that athletes' sport is also often appreciated and may encourage the athletes to more actively engage with the measures and what they can do to impact them.

How and when the results of physique assessments are distributed should be carefully considered prior to discussing them with the athlete or support staff. As a general rule, the athlete should be considered the owner of their results as they may have reasons for not wanting to disclose certain information to the wider support team. Under no circumstances should the results be made public by posting them in a public area or by sharing them inappropriately around other athletes or the support team. This practice has the potential to cause a great deal of undue stress, anxiety and ongoing compliance issues with your athletes. Keep in mind that athletes may not see their results in a positive way, and this can increase their level of anxiety. In addition, physique assessment should not be used as a means for selection as this does not take into account individual variability or other aspects of performance.

It is important to understand that the physique data that are collected are confidential. Outside of the formal processes of research institutions and ethical approval processes, you should consider the requirements for the safe and secure storage of confidential records. In most cases the storage of electronic copies in a password-protected and regularly backed up computer is considered suitable, whilst all hard copies should be stored in locked storage. A record of who has access to these files should also be kept.

In many programs it is common practice to obtain prior consent from the athlete to release their results to support staff (usually the coach/s, sports scientists and sports nutritionists). This process can often be beneficial to the athlete as the support staff can give guidance about when the athlete should receive feedback and what feedback will be beneficial. For example, physique assessment may be undertaken in the lead up to major competitions as a record of a peak in the athletes' physical preparation. If the athlete returns a result that is less than ideal, do they really need to know the results ahead of the competition? This could negatively impact their perception of their preparation and affect their subsequent performance. In this case it may be prudent to wait until the competition review to report the results back. In contrast, good results could be used as positive reinforcement for an athlete to support the assertion that they are ready to perform at a competition.

15.7 Frequency of Physique Assessment

As with any testing battery, the assessment of physique should be built into an athlete's larger training and competition calendar at times when benchmarking tests are completed and more importantly before and after periods when you may actively target changes in body composition as a training goal. There is likely to be a benefit in regularly obtaining a set of measures to track an athlete's progress as this allows you to track body composition changes over time relative to what is normal for each athlete rather than having to compare them to normative data. It also means that if an athlete has their body composition change in an unexpected way, you have a relatively recent record of what is normal for them. This change may be caused by a relative energy deficit, medical issues or because of some adaptive process that is being targeted by training (e.g. muscular hypertrophy).

In practice you will need to determine what is required for your program and individual athletes. In sports where body composition is less important for training and competition performance, or for individuals that fluctuate less, this may be relatively infrequent (i.e. every 3–6 months). However, with programmes where body composition is important (e.g. aesthetic, weight bearing and weight class sports) or with athletes that are actively making adjustments to their body composition, this may be more frequent (i.e. fortnightly to monthly). If you require regular measurements, you should consider the time frame that you expect a change to occur over and your ability to track meaningful change. It will be vital that you know your technical error of measurement (TEM) and confidence intervals to ensure that you can tell the difference between normal fluctuations in the measure and any real change.

15.8 Identifying Athletes Who Require Additional Support to Restore or Maintain Physique Status

As with much of the data we collect as health professionals, there is considerable value in considering the results of a physique assessment in the broader context of the athletes' current training load, goals, diet and health, since it is the interaction of these factors that will guide the interpretation. This may be achieved by simply talking with the athlete about their training, competition, health and personal life or may necessitate having a broader discussion with coaching, medical, sport science and sports nutrition staff to gain an overall insight into the factors currently affecting them. This highlights the importance of working inter-professionally to achieve the best outcome for athletes. During an assessment you may identify athletes who require additional support to restore or maintain physique status (e.g. at-risk athletes who have lost or gained weight rapidly).

Physique assessment can be an important screening tool for identifying issues indicating the need for further follow-up. Monitoring physique (specifically adipose tissue and muscle mass) will indicate when changes in the energy balance of the body have occurred. In healthy individuals, this reflects either a change in diet, a change in physical activity or both. By undertaking regular monitoring of physique, the healthcare practitioner will readily be able to identify changes in energy balance in both health and disease and help identify the need for further follow-up. For example, if an athlete is losing weight too quickly, this may indicate an underlying problem that needs further investigation by other health or medical professionals. The sports dietitian should be consulted to ensure that the athlete's diet meets their current energy usage requirements. This will also mean that you will need to consult the sports physiologist, coach and strength and conditioning coach to ensure that you are aware of the training load that is currently being prescribed to the athlete. As part of this discussion, you should consider environmental factors such as exercise in the heat or cold and travel to high altitudes or use of hypoxic environments, as these factors may affect body composition. It will also be worth consulting your athlete's sports physician or physiotherapist as they may have identified medical or injury issues that could explain changes in body composition. If assessing an athlete with injury to the right limbs which are usually measured with surface anthropometry, the left side will need to be measured instead, with notes made of the change in limb side.

You must consider that for an equal level of training history, athletes may have quite different physiques. This will impact what physique they naturally have, the body composition where they will be the healthiest and where they will perform the best. You will also find that the physique of athletes may respond to changes in training and diet differently. There is a significant component of our body composition that is hereditary, which will mean that our normal level of body fat, or lean tissue, relates to genetic factors, and how these factors change given a perturbation (i.e. training or changes to energy balance) will be different between people (Bouret et al. 2015). These factors need to be considered when interpreting changes in physique in athletes.

15.9 Summary

Physique assessment needs to be interpreted in conjunction with information on dietary intake and training load. The health professional needs to identify the reason for assessing physique. Knowledge of the sport and event that the athlete is competing in is important as some sports or events have greater tolerance to physique differences than others. Best practice techniques to assess physique need to be followed including consent of the athletes and confidentiality of results. It is important to consider cultural and gender issues that may be encountered whilst assessing physique. The timing for assessment of physique needs to be built into an athlete's training and competition calendar before and after periods when changes in body composition as a training goal are indicated.

References

Ackland TR, Ong KB, Kerr DA, Ridge BR (2003) Morphological characteristics of Olympic sprint canoe and kayak paddlers. J Sci Med Sport 6(3):285–294

Ackland TR, Elliot B, Bloomfield J (2009) Applied anatomy and biomechanics in sport, 2nd edn. Human Kinetics, Champaign, IL

Bouret S, Levin BE, Ozanne SE (2015) Gene environment interactions controlling energy and glucose homeostasis and the developmental origins of obesity. Physiol Rev 95(1):47–82

Carter JEL, Ackland TR (1994) Kinanthropometry in aquatic sports – a study of world class athletes. Human Kinetics, Champaign, IL

Keogh JWL, Hume PA, Pearson SN, Mellow P (2007) Anthropometric dimensions of male powerlifters of varying body mass. J Sports Sci 25(12):1365–1376

Kerr DA, Ross WD, Norton K, Hume P, Kagawa M, Ackland TR (2007) Olympic lightweight and open-class rowers possess distinctive physical and proportionality characteristics. J Sports Sci 25(1):43–45

Makhter R, Hume PA, Zakaria AZ, Mohd AM, Razali MR, Png W, Aziz AR (2008) Absolute size characteristics differences between 'best' and 'rest' world badminton players. In: Sport for all conference, Malaysia

Mountjoy M, Sundgot-Borgen J, Burke L, Carter S, Constantini N, Lebrun C et al (2014) The IOC consensus statement: beyond the female athlete triad – relative energy deficiency in sport (RED-S). Br J Sports Med 48:491–497

Ong K, Ackland T, Hume PA, Ridge B, Broad E, Kerr D (2005) Equipment set-up among Olympic sprint and slalom kayak paddlers. Sports Biomech 4(1):47–58

Ridge BR, Broad E, Kerr DA, Ackland TR (2007) Morphological characteristics of Olympic slalom canoe and kayak paddlers. Eur J Sport Sci 7(2):107–111

Slater GJ, Woolford SM, Marfell-Jones MJ (2013) Assessment of physique. In: Tanner RK, Gore CJ (eds) Physiological tests for elite athlete, 2nd edn. Human Kinetics, Champaign, IL

Sundgot-Borgen J, Meyer NL, Lohman TG et al (2013) How to minimize risks for athletes in weight-sensitive sports. Br J Sports Med 47:1012–1022

Chapter 16
Recommendations for Conducting Research on Athletes (Large-Scale Survey Case Studies)

Deborah A. Kerr, Patria A. Hume, and Timothy R. Ackland

Abstract Large-scale surveys of world-class athletes have been conducted at Olympic Games and World Championship events for over 60 years. These projects have provided valuable data for identifying the unique physique characteristics for sports and events. There are many challenges in undertaking these studies, and strong scientific rigour should always underpin such projects. Large-scale surveys of athletes should be conducted to address specific questions, rather than being an opportunistic data collection exercise. Considerable planning needs to go into a large-scale survey to ensure its success, including obtaining all the necessary approvals and support to conduct the project. This chapter outlines the practical steps in the process, including what should be in the research proposal, how to conduct large-scale surveys and how to report the results of the information gained.

Keywords Large-scale surveys • Olympic Games • World Championship Physique • Scientific rigour • Questions • Planning • Practical steps • Research Reporting • Feasibility • Equipment • Venue • Recruitment • Promotion • Media Budget • Funding • Data checking • Publishing

D.A. Kerr (✉)
School of Public Health, Curtin University, Perth, West Australia, Australia
e-mail: D.Kerr@curtin.edu.au

P.A. Hume
Sport Performance Research Institute New Zealand,
Auckland University of Technology, Auckland, New Zealand
e-mail: patria.hume@aut.ac.nz

T.R. Ackland
School of Sport Science, Exercise and Health, The University of Western Australia,
Crawley, WA 6009, Australia
e-mail: tim.ackland@uwa.edu.au

© Springer Nature Singapore Pte Ltd. 2018
P.A. Hume et al. (eds.), *Best Practice Protocols for Physique Assessment in Sport*,
https://doi.org/10.1007/978-981-10-5418-1_16

191

16.1 Why Do You Want to Conduct a Large-Scale Survey?

16.1.1 Opportunity and Addressing the Research Question

Historically, the impetus for conducting large-scale surveys has been mostly opportunistic, where a unique occasion presents for researchers to collect data on a quality sample in one place and at one time. However, it is very easy to fall into the trap of collecting large amounts of data on athletes without starting with a good research question that will ensure the data are useful and will ultimately make a difference to sports performance. For example, is the particular sport or event lacking recent normative data, or is it a sport where there are clear links between physique and performance? If the question requires measurements on the best performing athletes, then you must ask if the event opportunity will provide this quality sample. World Championships may provide more events and superior quality competitors than an Olympic Games, where the number of events may be restricted in some sports and the top athletes may not be present due to restrictions placed on the permitted number of national representatives. For those who are starting out in research on physique assessment, it is important to seek advice from more experienced researchers to help refine the research question and write a compelling research proposal.

16.1.2 Feasibility

A well-designed study also needs to consider how feasible the project will be. First, consider how easy it will be to access the athletes prior to competition. Will the athletes be in one place and at one time? Contacting sporting officials to find out background information early will help guide how feasible it will be to conduct the study. Allowing sufficient time is important with the realisation that it takes several years of planning to put everything in place prior to an event.

Olympic Games can be difficult as athletes may train in other countries prior to arriving at the games venue. There may not be sufficient time to conduct the survey prior to their event starting. Data collection needs to be completed prior to the games commencing as obtaining accreditation for the research team during the Olympics can be challenging as these are often restricted in number. Athletes may be unwilling to participate once competition commences. At the time of publication of this book, the International Olympic Committee (IOC) has withdrawn support for all research during both summer and winter games that involves an athlete's physical participation in data collection during the games themselves.

It is also tempting to collect more data than needed. This is where having a strong research question will ensure the research is focused, and only data required to answer the research question are collected. By being focused, this will ensure the time for data collection is kept to a minimum. From our experience, we aim to collect all individual data in less than 45 min.

16.2   What Is a Large-Scale Survey?

There are no recommended minimum participant numbers for a survey to be considered large; however, surveys with over 100 participants could be considered a starting point. The nature of the data collection for large-scale surveys is often complex; therefore, attention to detail in planning is required.

16.2.1   Research Proposal

Having defined the research question, the next step is to write a research proposal. A proposal is needed for most institutional ethics applications and will require details of the recruitment process, protocols and methods of data collection to be used. Table 16.1 contains a checklist of items to consider when planning a large-scale survey. Consideration of these items needs to be thorough and achieved well in advance of the intended date of data collection.

16.3   How Do You Conduct Large-Scale Surveys for Athletes?

There are many factors that need to be addressed when designing how the survey will be conducted. This section provides advice on key factors.

16.3.1   Consent to Conduct Measurements: Ethics Approval

Athletes must derive benefit from the study rather than being 'experimented on' for an 'interesting to know' approach to the research question. It is now the case that institutional ethics committees will not give approval unless there is a focused research question demonstrating a clear benefit to the athlete participating in the research. The ethics committee will consider the time commitment for the athletes, safety aspects such as exposure to ionising radiation with dual energy X-ray absorptiometry and information provided in the informed consent documentation. Approval for incentives provided to athletes may vary from country to country. In some countries, ethics committees will only allow reimbursement for an athlete's time, so the incentive needs to be appropriate to the time commitment. Incentives could include athlete appropriate gifts such as water bottles, caps or towels with the study logo. For example, in the Sydney 2000 Olympic Games Project (Kerr et al. 2007; Ong et al. 2005; Ackland et al. 2003), athletes were offered breakfast cereal as an incentive to participate.

Table 16.1 Checklist for conducting large-scale surveys in physique assessment

Topic	Checklist
Opportunity	– What is the opportunity to measure? – Is the sport or event lacking in recent normative data? – How easy will it be to access the athletes? – Will the athletes be in one place at one time? – Is there sufficient time to put everything in place prior to the event?
Research question	– What is the research question you want to answer? – Will answering this question contribute to improving the sport and sporting performance (i.e. what is the impact)? – What is the quality of the sample (e.g. national, world-class competitors)? – Have you written a research proposal? – Have you sought feedback from experienced researchers regarding the project and the feasibility of the proposed study?
Feasibility	– Is the study feasible in the time available to collect the data? – How long will the data collection take, and is this feasible for individual athletes?
Ethics approval	– Have you obtained ethics approval? – Are there other organisations that you need to seek approval from? – Will you need consent forms translated into several languages? – What incentives or participant reimbursement will you provide?
Permissions	– What permissions are required to conduct the survey (e.g. international and external organisations)? – What are the key organisations you need to contact and seek permission from? – How will you obtain any necessary permits and passes?
Budget	– Will the survey require funding, and is the success of the project dependent on obtaining this funding? – What funding opportunities exist? – Will you seek sponsorship? – If you seek sponsorship, is this sponsorship ethical and appropriate? – Will you need to employ research staff or pay honorariums (e.g. Level 4 criterion anthropometrists)? – Will there be travel costs (e.g. airfares, accommodation and transport)? – What consumables are needed? – Is there equipment you will need to purchase or lease? – Will you provide catering for research staff? – Will research staff wear a uniform? – Have you budgeted for athlete incentives and gifts (e.g. water bottles)?
Equipment	– What equipment is needed to conduct the study? – Has the equipment been calibrated?

(continued)

Table 16.1 (continued)

Topic	Checklist
Research staff	– Do you have research staff/students available and willing to take part in the data collection? – What size of research team will you need to ensure data collection occurs efficiently? – What skills/qualifications are required? – Do you need staff who can speak multiple languages? – How will you assign roles before, during and after the data collection phase?
Training	– What training of staff will need to be undertaken prior to the commencement of data collection? – Who will conduct the training? – Does the training address issues of confidentiality of the data and the athletes being assessed?
Recruitment	– How do you intend to recruit the athletes? – How will participant information be delivered to the coach and athletes? – Do you intend to set up a study website? – What incentive/participant reimbursement will you provide?
Promotion	– Do you have a study name and logo? – Do you have a pull up banner for use as a backdrop during interviews? – Do you have a media plan in place to help with recruitment of participants and to disseminate findings after the project is completed? – Have media statements been prepared? – Has a media relations person been appointed? – Think of interesting pictures and statements that the media can use – Ensure the research team are well versed on what they can and cannot say to media – Try to find an athlete who is willing to have their photo taken or be interviewed about the study and the implications for them
Data checking, collation and security	– Have you created a database management system? – What software and protocols do you have in place for rapid data entry? – Do you have a method for checking that the entered data are correct and free of errors? – Have you a plan for dealing with detected systematic measurement errors? – What systems are in place for keeping the data (both physical and electronic) confidential and secure? – What systems are in place to ensure data are regularly backed up?

(continued)

Table 16.1 (continued)

Topic	Checklist
Athlete, coach and organisation reports	– Do you have a plan for rapid reporting of individual results back to the athlete? – What normative data do you have available so that the individual results can be compared to? – Will the reporting of normative data be consistent with ethical guidelines? – Do you have report templates ready to provide summary information back to coaches and sports organisations?
Publishing in journals	– Do you have a publishing agreement in place with the research team covering authorship and access to the data?

16.3.2 Sports Organisation Approvals and Permissions

Start early in obtaining approval for the study as the approval process to access elite athletes at World Championships and Olympic Games may take several years of negotiations. The Sydney 2000 Olympic Games Project received approval from the IOC; however, data could only be collected prior to the commencement of the games. This was only possible because athletes had arrived in Australia before the games to acclimatise to the conditions. There were many challenges as the athletes were spread out across several states in Australia, necessitating the need for two teams, one of which was a mobile team.

16.3.3 Equipment

Create a list of all equipment needed for the study. It may be possible to loan some equipment rather than purchase new equipment. Maintenance of the equipment is very important; particularly with the daily use of anthropometric equipment, the risk of damaging equipment becomes high. Always have extra equipment and a toolkit available should repairs be needed. Calibration of the scales and skinfold calipers will need to be done prior to the study.

16.3.4 Venue Choice and Set-Up

Create a plan for how your athlete will proceed through the data collection. Most large-scale surveys result in athletes attending data collection in groups, so a plan to move athletes from station to station is needed. It may be important to have stations with specific staff trained in the requirements of the station to ensure quality data are collected in a timely fashion for groups of athletes. For example, for an anthropometric project, there may be stations for registration and consent, landmarking, measurement (e.g. skinfolds, girths, breadths, lengths, height/weight) and data checking, with those anthropometrists having better technical error of measurement on particular measurement stations. Ideally, there should also be an additional person to marshal athletes to stations that are free. In previous anthropometric projects, two stations for collecting girth measurements helped ensure rapid data collection that could occur. Trained data recorders should also be considered. It is also ideal to have enough space and good lighting in which to measure. However, often athletes/ coaches dictate where measurements can be done, and therefore measurements in hotel rooms, lobbies and by the poolside have occurred during past surveys.

16.3.5 Research Staff

There are myriad roles for personnel before, during and after the data collection phase. Prior to data collection, the organising and scientific committees must work on all aspects of logistics, human resources, permissions and accreditation, in addition to establishing the methods and protocols and attending to quality assurance matters. During the data collection phase, various personnel will be responsible for recruitment, logistics, equipment, measurement quality, data checking and collation and data security. And finally, there are many tasks to be performed after the event, including the provision of feedback to participants, reporting to event hosts and sport governing bodies as well as preparations for data analysis and publication. Below are some important considerations related to the staff:

- Do you have research staff/students available and willing to take part in the data collection?
- What size of research team will you need to ensure data collection occurs efficiently?
- What skills/qualifications are required by the research staff?
- Do you need research staff who can speak multiple languages?
- How will you assign roles before, during and after the data collection phase?
- Do you need both male and female research staff to conduct the measurements?
- How will research staff be identified by the athletes (e.g. shirts and name badges)?
- How will research staff fund their attendance at the survey data collection sessions?
- Do you have research staff who are 'team players' and good communicators?
- Do you have research staff who can respond well to pressure situations?
- Do you have research staff who are able to work long hours and still remain accurate in data collection and pleasant to athletes and other staff?

16.3.5.1 Training and Quality Assurance of Staff

Training, upskilling and refreshing the measurement team are vital regardless of their prior level of experience. This helps to minimise measurement errors and ensures all personnel use an agreed, standardised methodology. It also provides a good opportunity to discuss other aspects of measurement sessions, such as schedules, health and safety, appropriate clothing, personal hygiene, professionalism and rules related to the provision of informal feedback to participants. Use this opportunity to record the technical error of measurement for all members of the team—an essential reporting element for future publications. In our experience, it is also important to train the data recorders in aspects such as not commenting on the measurements. For the Sydney 2000 Olympic Games Project, the data recorders were all ISAK Level 1 anthropometrists. Further considerations must be addressed in regard to training, as follows:

- What training of staff will need to be undertaken prior to the commencement of data collection?
- Who will conduct the training?
- Where will you train the research staff?
- Will there be training for both those conducting the measurements and for data recorders?
- Does the training address issues of confidentiality of the data and the athletes being assessed?

16.3.6 Recruitment of Athletes and Endorsement by Sports Organisations and Coaches

It is important to gain endorsement by sports organisations and coaches for the study. Without this early support for the study, based on the governing body's ability to see the rationale and benefit of the survey, later recruitment of athletes will be very difficult.

Promotion of the study prior to the data collection phase is paramount to ensure the athletes and coaches are already aware of the project. A study website can be set up where there is an opportunity to register interest in participating or to book an appointment. Letters of invitation can be mailed to the appropriate person for distribution. However, even with the best made plans, the information may not always get to the athletes. So be prepared to put effort into face-to-face recruitment at the venue. Consider setting up a registration system so that athletes can be booked in to ensure a quick and efficient measurement process. 'Word of mouth' promotion of the project is important, so make sure the process is enjoyable for the athlete. Participant incentives can also be very helpful in the recruitment effort.

16.3.7 Promotion and Media

Interest in your project will increase markedly during the data collection phase from many quarters, including the media. Being prepared for the barrage of interest and requests for information allows you to continue collecting data whilst dealing with this added distraction. Here are some useful checklist items to consider:

- Do you have a study name and logo?
- Do you have a pull up banner for use as a backdrop during interviews?
- Have media statements been prepared?
- Has a media relations person been appointed?
- Think of interesting pictures and statements that the media can use.
- Ensure the research team are well versed on what they can and cannot say to the media.
- Try to find an athlete who is willing to have their photo taken or be interviewed about the study and the implications for them.

16.3.8   Budget and Funding

Most large-scale surveys will require funding. Funding success, however, can be difficult as these projects may not fit the criteria or timeline for standard funding applications. Starting the planning early is important, particularly if the success of the project is dependent on obtaining financial support.

Begin by exploring what funding opportunities may exist to support the project. This may include any local government sporting organisations where the project is to take place. For example, in the Kinanthropometry in Aquatic Sports Project (KASP) (Carter and Ackland 1994), the Department for Sport and Recreation in Western Australia provided funding for the project. Sponsorship from companies may also be an avenue for funding. However, consider if the sponsorship is ethical and appropriate, particularly if the sponsorship involves the provision of food or nutritional supplements.

As shown in Table 16.1, there are many potential costs to consider when planning a budget. These include the need to employ research staff, pay honorariums or provide accommodation and meals. Depending on the location of the data collection (e.g. if there are multiple sites over several locations), there may be travel costs to consider. As an example, during the Sydney 2000 Olympic Games Project, there were two data collection teams of approximately six to eight members during the 2-week period prior to the games. In total, the measurement team consisted of approximately 40 volunteers. One team was located in Penrith near the rowing and canoeing venue, whilst the other team was a mobile team that visited several locations across two states where the teams were located for pregames training camps. The budget included car hire, fuel, accommodation and meals for the two teams. Many of the volunteers were students who were prepared to fundraise for their airfares and volunteered their time for the opportunity to take part in the data collection.

Equipment costs may also need to be included in the budget (e.g. a portable stadiometer if a mobile data collection team is to be used). Laptop computers and printers may need to be purchased or leased. Consumable items, such as marker pens, clip boards and hand gel, are needed, and uniforms or a standard polo shirt can be helpful in making the study more visible. Other budget considerations include athlete incentives and small gifts for those participating in the project.

16.4   How Do You Report the Large-Scale Survey Data?

When conducting a large-scale survey, you need to consider how you will report the data to athletes, coaches, sports organisations, media and journals.

16.4.1   Data Checking, Collation and Security

Data checking, collation and security are important aspects of the project and must be pre-planned with particular attention to detail. Much time, energy and expense will have been invested in the project, so the collected data are precious and irreplaceable. These data might be considered valuable to others, so keeping the results confidential and secure from rival athletes and teams, as well as the media, must be a priority in your planning. Several important considerations in this regard include:

- Have you created a database management system?
- What software and protocols do you have in place for rapid data entry?
- Do you have a method for checking that the entered data are correct and free of errors?
- Have you a plan for dealing with detected systematic measurement errors?
- What systems are in place for keeping the data (both physical and electronic) confidential and secure?
- What systems are in place to ensure data are regularly backed up?

16.4.2   Athlete, Coach and Sports Organisation Reporting

Ensuring the athletes receive their individual report in a timely manner is critical. Athletes have often commented that they never received their results following a large survey. This then impacts on their willingness to participate in future studies. It is vital to ensure a system is in place for rapid reporting of results back to the athletes and coaches. Most athletes will want to see how their data compares against others. Therefore, find out what normative data are available for the sport or event. In some circumstances, if comparison data are not available, or they are dated, you might need to create a set of normative data from the (de-identified) information you have collected.

During the Sydney 2000 Olympic Games Project, athletes were surprised that they received their feedback report during the Olympic competition as had been promised. This report showed their individual results compared to the group means and percentiles for their sport and gender. Although athletes and coaches wanted to see the data on their competitors, we did not provide this as it would have been unethical to do so. It is important to provide summary of information to the organisations who supported the study. This will help future collaborative efforts for large-scale surveys, when you are able to show outcomes from the study.

16.4.3   Media Reporting

It is important when presenting results to the media that confidentiality is not breached for the athletes or that any agreements with funding organisations or collaborative sports organisations are revealed. Media can be very helpful in recruiting participants for large-scale surveys and reporting key outcomes of the study to the general public. During the KASP study (Carter and Ackland 1994), we were permitted to access to the onsite media centre, which allowed us to gather competition results, placings and times for use in subsequent publications. When dealing with large events or professional sports, there can be pressure on researchers to release results as soon as possible. Usually it is recommended that a summary of results is made into a press release for distribution once the journal article is published—ensuring that the research has undergone peer review. Researchers have ethical responsibility to report results back to the participants and to the general public where there is heightened interest in the project or if the results have significant impact for the sport and society.

16.4.4   Publishing: Journals and Conferences

We stress highly, the importance of discussion and agreement by members of the team on matters of data ownership and authorship rights. Having a publishing agreement in place before the event is wise, with members of the research team agreeing to rules about data access and covering aspects of authorship for planned publications and presentations. Taking part in data collection alone would not be considered sufficient to gain authorship rights on a paper. Unless this is made clear before the event, unrealistic expectations around authorship may occur. It is important to consider journal statements of authorship contribution that are now required by most journals. For example, to fulfil all of the criteria for authorship for a publication in the journal *Sports Medicine*, every author of the manuscript must have made substantial contributions to all of the following aspects of the work:

- Conception and planning of the work that led to the manuscript or acquisition, analysis and interpretation of the data or both.
- Drafting and/or critical revision of the manuscript for important intellectual content.
- Approval of the final submitted version of the manuscript.

16.5   Examples of Large-Scale Surveys

Several examples of large-scale surveys that relate to the physique of elite sports performers are shown in Table 16.2. This table is not meant to be an exhaustive list; however, it does cover some of the projects we feel added substantially to the body

Table 16.2 Important large-scale surveys of the physique and performance of elite athletes

Project name	Year	Chief investigators	Sample
The Physique of the Olympic Athlete (Tanner 1964)	1960	Tanner JM, Whitehouse RH, Jarman S	137 track and field athletes at the XVII Olympic Games in Rome and a comparison with weight lifters and wrestlers
Genetic and Anthropological Studies of Olympic Athletes (De Garay et al. 1974)	1968	De Garay AL, Levine L, Carter JEL, Hebbelinck M	1265 athletes across multiple sports at the 1968 Mexico Olympic Games
Montreal Olympic Games Anthropological Project (Carter et al. 1982)	1976	Bouchard C, Carter, JEL, Hebbelinck M, Lariviere G, Malina R, Ross WD	487 athletes from 87 countries were measured over a 3-week period before and during competition at the 1976 Montreal Olympic Games
Kinanthropometry in Aquatic Sports (Carter and Ackland 1994)	1991	Carter JEL, Ackland TR, Mazza JC, Ross WD	919 athletes from 52 countries across four sports were measured in 2 weeks on the full ISAK anthropometry profile at the World Swimming Championships in Perth, Australia
Women's World Basketball Championships (Ackland et al. 1997)	1994	Kerr DA, Schreiner AB, Ackland TR	168 basketball players from 14 of the 16 competing teams were stratified according to player position (guards, forwards and centres) and measured on the full ISAK anthropometry profile
World Triathlon Championships (Ackland et al. 1998; Landers et al. 2000)	1997	Landers G, Ackland TR, Blanksby BA, Smith D	71 elite and junior triathletes from 11 nations competing at the 1997 World Triathlon Championships in Perth, Australia, were measured on a battery of 28 anthropometric dimensions
OZ^{2000}Sydney Olympic Games Project (Ackland et al. 2003; Kerr et al. 2007; Ong et al. 2005)	2000	Kerr DA, Ackland TR, Hume PA, Norton K, Ross WD	423 rowing and canoe/kayak athletes were measured on the full ISAK anthropometry profile in the 2 weeks prior to the Sydney 2000 Olympic Games
Oceania Powerlifting Championships, New Zealand (Keogh et al. 2007)	2002	Keogh J, Hume PA, Pearson S, Mellow P, Sheerin K	68 Australasian and Pacific powerlifters (54 males and 14 females) were measured for 42 ISAK anthropometric dimensions during the Oceania Powerlifting Championships and the New Zealand Bench Press Championships

Project name	Year	Chief investigators	Sample
Malaysian World Badminton Championships (Makhter et al. 2008)	2008	Makhter R, Hume PA, Zakaria AZ, Mohd AM, Razali MR, Png W, Aziz AR	109 players from 23 participating countries competing in five events (18 men's singles, 20 women's singles, 25 men's doubles, 29 women's doubles and 17 mixed doubles) were measured for 40 body dimensions according to ISAK at the 2007 Kuala Lumpur Proton-BWF World Championships

of knowledge. Showing great foresight, Dr. James (Jim) Tanner (1964) wrote the following in his foreword to the publication of the first of these large-scale surveys:

> In a sense this book is written for my colleagues of the year 2000. I hope it will appeal to present day athletes, coaches, physical educationalists and sports doctors; that it will stimulate their thoughts, sharpen their criticism and even improve their practice. But especially I hope it will serve as a faithful record of what track and field athletes were like in 1960, so that, looking back from 2000, coaches will be able to see to what extent higher standards are due to physical improvement and to what extent the evolution of techniques of training and performance have modified the relationship between event and body build described here.

16.6 Summary

Large-scale surveys of world-class athletes provided valuable data for identifying the unique physique characteristics for sports and events. Large-scale surveys of athletes should be conducted to address specific questions. Considerable planning needs to go into a large-scale survey to ensure its success.

References

Ackland TR, Schreiner AB, Kerr DA (1997) Absolute size and proportionality characteristics of World Championship female basketball players. J Sports Sci 15(5):485–490

Ackland TR, Blanksby BA, Landers G, Smith D (1998) Anthropometric profiles of elite triathletes. J Sci Med Sport 1(1):52–56

Ackland TR, Ong KB, Kerr DA, Ridge B (2003) Morphological characteristics of Olympic sprint canoe and kayak paddlers. J Sci Med Sport 6(3):285–294

Carter JEL, Ackland TR (1994) Kinanthropometry in Aquatic Sports - A Study of World Class Athletes. Human Kinetics, Champaign, IL

Carter JEL, Ross WD, Aubry SP, Hebbelinck M, Borms J (1982) Physical structure of Olympic athletes. Part 1: the Montreal Olympic Games Anthropological Project. S Karger, Basel

De Garay AL, Levine L, Carter JEL (1974) Genetic and anthropological studies of Olympic athletes. Academic, Cambridge, MA

Keogh JW, Hume PA, Pearson SN, Mellow P (2007) Anthropometric dimensions of male power-lifters of varying body mass. J Sports Sci 25(12):1365–1376

Kerr DA, Ross WD, Norton K, Hume P, Kagawa M, Ackland TR (2007) Olympic lightweight and open-class rowers possess distinctive physical and proportionality characteristics. J Sports Sci 25(1):43–45

Landers GJ, Blanksby BA, Ackland TR, Smith D (2000) Morphology and performance of world championship triathletes. Ann Hum Biol 27(4):387–400

Makhter R, Hume PA, Zakaria AZ, Mohd AM, Razali MR, Png W, Aziz AR (2008) Absolute size characteristics differences between 'best' and 'rest' world badminton players. In: Sport for all conference, Malaysia

Ong K, Ackland T, Hume PA, Ridge B, Broad E, Kerr D (2005) Equipment set-up among Olympic sprint and slalom kayak paddlers. Sports Biomech 4(1):47–58

Tanner JM (1964) The Physique of the Olympic Athlete. George Allen and Unwin Limited

Chapter 17
Physique Characteristics Associated with Athlete Performance

Patria A. Hume

Abstract Profiling of athletes at levels of participation in sport can help determine potential suitability for sport and effectiveness of interventions such as diet and training. As scientists and clinicians, we ask what physique characteristics are important for athletes in the sports we work with to help improve performance or reduce injury risk; what should we measure and monitor? Athletes, and their coaches, often ask how the athletes' physique compares to elite athletes in their sport. Accessing normative data for athletes at levels of participation from development to elite can be difficult. Consideration of secular trends for physique characteristics in normative databases is needed. Where possible current research data should be gained to enable comparisons of physique characteristics for athletes of similar age, gender, ethnicity and sports participation level. This chapter aims to highlight important physique characteristics for selected sports that aim to optimise power and leverage or have a high metabolic demand, based on studies report in recent published literature.

Keywords Physique • Assessment • Best practice • Profile • Talent identification Talent development • Secular trend • Normative data • Participation level Performance

P.A. Hume
Sport Performance Research Institute New Zealand,
Auckland University of Technology, Auckland, New Zealand
e-mail: patria.hume@aut.ac.nz

© Springer Nature Singapore Pte Ltd. 2018
P.A. Hume et al. (eds.), *Best Practice Protocols for Physique Assessment in Sport*,
https://doi.org/10.1007/978-981-10-5418-1_17

17.1 Introduction

Anticipating adult morphology in the growing child (morphological prediction) has implications for athlete talent identification and development for sports performance (Hume and Stewart 2012). During growth, segment breadths are most useful for predictive purposes because they remain stable in relation to stature throughout adolescence. By contrast, changes in soft tissue for maximum functional effectiveness (morphological prototype) respond to training. Alignment of morphology to performance, and recognition of the wide individual variability in maturation rate, helps avoid biasing athlete selection or overlooking individuals with athletic potential.

Physique assessment (e.g. body composition, proportionality) is only one indicator of an athlete's suitability to perform at a high level and must be combined with other capacities such as strength and power, flexibility, posture, speed, agility, level of skill, cardiovascular fitness and psychological profile. Many sports share a common influence of the pressure for leanness, minimising fat levels and optimising power to weight ratio. Profiling of athletes at levels of participation in sport can help determine potential suitability for sport and effectiveness of interventions such as diet and training. Optimum equipment set-up for sports usually needs to take into account absolute size and proportionality characteristics of the athlete.

Athletes, and their coaches, often ask how the athletes' physique compares to elite athletes in their sport. Accessing normative data for athletes at levels of participation from development to elite can be difficult. Large-scale surveys of Olympic and world champion athletes have provided some normative data; however, many data sets can be considered historical and not able to reflect the secular increases in body size (Sorkin et al. 1999) due to changes in environmental conditions, nutrition and health care which have reduced growth-inhibiting factors (van Wieringen 1986). For example, adult height has increased over the last 150 years but has slowed since the mid-1990s. Body mass and mass for height indices have increased and in some countries accelerated since the 1990s (Tomkinson et al. 2017). Data for other body dimensions such as girths, lengths, breadths and segmental heights are limited. Where possible current research data should be gained to enable comparisons of physique characteristics for athletes of similar age, gender, ethnicity and sports participation level.

17.2 What Physique Characteristics Are Associated with Performance?

Knowledge of the physique characteristics that are important for athletes in the sports we work with as scientists and clinicians will enable us to help improve performance or reduce injury risk. We need to know what physique characteristics we should measure and monitor. For example, the relative contributions of a comprehensive range of physical, psychological and training measures to performance in 106 female rhythmic gymnasts aged 7–27 years showed that lean body mass was significantly related to attainment (Hume et al. 1993). Anthropometry has been reported as an injury risk factor in gymnastics (Hume 1999). Examples of important physique characteristics for selected sports that aim to optimise power and leverage or have a high metabolic demand are provided in this chapter based on studies reported in the literature since 2000.

17.2.1 Powerlifting

Powerlifting is a sport that aims to optimise power to weight ratios to improve performance. The anthropometric dimensions of powerlifters across various body mass (competitive body weight) categories have been described (Keogh et al. 2007). Fifty-four male Oceania competitive powerlifters (9 lightweight, 30 middleweight and 15 heavyweight) were recruited from one international and two national powerlifting competitions held in New Zealand. Powerlifters were assessed for 37 anthropometric dimensions using ISAK surface anthropometry protocols. The powerlifters were highly mesomorphic and had large girths and bony breadths, both in absolute units and when expressed as Zp-scores compared through the Phantom (Ross and Wilson 1974). These anthropometric characteristics were more pronounced in heavyweights, who were significantly heavier, had greater muscle and fat mass, were more endo-mesomorphic and had larger girths and bony breadths than the lighter lifters. Although middleweight and heavyweight lifters typically had longer segment lengths than the lightweights, all three groups had similar Zp-scores for the segment lengths, indicating similar segment length proportions.

Absolute and proportional anthropometric characteristics can distinguish stronger and weaker powerlifters (Keogh et al. 2009a). However, the anthropometric profiles of 17 weaker and 17 stronger Oceania competitive powerlifters of the same cohort showed that because all powerlifters were highly mesomorphic and possessed large girths and bone breadths, both in absolute terms and when expressed as Phantom Z-scores compared through the Phantom, only a few significant anthropometric differences were observed. Stronger lifters were defined as those having a Wilks score greater than 410, whereas those in the weaker group had a Wilks score less than 370. Stronger lifters had significantly greater muscle mass and larger muscular girths in absolute terms as well as greater Brugsch index (chest girth/height) and 'Phantom'-normalised muscle mass, upper arm, chest and forearm girths. In terms of the segment lengths and bone breadths, the only significant difference was that stronger lifters had a significantly shorter lower leg than weaker lifters. Because the majority of the significant differences were for muscle mass and muscular girths, it would appear likely that these differences contributed to the stronger lifters' superior performance. Powerlifters therefore need to devote some of their training to the development of greater levels of muscular hypertrophy if they wish to continue to improve their performance.

Although competitive powerlifters exhibit sexual dimorphism for many absolute anthropometric measures, little dimorphism is found for measures of adiposity and for proportional segment lengths and bone breadths (Keogh et al. 2008). Data from 68 (14 females, 54 males) of the Oceania competitive powerlifters of the same cohort were analysed further. When normalised through the Phantom, the female and male powerlifters had relatively similar segment lengths and bone breadths, indicating that regardless of gender, competitive powerlifters possess comparable skeletal proportions.

From Keogh and colleagues' series of journal articles presenting analysis of powerlifters, it was concluded that while population comparisons would be required to identify any connection between specific anthropometric dimensions that confer a competitive advantage to the expression of maximal strength, anthropometric profiling may prove useful for talent identification and for the assessment of training progression in powerlifting.

17.2.2   Rowing

Rowing is a sport with a high metabolic demand and ergonomic relationships between the athletes and the boat set-up. Researchers trying to identify the key predictors of performance in rowing have compared a rowing population to a normative population (Bourgois et al. 2001, 2000) or compared the population based on rowing class (Jurimae and Jurimae 2002) or athlete skill level (Bourgois et al. 2000, 2001; Hahn 1990). Assessment of 383 elite male juniors at the 1997 World Junior Rowing Championships (Bourgois et al. 2000) indicated that finalists were taller and heavier and had greater limb lengths, breadths and girths. The junior male rowers were 7% taller and 27% heavier and had significantly greater limb lengths and breadths than the normative population. It is assumed that this greater limb length gives a rower a mechanical advantage by increasing their lever length and time available for force application.

Olympic lightweight and open-class rowers possess distinctive physical and proportionality characteristics (Kerr et al. 2007). The 140 male open-class rowers, 69 female open-class rowers, 50 male lightweight rowers and 14 female lightweight rowers competing at the 2000 Olympic Games were measured for 38 anthropometric dimensions using ISAK surface anthropometry protocols. Body mass, stature and sitting height were different between the open-class and lightweight rowers, as well as a comparison group of healthy young adults (non-rowers, 42 males, 71 females), for both genders. After scaling for stature, the open-class rowers remained proportionally heavier than the non-rowers, with greater proportional chest, waist and thigh dimensions. Rowers across all categories possessed a proportionally smaller hip girth than the non-rowers which suggested the equipment places some constraints on this dimension. Top-ranked male open-class rowers were significantly taller and heavier and had a greater sitting height than their lower-ranked counterparts. They were also more muscular in the upper body, as indicated by a larger relaxed arm girth and forearm girth. For the male lightweight rowers, only proportional thigh length was greater in the best competitors. In the female open-class rowers, skinfold thicknesses were lower in the more highly placed competitors. A study of New Zealand junior rowers showed that after identification of desirable anthropometry, the 2000-m rowing ergometer potential of the juniors could be accounted for by upper body strength and endurance (Lawton et al. 2012).

Anthropometry profiling can be used for ergonomic applications where athletes' relationships to the equipment they use are examined to optimise performance. To maximise rowing performance, it appears important to tune the rigging of the boat to match the rower's size and strength (Soper and Hume 2004). In a study of 15 Australian elite single scullers (Barrett and Manning 2004), the fastest rowers tended to be the largest and strongest, and these larger body dimensions were reflected in their choice of rigging settings (oar length, inboard, span, gearing ratio, swivel-seat height, foot stretcher-seat height and distance and foot stretcher angles). Rigging set-up itself was not considered to be a primary determinant of rowing performance but a consequence of faster rowers being larger and stronger and scaling their rigging set-up accordingly. However, in an earlier study of New Zealand elite rowers (Hume et al. 2000), an individual's lower limb anthropometry was shown to affect the optimal foot stretcher position used to position the feet in a skiff. Adjustment of the foot stretcher position can optimise the work angle of the knees and ankles to obtain maximum efficiency for the leg drive.

Based on the rowing studies to date, specific anthropometric parameters distinguish between ability levels and successful or unsuccessful techniques. These attributes can be considered when modifying technique or predicting future rowing performance.

17.2.3 Kayak

Performance time varies among individual kayak paddlers based on technique style, strength, equipment and anthropometric characteristics (McDonnell et al. 2013). Indirect evidence from studies on anthropometry (Fry and Morton 1991; Van Someren and Howatson 2008) and equipment set-up (Ong et al. 2005) shows these characteristics may influence stroke rate or stroke displacement for sprint kayak performance. Given that high stroke rates and faster kayak velocity occur in shorter race distances, large upper body musculature may be required to produce enough power to achieve or sustain high stroke rates without decreasing stroke displacement excessively. Relaxed biceps girth, flexed biceps girth and humerus breadth have been correlated with 200- and 500-m average race velocity, but not 1000-m average race velocity (Akca and Muniroglu 2008). The strongest correlation was between flexed biceps girth and race time. In contrast, paddlers with longer segment lengths may emphasise greater forward reach, which would enhance the stroke displacement more than the stroke rate. Body mass and body fat percentage had a strong correlation with 500- and 1000-m average kayak velocity. Greater mass of the system may affect the surface area of the kayak exposed to the water, which would increase the surface drag. Subsequently, stroke displacement would decrease. Reducing body fat within a healthy range may help enhance performance via increasing stroke displacement, particularly for longer distance events.

At the 2000 Olympic Games, the morphological characteristics of 31 male and 12 female Olympic slalom kayak and canoe paddlers were measured using 36 anthropometric dimensions (Ridge et al. 2007). Compared with Olympic sprint paddlers, male slalom paddlers were older, lighter and shorter and had similar body fat and almost identical proportionality characteristics. While a high brachial index was reported for both male and female slalom paddlers, the best male paddlers (those ranked in the top 10 placings) were more compact, had smaller proportional hip girth and showed a tendency for smaller proportional hip breadth but a larger proportional waist girth than the rest (those not ranked in the top 10 placings).

The optimum boat set-up for sprint or slalom paddlers should require the internal structure of the kayak to be designed to fit the participant's body dimensions. Knowledge of an individual's body segment dimensions may provide important information to assist coaches and athletes to adjust certain aspects of the boat and paddle to maximise comfort and performance yet minimise the potential for injury. Equipment set-up (kayak and paddle characteristics) among the Sydney 2000 Olympic Games sprint and slalom kayak paddlers (Ong et al. 2005) was analysed. Sixty percent of the variance in the model to predict performance based on equipment set-up was accounted for based on the paddler's physical structure. There was moderate association with footbar distance with height, thigh length, leg length and foot length. Paddler height accounted for over half of the variance in footbar distance and paddle grip width. However, the 31 male and 11 female sprint paddlers, as well as 12 male and 12 female slalom competitors, exhibited little variability in absolute or relative body dimensions (Ackland et al. 2002).

17.2.4   Cycling

The most frequently suggested strategy to reduce injuries in cyclists is to optimise body position by adjusting the bicycle configuration to fit the cyclist's anthropometry. A cyclist is in contact with the bicycle via the handlebars, saddle and pedals. Consequently, the way a bicycle is configured can change a cyclists' body position. The position of the saddle can be measured relative to the cyclist (e.g. saddle height relative to the trochanteric length). For a proper configuration, the saddle height measurement must be completed with the crank in line with the seat tube and the measurement taken from the pedal surface to the top of the saddle. When using the length of body segments to configure the saddle height, the distance from the greater trochanter to the floor, the distance from the pubis to the floor and the distance from the ischial tuberosity to the floor have all been used (Bini et al. 2011a). For example, the Greg LeMond method involves the measurement of the inseam leg length and the configuration of the saddle height based on 88.3% of the distance between the top of the saddle and the centre of the bottom bracket. If the saddle height is too low, then the larger knee flexion angle close to peak pedal force may increase knee joint forces and lead to overuse injuries (Bini et al. 2011b). Increases in saddle height by 5% of preferred saddle height have resulted in large increases in index of effectiveness measured via pedal forces, joint mechanical work and kinematics for 12 cyclists and 12 triathletes (Bini et al. 2012). However, changes in saddle height smaller than 94% of trochanteric leg length appear not to result in substantial differences in pedal forces and joint mechanical work, and on this basis, cycling performance may not be affected (Bini et al. 2011b).

17.2.5 Rugby League

The anthropometric and physiologic capacities of rugby league players and the physiologic demands of rugby league participation generally increase as the participation levels increase. However, there is evidence that player physiologic capacities may deteriorate as the season progresses (King et al. 2009). This occurs with increases in skinfold thickness and some decrement in players' maximal aerobic power and muscular power over a season. Rugby league forwards usually have a higher body mass than backs. Amateur forwards had a higher estimated body fat percentage (19.9%), lower body mass (90.8 kg), lower vertical jump height (38.1 cm) and lower estimated maximum oxygen uptake (38.1 ml kg^{-1} min^{-1}) than semi-professional and professional players.

The index of lean mass based on body mass and sum of seven skinfolds is a useful tool for assessing body composition of athletes (Duthie et al. 2006). Athletes can show substantial individual variation in lean mass within and between seasons. Elite rugby players (40 forwards and 32 backs) between 1999 and 2003 were assessed on 13 ± 7 occasions over 1.9 ± 1.3 years. The forwards had a small 5.3% decrease in skinfolds between preseason and competition phases and a small 7.8% increase during the club season. A small 1.5% decrease in lean mass index occurred after 1 year in the programme for forwards and backs, whereas increases in skinfolds for forwards became substantial (4.3%) after 3 years. Individual variation in body composition was small within a season (1.6% body mass, 6.8% skinfolds, 1.1% lean mass index) but greater for body mass (2.1%) and lean mass index (1.7%) between seasons.

Research on tackles in rugby league has shown anthropometric (stature, body mass, skinfold thickness, somatotype) and physiological (fast acceleration and change-of-direction speed) factors are associated with tackling ability (King et al. 2012). In an investigation of 12 rugby league players, better rugby league tacklers were older, more experienced, shorter, lighter and leaner than players with poor tackling proficiency (Gabbett 2009b). Better tacklers also had greater levels of mesomorphy, acceleration and change-of-direction speed than poor tacklers. The strongest correlates of tackling ability were age, skinfold thickness, body mass, waist girth, gluteal girth and level of endomorphy. An additional study (Gabbett 2009a) of physiological and anthropometric characteristics of 88 junior rugby league players showed the starters in the competition (compared with non-starters who were tested preseason but did not start in the competition) were taller and had faster change of direction speed.

17.2.6 Badminton

The anthropometry of badminton players may be different due to the requirements for singles versus doubles play (Hume et al. 2009). Analysis of the 2007 Proton-BWF World Badminton Championships doubles versus singles players by gender (109 players in total: 18 men's singles, 20 women's singles, 35 men's doubles, 36 women's doubles players) showed that both male and female singles badminton players were taller and had a smaller body mass and had longer segments than the doubles badminton players. The sum of eight skinfolds was smaller for singles than doubles for both males and females. Males had significantly greater corrected muscle mass than females, but there were no differences between singles and doubles as event groups or any differences for group by event comparisons. There were differences by gender and event separately for Cormic index, but no gender by event differences. There was only one variable: leanness ratio score (body mass/sum of eight skinfolds) showed differences for gender, event and gender by event. Men's and women's singles badminton players had a higher leanness ratio score (over 1.0) than their doubles counterparts. Therefore, leanness ratio score may be a possible variable to help determine whether a player should play in doubles or singles, with higher leanness ratio scores (i.e. being more lean) being more desirable. Additional analysis of absolute size characteristic differences showed that a high brachial index (the ratio of lower arm length to upper arm length) and a low acromioilliac index (the ratio of bi-illiocristale breadth to biacromial breadth) were evident for 'best' (a world ranking of better than 20) than 'rest' world badminton players (Makhter et al. 2008). Measurements of forearm length, upper arm length, bi-illiocristale breadth and biacromial breadth may be used for talent identification and development screening purposes in badminton.

17.2.7 Other Sports Examples

There is increasing evidence from a number of studies of the importance of physique characteristics for performance optimisation. For example, lower body mass, lower body mass index and lower body fat have been associated with both a faster ironman race and a faster run split in 184 recreational male ironman triathletes.

Lower circumferences of the upper arm and thigh were also related with a faster run split (Knechtle et al. 2011).

Golfers with high strength and longer arms may be at a competitive advantage, as these characteristics allow the production of greater clubhead velocity and resulting ball displacement. Ten low handicap (best) golfers had 28% greater strength, 5% longer upper arms and 4% longer total arm length and 24% less right hip internal rotation than ten high handicap golfers (Keogh et al. 2009b).

Anthropometry (height/hip width ratio, body weight, body mass index and torso length) was an important predictor of front squat performance in 18 American college football players (Caruso et al. 2009).

Levels of success in 24 male handball teams (409 handball players) in the 2013 world championships were differentiated by standing stature and body mass (Ghobadi et al. 2013). Anthropometry of 33 female handball players, independent of competitive level (elite/sub-elite) and playing position, did not change significantly over a competitive season. However, postseason, the bone mineral content increased in the limbs, and lean mass increased in the upper limbs (Milanese et al. 2012). These results can help in the development of guidelines optimising in-season training programmes for team handball.

Within team sports, body composition can vary substantially based on position in the team. America's Cup sailors with a primary on-board function of grinding have significantly different anthropometric dimensions to the other sailors. The different anthropometric dimensions (e.g. height, body mass, various limb and bone measurements and skinfolds) of the grinders from 35 male team New Zealand America's Cup sailors (12 grinders, 7 trimmers, 11 afterguard, and 5 bowmen) reflect the physical tasks required of them during a sailing race. The larger standing height for the grinders was due to a longer tibia and not from a longer femur or longer trunk. Grinders had significantly more lean muscle mass than all other sailing groups. The largest lean muscle mass was 103.8 kg for a grinding sailor of 117.1 kg (11.3% body fat). Sailors in afterguard, trimming and bow groups showed very few differences in anthropometric characteristics between them (Pearson et al. 2006).

Relationships between body mass index, body mass and height and sports competence among participants of the 2010 winter Olympic games were measured to assess whether sport metabolic demand differentiated between the best and the rest athletes (Stanula et al. 2013). Athletes in the top 20 places of 14 sports disciplines (1460 cases) were grouped according to the predominant type of energy metabolism during competition. The large differences in body mass among the groups of athletes appeared to be related to the predominant type of metabolism during competition and the level of sports competence. The male athletes in the speed discipline (anaerobic-alactic) sports were the tallest, and those in the anaerobic-glycolytic sports such as cross-country sprint, figure skating, short track and speed skating were the shortest. In the speed disciplines (anaerobic-alactic), the female athletes were the tallest.

17.3 Summary

Physique characteristics play an important role in the self-selection of individuals for competitive sport. However, as a large number of factors are involved in the physical make-up of a champion sportsman or sportswoman, there is not necessarily one perfect body shape for a particular sport or event within that sport. Anthropometric tools have been used in profiling athletes' trajectory thereby optimising the trainable parameters at the times that matter most. This has important implications for weight category sports, where athletes may be at risk of employing unsafe weight control practices in order to 'make weight'. Rowing and powerlifting are two sports that require body mass to meet weight class categories for competition. Gymnastics is a sport that has pressure for leanness due to aesthetic reasons. As scientists and clinicians, we should have a good understanding of what physique characteristics are important for athletes in the sports we work with to help improve performance or reduce injury risk. Keeping up to date with current research data to enable comparisons of physique characteristics for athletes of similar age, gender, ethnicity and sports participation level is important.

References

Ackland T, Kerr D, Hume PA, Ross B (2002) Anthropometric normative data for Olympic rowers and paddlers. In: Sport medicine Australia conference, Melbourne

Akca F, Muniroglu S (2008) Anthropometric-somatotype and strength profiles and on-water performance in Turkish elite kayakers. Int J Appl Sports Sci 20(1):22–34

Barrett RS, Manning JM (2004) Relationships between rigging set-up, anthropometry, physical capacity, rowing kinematics and rowing performance. Sports Biomech 3(2):221–225

Bini RR, Hume PA, Croft J (2011a) Effects of saddle height on pedal force effectiveness. Proc Eng 13:51–55

Bini RR, Hume PA, Croft JL (2011b) Effects of bicycle saddle height on knee injury risk and cycling performance. Sports Med 41(6):463–476

Bini RR, Hume PA, Kilding AE (2012) Saddle height effects on pedal forces, joint mechanical work and kinematics of cyclists and triathletes. Eur J Sport Sci 14(1):44–52. https://doi.org/10.1080/17461391.2012.725105

Bourgois J, Claessens AL, Vrijens J, Philippaerts R, Van-Renterghem B, Thomis M, Janssens M, Loos R, Lefevre J (2000) Anthropometric characteristics of elite male junior rowers. Br J Sports Med 34(3):213–216

Bourgois J, Claessens AL, Janssens M, Van-Renterghem B, Loos R, Thomis M, Philippaerts R, Lefevre J, Vrijens J (2001) Anthropometric characteristics of elite female junior rowers. J Sports Sci 19(3):195–202

Caruso J, McLagan J, Shepherd C, Olson N, Taylor S, Gilliland L, Kline D, Detwiler A, Griswold S (2009) Anthropometry as a predictor of front squat performance in American college football players. Isokinet Exerc Sci 17(4):243–347

Duthie GM, Pyne DB, Hopkins WG, Livingstone S, Hooper SL (2006) Anthropometry profiles of elite rugby players: quantifying changes in lean mass. Br J Sports Med 40(3):202–208

Fry R, Morton A (1991) Physiological and kinanthropometric attributes of elite flatwater kayakists. Med Sci Sports Exerc 23:1297–1301

Gabbett T (2009a) Physiological and anthropometric characteristics of starters and non-starters in junior rugby league players, aged 13–17 years. J Sports Med Phys Fitness 49(3):233–239

Gabbett T (2009b) Physiological and anthropometric correlates of tackling ability in rugby league players. J Strength Cond Res 23(2):540–548

Ghobadi H, Rajabi H, Farzad B, Bayati M, Jeffreys I (2013) Anthropometry of world-class elite handball players according to the playing position: reports from men's handball world championship 2013. J Hum Kinet 39:213–218

Hahn A (1990) Identification and selection of talent in Australian rowing. Excel 6(3):5–11

Hume PA (1999) Minimising injuries in gymnastics activities. In: International society of biomechanics in sport applied proceedings: acrobatics, Perth, WA, Australia, 1999. Edith Cowan University, School of Biomedical and Sports Science, pp 23–36

Hume PA, Stewart AD (2012) Body composition change. In: Stewart AD, Sutton L (eds) Body composition in sport, exercise and health, 1st edn. Taylor and Francis, London, pp 147–165

Hume PA, Hopkins WG, Robinson DM, Robinson SM, Hollings SC (1993) Predictors of attainment in rhythmic sportive gymnastics. J Sports Med Phys Fitness 33(4):367–377

Hume PA, Soper C, Joe GM, Williams TR, Aitchison DR, Gunn S (2000) Effects of foot-stretcher angle on the drive phase in ergometer rowing. In: 2000 Pre-Olympic congress, Brisbane, Australia, 2000, p 197

Hume PA, Png W, Aziz AR, Makhtar R, Zakaria AZ, Mohd MA, Razali MR (2009) Differences in world badminton players' physical and proportionality characteristics between singles and doubles players. In: Hume PA, Stewart AD (eds) Kinanthropometry XI: 2008 pre-olympic congress anthropometry research. Sport Performance Research Institute New Zealand, Auckland University of Technology, Auckland, pp 80–91

Jurimae J, Jurimae T (2002) A comparison of selected anthropometric, metabolic and hormone parameters in lightweight and open-class rowers. Biol Sport 19(2):149–161

Keogh JWL, Hume PA, Pearson SN, Mellow P (2007) Anthropometric dimensions of male powerlifters of varying body mass. J Sports Sci 25(12):1365–1376

Keogh JWL, Hume PA, Pearson SN, Mellow P (2008) To what extent does sexual dimorphism exist in competitive powerlifters? J Sports Sci 26(5):531–541

Keogh JWL, Marnewick M, Maulder P, Nortje J, Hume PA, Bradshaw EJ (2009a) Are anthropometric, flexibility and muscular strength and endurance variables related to clubhead velocity in low- and high-handicap golfers? J Strength Cond Res 23(6):1841–1850

Keogh JWL, Hume PA, Mellow P, Pearson SN (2009b) Can absolute and proportional anthropometric characteristics distinguish stronger and weaker powerlifters? J Strength Cond Res 23(8):2256–2265

Kerr DA, Ross WD, Norton K, Hume P, Kagawa M, Ackland TR (2007) Olympic lightweight and open-class rowers possess distinctive physical and proportionality characteristics. J Sports Sci 25(1):43–45

King D, Hume PA, Milburn P, Guttenbeil D (2009) A review of the physiological and anthropometrical characteristics of rugby league players. S Afr J Res Sport Phys Educ Recreation 31(2):49–67

King D, Hume PA, Clark T (2012) Nature of tackles that result in injury in professional rugby league. Res Sports Med 20(2):86–104

Knechtle B, Wirth A, Rüst CA, Rosemann T (2011) The relationship between anthropometry and split performance in recreational male ironman triathletes. Asian J Sports Med 2(1):23–27

Lawton TW, Cronin JB, Mcguigan MR (2012) Anthropometry, strength and benchmarks for development: A basis for junior rowers' selection? J Sports Sci 30(10):995–1000

Makhter R, Hume PA, Zakaria AZ, Mohd AM, Razali MR, Png W, Aziz AR (2008) Absolute size characteristics differences between 'best' and 'rest' world badminton players. In: Sport for all conference, Malaysia, 2008

McDonnell LK, Hume PA, Nolte V (2013) A deterministic model based on evidence for the associations between kinematic variables and sprint kayak performance. Sport Biomech 12(3):205–220

Milanese C, Piscitelli F, Lampis C, Zancanaro C (2012) Effect of a competitive season on anthropometry and three-compartment body composition in female handball players. Biol Sport 29(3):199–204

Ong K, Ackland T, Hume PA, Ridge B, Broad E, Kerr D (2005) Equipment set-up among Olympic sprint and slalom kayak paddlers. Sports Biomech 4(1):47–58

Pearson SN, Hume PA, Mellow P, Slyfield D (2006) Anthropometric dimensions of Team New Zealand America's Cup sailors. N Zeal J Sports Med 33(2):52–57

Ridge BR, Broad E, Kerr DA, Ackland TR (2007) Morphological characteristics of Olympic slalom canoe and kayak paddlers. Eur J Sport Sci 7(2):107–111

Ross WD, Wilson NC (1974) A stratagem for proportional growth assessment. Acta Paediatrica Belgica, 28(Suppl):169–182

Soper C, Hume PA (2004) Towards an ideal rowing technique for performance: the contributions from biomechanics. Sports Med 34(12):825–848

Sorkin JD, Muller DC, Andres R (1999) Longitudinal change in height of men and women: implications for the interpretation of the body mass index. Am J Epidemiol 150:969–977

Stanula A, Roczniok R, Gabryś T, Szmatlan-gabryś U, Maszczyk A, Pietraszewski P (2013) Relations between BMI, body mass and height, and sports competence among participants of the 2010 winter olympic games: does sport metabolic demand differentiate? Percept Motor Skills 117(3):837

Tomkinson GR, Daniell N, Fulton A, Furnell A (2017) Time changes in the body dimensions of male Australian Army personnel between 1977 and 2012. Appl Ergon 58:18–24

van Wieringen JC (1986) Secular growth changes. In: Falkner F, Tanner JM (eds) Human growth, vol 3, 2nd edn. Plenum, New York, NY

Van Someren KA, Howatson G (2008) Prediction of flatwater kayaking performance. Int J Sports Physiol Perform 3:207–218

Chapter 18
Body Image for Athletes

Duncan J. Macfarlane

Abstract The concept of body image includes how we perceive, think, feel and ultimately behave due to our own conception of our physical image. Body image dissatisfaction is when there is a difference between our perceived body image and our desired body image. The prevalence of body image disorders in athletic populations remains worryingly high, although rather poorly documented. Unfortunately the assessment of body image, especially in athletic populations, has not progressed significantly, and many researchers still rely on traditional/out-dated instruments. Modern 3D scanning technology together with volumetric assessment gives potential for body image assessment to be conducted. The novel iPad SomatoMac application uses male and female somatotype photographs that allow for more comprehensive estimates of body image dissatisfaction than existing figural images/ silhouettes and photographic/pictorial scales.

Keywords Body image • Physical image • Body image dissatisfaction • Perceived • Desired • Disorders • 3D scanning • Volumetric assessment • iPad SomatoMac • Somatotype • Images • Photographic scales

18.1 Introduction

The concept of body image includes how we perceive, think, feel and ultimately behave due to our own conception of our physical image. Body image disturbances are only one part of this generic area, but one that is commonly reported, especially body image dissatisfaction and body image distortion. Body image dissatisfaction is typically defined as when there is a difference between our perceived body image and our ideal (or desired) body image, and this is relatively easy to assess. This should not be confused with body image distortion, which is considered to be the difference between perceived and true (measured) body shape/image (Liechty 2010) and is relatively difficult to assess. Such disturbances and a negative body image are

D.J. Macfarlane
University of Hong Kong, Pok Fu Lam, Hong Kong
e-mail: djmac@hku.hk

© Springer Nature Singapore Pte Ltd. 2018   217
P.A. Hume et al. (eds.), *Best Practice Protocols for Physique Assessment in Sport*,
https://doi.org/10.1007/978-981-10-5418-1_18

critical risk factors for the development of eating disorders (e.g. bulimia/anorexia nervosa) and likely causes of relapse for those with these conditions and depression, social anxiety, poor self-esteem and a lower quality of life (Cash et al. 2004). In men, these risk factors may also lead to reverse anorexia, sexual dysfunction, abuse of steroids and other illegal performance-enhancing drugs (Burlew and Shurts 2013).

The field of body image research is considerable and involves many multidimensional constructs. Data collection on body image can assess the cognitive and affective dimensions typically using self-reported/subjective questionnaires, or it can focus on the perceptual components using quasi-objective instruments. This later component will be the focus of this chapter, with currently available perceptual methods having several benefits, but also significant limitations. Until recently, no methodology had adapted to the modern era using ubiquitous portable digital technologies. Most still rely on pen/pencil formats of simple and often unrealistic figural images/silhouettes or single 2D photos that take little consideration of muscularity/mesomorphy, thus not well-suited for athletic populations, or are inappropriately based on body mass index as a poor proxy of body shape/composition. Few of these current methods can rapidly assess both body image dissatisfaction and body image distortion and take into consideration the need for a 3D-type approach for the realistic portrayal of the human body (Mutale et al. 2016).

A revolutionary approach developed recently (Macfarlane et al. 2016) relies on a wide range of more than 50 somatotype images for both men and women, thus incorporating the three important physical components of body image (endomorphy, mesomorphy, ectomorphy). Uniquely, this permits use with both athletic and nonathletic populations, and the three somatotype images (front, side, rear) provide a quasi-3D realistic view of the human form. This iPad-based SomatoMac application allows portable, rapid and reliable data collection and storage, plus the ability to obtain/calculate objectively both body image distortion using the true body shape and body image dissatisfaction. It is planned to make this iPad application available to health and medical professionals, not only to dramatically enhance the rapid assessment of body image perception, especially in athletic populations, but also as an aid to helping treat those with body image disorders.

18.2   Why Measure Physique Using Body Image?

It is known that a considerable portion of the Western population is unhappy with their body size, shape and/or appearance, with percentages of >20% for men and 40–50% for women often reported (Drewnowski and Yee 1987; Grabe et al. 2008; Pidgeon and McNeil 2013). However, in some groups of adolescents, the levels of body image dissatisfaction are reported to be as high as 80% in men and 82% in women (Furnham et al. 2002). In some Asian countries, levels of body image dissatisfaction have also been reported to be above 80% for young women and in adolescent boys (Fung and Yuen 2003; Fung et al. 2010; Lai et al. 2013). One clear caveat is that since there is no widely agreed criterion measure to assess body image disorders, its prevalence will vary according to the wide range of available methodologies. But even so, these data clearly suggest that body image disorders are a significant issue within the population, especially as research indicates that those with body image issues are less likely to engage in healthy eating and exercise behaviours (Furnham et al. 2002; Kruger et al. 2008). Problems with body image disorders appear to have grown in recent decades (Cash et al. 2004; Feingold and Mazzella 1998; Grabe et al. 2008), to the extent that they now appear to influence children as young as 3–5 years (Tremblay et al. 2011).

The prevalence of body image disorders in athletic populations remains worryingly high, although rather poorly documented. If eating disorders/disordered eating and weight control behaviours are a reasonable proxy of distorted body image, then the research evidence appears somewhat consistent especially when related to weight-sensitive or leanness-focussed sports. One consensus statement suggested that elite athletes may be at greater risk than lower-tier athletes and non-elite athletes (Sundgot-Borgen et al. 2013) and particularly in the aforementioned weight-sensitive or leanness-focussed sports and among elite female athletes (Kong and Harris 2015). In contrast, one systematic review suggested comparable levels of pathogenic weight control behaviours existed between athletes and controls and that participation in elite sports may be somewhat protective. Yet in leanness sports, the authors concluded the prevalence may be higher in elite athletes than in controls (Werner et al. 2013). A similar finding comes from a systematic review of body image concerns of women (Varnes et al. 2013), in which the authors concluded that participation in collegiate sport was somewhat protective against body image concerns compared to nonathletes, but noted this was not so in appearance-focussed sports and for higher-tier athletes. In male athletes, levels of eating and body image disorders appear generally lower than their female counterparts, but in some sports where a drive towards muscularity is dominant (e.g. weightlifting, bodybuilding), such disorders are high, along with concerns of associated muscle dysmorphia and anabolic-androgenic steroid use (Bratland-Sanda and Sundgot-Borgen 2013).

Body image disorders, therefore, remain a significant public health issue that should be addressed more seriously and are also an important issue for many athletic populations. Unfortunately the assessment of body image, especially in athletic populations, has not progressed significantly, and many researchers still rely on traditional/out-dated instruments. These include the use of unrealistic figural drawings/silhouettes, or images that are based on the inappropriate use of body mass index. Most current methods are also clearly limited to assessing only one, or at most two, of the three physical components necessary for assessing the total perceptual component of body image in athletes: adiposity (endomorphy), muscularity (mesomorphy) and leanness/linearity (ectomorphy).

18.3   What Is the Body Image Technique and Technology?

18.3.1   Traditional Methods of Measuring the Perception of Whole Body Image

A wide range of figural rating scales, silhouettes, photographic and pictorial representations, distorting mirrors and computer morphing techniques have been developed in attempt to quantify the perceptual components of body image. It is not possible to examine/review each of these in detail here, and the reader is, therefore, recommended to some other excellent articles pertaining to these methodologies (Cafri and Thompson 2004; Cash and Brown 1987; Cash and Pruzinsky 2004, 1990; Cash and Smolak 2011; Gardner 1996; Gardner and Brown 2010a; Gardner et al. 1998; Grogan 2007; Krawczyk et al. 2012; Norton and Olds 1996; Thompson 2001, 2004; Thompson et al. 2012).

Most of these methodologies have served the area well, yet with the passage of time, these existing instruments contain a range of well-recognized limitations (see below), not the least that they were devised primarily for nonathletic populations. In particular, many methods do not assess all three necessary body image components (endomorphy, mesomorphy, ectomorphy) along a comprehensive continuum, which is important for accurate and realistic assessment in athletic populations.

Each of the traditional body image assessment methods has clear benefits. For example, the basic Stunkard figural scale is very well known and simple to apply and to interpret, and the photographic and pictorial models appear more realistic than simple figural scales with potentially higher content validity. In addition, computer-morphing techniques allow an infinite range of modifications and refinements, but each assessment method is not without some significant limitation, as follows.

18.3.1.1   Figural Images/Silhouettes

Although frequently used in the body image literature and possessing reasonable reliability, figural drawings such as the original Stunkard images (Stunkard et al. 1983) and more recent variations (Gardner et al. 2009) still have a recognized range of weaknesses (Gardner and Brown 2010a; Gardner et al. 1998; Mutale et al. 2016; Stewart et al. 2009). Some of the key weaknesses include the following factors:

- Very coarse response scales and restriction of scale range. When using figural drawings/silhouettes, the respondent is asked to select a figure from a finite number of drawings, typically in the range of 5–12 images. Studies have shown that information can be restricted when a coarse response scale is used to assess a more finely detailed, continuous variable (Gardner et al. 1998). The limited number of figures presented means that 85–90% of patients only select one of three images, out of a range of 10–12 presented images, when asked to rate their perceived size (Gardner and Brown 2010a). This artificially reduces the standard deviations in the response range and can also lead to spurious inflation in the test-retest reliability (Thompson and Gray 1995), in part due to an increased likelihood of remembering the previous selection due to the restricted range.

- Inability to assess body distortion and body dissatisfaction. The assessment of body image is multidimensional and can involve disturbances in two key areas: body dissatisfaction (difference between perceived and ideal/desired image) and body distortion (difference between perceived and true body image)—which is especially important for clinical patients with eating disorders. Figural silhouettes are, typically, only used to assess body dissatisfaction and generally cannot assess body distortion (which computer-morphing techniques attempt—see below). This is a significant limitation since body dissatisfaction and body distortion are independent constructs (Gardner and Brown 2010a).
- Questionable content validity. Figural silhouettes have been heavily criticized as unrealistic representations of the human form, including disproportionately sized arms and legs and poorly defined bodily features (Thompson and Gray 1995). This criticism was supported by Stewart and colleagues (Stewart et al. 2009), stating these images are typically animated-type drawings or grossly unrealistic sketches of human figures, and it is difficult for individuals to relate to in reference to their own body. Consequently, they are considered to have insufficient content validity, thus underscoring the need for improved (realistic) images. Others have commented that these scales lack documentation on their psychometric properties and have questionable validity and reliability (Gardner and Brown 2010a).

18.3.1.2   Photographic and Pictorial Scales

To counter some of the known issues of figural silhouettes, a novel Photographic Figure Rating Scale (PFRS) was devised by Swami et al. (2008), incorporating ten standardized photographs of women with a varying body mass index from 12.5 (emaciated) to 41 (obese). The presentation of consistent views and the lack of extraneous features are potential strengths; however, this PFRS has only been created for women. It also contains only ten images (arguably a lack of scale range) and was based on variations only in body mass index, which takes no account for true variations in levels of adiposity compared to muscularity—which has been previously criticized in the body image literature (Cohn and Adler 1992). Thus, the PFRS appears not to account sufficiently for levels of muscularity between images and only uses a 2D frontal view image (no side nor rear view).

A recent addition to the body image scales (Mutale et al. 2016) used computer-generated 2D pictorial images of nine male/female stimuli—each varying by body mass index alone and with no apparent element of muscularity or linearity. It should be remembered that body mass index is only a measure of ponderosity (heaviness) (Norton and Olds 1996; Sundgot-Borgen et al. 2013) and certainly not a measure of body composition, as it cannot differentiate between levels of fat or muscle within an individual. Novella et al. (2015) recently introduced a new range of stimuli, the

Presentation of Images on a Continuum Scale (PICS) showing pictorial drawings of eight thin to obese figures plus eight thin to muscular images for both men and women. Although undoubtedly more realistic and an improvement on the more basic Stunkard-type silhouettes, and attempting to include an element of muscularity, these images do not allow for some important athletic body shape combinations, such as moderate adiposity plus strong muscularity, that can be associated in many collision-type sports (rugby/league, wrestling, ice hockey) or throwing events (shot-put, discus, hammer).

18.3.1.3 Computer Programmes

There have been a small number of computer programmes to morph images in an attempt to overcome many of the limitations of figural silhouettes (Gardner and Boice 2004; Gardner and Brown 2010b; Shibata 2002; Stewart et al. 2009) and provide an opportunity to examine both body distortion and body dissatisfaction. However, these programmes are not generally suited for routine use by health professionals as they require specialist equipment (digital camera/specialist software), plus significant analysis time and training. One computer programme, the somato-morphic matrix, was a novel attempt to incorporate both the level of adiposity and muscularity in the assessment (Gruber et al. 1999). Unfortunately, it was shown to be unreliable (Cafri and Thompson 2004) and also seems no longer available, although an adapted paper version is available (Cafri and Thompson 2004). The most recent Body Morph Assessment version 2 (BMA 2.0) (Stewart et al. 2009) has been a major step forward, attempting to overcome many of the numerous limitations when using figural images/silhouettes. The BMA 2.0 used a specialist computer programme to morph a body movie over 100 increments from an extremely thin person into an extremely obese person. Yet this programme also has several limitations, in that:

- It is not readily available, nor directly portable, nor able to be used routinely for clinical work
- It fails to consider the component of muscularity (only morphs the image from extreme thinness to extreme obesity)
- The actual body size/measures of the morphed image is typically not actually known

Most of these traditional instruments only assess body image along a thin-to-obese (ectomorphy-endomorphy) continuum and without adequate consideration of muscularity (mesomorphy). Until recently there has been limited availability of body image instruments to assess muscularity for men (Galli and Reel 2009), and almost none allow specific assessment of muscularity in women (Novella et al. 2015). Consequently, most existing body image instruments remain poorly designed for use on athletic populations. The ectomorphy component of leanness/linearity is important in athletes and is also poorly assessed using traditional measures. Leanness/linearity is not just the opposite of adiposity as is assumed by some scales.

In kinanthropometry measurements, ectomorphy contains a critical element of linearity (and not just leanness alone), which is a vital capacity in some sports such as high jump, netball, volleyball and basketball. Thus, enhanced measures are needed for body image assessment both for body dissatisfaction and distortion and particularly instruments that can be applied to athletes.

Currently there are no standards for training and accreditation systems or equipment/software for body image analysis.

18.3.2   How Can These Traditional Body Image Assessments Be Improved, Especially for Athletes?

Modern 3D scanning technology together with volumetric assessment gives the potential for semi- or fully automated somatotype determination that may provide extremely detailed information for future body image research (Stewart et al. 2014, 2012; Olds et al. 2013). Although promising, this modern technology will be most likely restricted to laboratory studies since although semi-mobile, the hardware is not fully portable and cannot be used for rapid body image assessments in multiple chosen venues. The software for such systems remains expensive and complex. Therefore, for the foreseeable future, it will remain a research-only instrument rather than a rapid measure of body image for athletes or nonathletes by health professionals such as trainers, psychologists and psychiatrists who may wish to measure/monitor body image routinely as part of client management and treatment.

18.4   How Do You Use Body Image Technique for Your Athlete?

To try to counter many of the limitations with existing body image methodologies and to satisfy the need for a unique instrument equally suited to both nonathletic and athletic populations, we developed a novel iPad SomatoMac application (Macfarlane et al. 2016) (www.somatomac.com). This uses more than 50 male and female somatotype photographs (see Fig. 18.1a, b) that allow for more comprehensive estimates of body image dissatisfaction than existing figural images/silhouettes and photographic/pictorial scales. We have piloted the SomatoMac application with over 20 adults who rated their perceived and desired body images from the somatotype photographs (>3 days between tests). Pearson reliability correlation coefficients were determined for perceived endomorphy $r = 0.91$ (68% chose the identical rating), perceived mesomorphy $r = 0.84$ (71% identical) and perceived ectomorphy $r = 0.93$ (61% identical) and for desired endomorphy $r = 0.78$ (85% identical), desired mesomorphy $r = 0.93$ (65% identical) and desired ectomorphy $r = 0.88$ (70% identical). Overall, on retest, 45% chose the identical perceived somatotype and 50% the identical desired somatotype. These data suggest this new iPad-based assessment method has high levels of reliability for both perceived and desired body image whilst offering a much wider range of real body shapes from which to select. The method takes about 5 min to conduct an assessment for a client when recording perceived, desired and true photo images, but approximately 10 min further if the ISAK-determined anthropometric somatotype is required using skinfolds/girths/ breadths by a trained anthropometrist.

Developing a rapid, reliable and portable digital body image assessment scale that can be applied to both athletic and nonathletic populations has benefits including:

- The use of anonymized images taken from existing human somatotype photographs (including many athlete images) allows the use of true anatomical images, rather than artificial silhouettes or figural drawings (see Fig. 18.1a: only 9 of >50 images shown).
- A large range of images to choose from (e.g. approximately 50 images for both men and women).
- The quasi-3D images help provide more information on body shape (as the somatotype photo shows front, side and rear images), rather than just a single 2D image.
- The somatotypes are presented on a typical somatochart or Reuleaux triangle— with the three traditional apices for endomorphy (adiposity), mesomorphy (muscularity) and ectomorphy (leanness/linearity), thus allowing the user to select/ quantify a body image using all three important anatomical/body-build axes (endo-ecto, endo-meso, meso-ecto: Fig. 18.1a and Fig. 18.1b). Currently, no comparable body image scale allows this fine degree of quantification in all three dimensions/axes.
- The ability to assess true body image (necessary for determining body image distortion) by the use of either (a) Heath-Carter anthropometric calculations of somatotype (Carter and Heath 1990; Norton and Olds 1996) or (b) simple but near instantaneously assessed on-screen comparisons (via built-in iPad camera and software) between their true real life body shape and their perceived body image (see Fig. 18.1c). This feature provides the potential to help reduce pathogenic levels of body image distortion.
- The ability to objectively obtain/calculate both body image distortion using the true body shape via anthropometric measures and body image dissatisfaction and to report these using simple three-component histograms or more advanced somatotype attitudinal distances (Carter and Heath 1990; Norton and Olds 1996).
- All selections/data/history are stored electronically for easy retrieval (with password security protection) and downloadable to a desktop as a CSV/Excel file format.
- The final iPad SomatoMac application is planned to be made available worldwide in multiple languages via the Apple app store (if acceptable to Apple's quality control system).

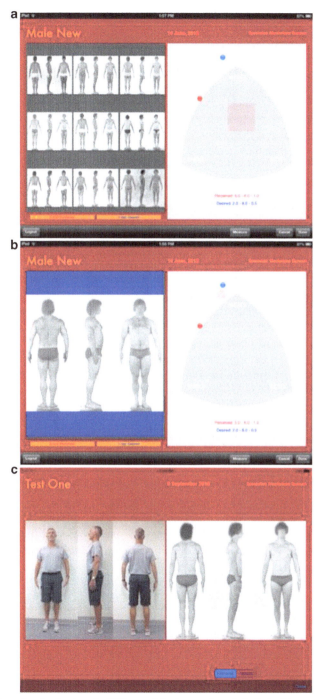

Fig. 18.1 Example of only nine of >50 SomatoMac images (panel **a**), desired image chosen (panel **b**), photo comparison of true versus perceived images (panel **c**)

18.5   How Do You Report the Data to Your Athlete and Coach?

Considerable care needs to be exercised when providing feedback to a coach, and especially any athlete, as the athlete may be at risk of an adverse psychological event when they realize their perceived (or even desired) image is considerably different from their true photo image or true ISAK-determined somatotype. For example, issues may arise if the person is shown to be considerably more endomorphic (higher body fat) than they perceived themselves to be, or for some individuals with eating disorders, realizing they are considerably more ectomorphic (leaner) than they had perceived. Seeking the professional advice of trained staff such as clinical psychologists or medical psychiatrists is recommended if the results have potential to be significantly traumatic to the athlete. These feedback issues need to be dealt with in a very sensitive manner, using appropriate language and including cultural/gender awareness.

A range of comparative body image data is provided by the SomatoMac application that can be used to enhance feedback. This feedback may be provided in the form of simple histograms that compare each of the endomorph, mesomorph and ectomorph ratings of perceived, desired and true somatotype or by showing all three ratings on the Reuleaux somatochart. Alternatively, feedback can be provided using the more detailed somatotype attitudinal distance (SAD), which can be provided for those with advanced anthropometric knowledge. For relatively simple supplementary background information on somatotypes, the athletes can also be referred to a myriad of web-based resources such as Wikipedia.

18.6   Summary

Body image includes how we perceive, think, feel and ultimately behave due to our own conception of our physical image. Body image dissatisfaction is when there is a difference between our perceived body image and our desired body image. The assessment of body image in athletic populations may progress with the use of modern 3D scanning technology together with volumetric assessment. The novel iPad SomatoMac application may be useful for estimates of body image dissatisfaction and distortion, especially in athletes.

Funding Acknowledgements and Disclaimer The iPad SomatoMac application was developed using funding from Hong Kong University's Knowledge Exchange Fund and Seed Funding Programme #201411159144 and the J.E. Lindsay Carter Kinanthropometry Clinic and Archive New Zealand funding programme #KAPHK1.

References

Bratland-Sanda S, Sundgot-Borgen J (2013) Eating disorders in athletes: overview of prevalence, risk factors and recommendations for prevention and treatment. Eur J Sport Sci 13(5):499–508

Burlew LD, Shurts WM (2013) Men and body image: current issues and counseling implications. J Couns Dev 91(4):428–435

Cafri G, Thompson JK (2004) Measuring male body image: a review of the current methodology. Psychol Men Masculinity 5(1):18

Carter JL, Heath BH (1990) Somatotyping: development and applications. Cambridge University Press, Cambridge

Cash TF, Brown TA (1987) Body image in anorexia nervosa and bulimia nervosa: a review of the literature. Behav Modif 11(4):487–521

Cash TF, Pruzinsky T (1990) Body images: development, deviance, and change. Guilford Press, New York, NY

Cash TF, Pruzinsky T (2004) Body image: a handbook of theory, research, and clinical practice. Guilford Press, New York, NY

Cash TF, Smolak L (2011) Body image: a handbook of science, practice, and prevention. Guilford Press, New York, NY

Cash TF, Morrow JA, Hrabosky JI, Perry AA (2004) How has body image changed? A cross-sectional investigation of college women and men from 1983 to 2001. J Consult Clin Psychol 72(6):1081–1089

Cohn LD, Adler NE (1992) Female and male perceptions of ideal body shapes: distorted views among Caucasian college students. Psychol Women Q 16(1):69–79

Drewnowski A, Yee DK (1987) Men and body image: are males satisfied with their body weight? Psychosom Med 49(6):626–634

Feingold A, Mazzella R (1998) Gender differences in body image are increasing. Psychol Sci 9(3):190–195

Fung MSC, Yuen M (2003) Body image and eating attitudes among adolescent Chinese girls in Hong Kong. Percept Mot Skills 96(1):57–66

Fung SSW, Stewart SM, Ho SY, Wong JPS, Lam TH (2010) Body dissatisfaction, maternal appraisal, and depressive symptoms in Hong Kong adolescents. Int J Psychol 45(6):453–460

Furnham A, Badmin N, Sneade I (2002) Body image dissatisfaction: gender differences in eating attitudes, self-esteem, and reasons for exercise. J Psychol 136(6):581–596

Galli N, Reel JJ (2009) Adonis or Hephaestus? Exploring body image in male athletes. Psychol Men Masculinity 10(2):95–108

Gardner RM (1996) Methodological issues in assessment of the perceptual component of body image disturbance. Br J Psychol 87(2):327–337

Gardner RM, Boice R (2004) A computer program for measuring body size distortion and body dissatisfaction. Behav Res Methods Instrum Comput 36(1):89–95

Gardner RM, Brown DL (2010a) Body image assessment: a review of figural drawing scales. Pers Individ Dif 48(2):107–111

Gardner RM, Brown DL (2010b) Comparison of video distortion and figural drawing scale for measuring and predicting body image dissatisfaction and distortion. Pers Individ Dif 49(7):794–798

Gardner RM, Friedman BN, Jackson NA (1998) Methodological concerns when using silhouettes to measure body image. Percept Mot Skills 86(2):387–395

Gardner RM, Jappe LM, Gardner L (2009) Development and validation of a new figural drawing scale for body-image assessment: the BIAS-BD. J Clin Psychol 65(1):113–122

Grabe S, Ward LM, Hyde JS (2008) The role of the media in body image concerns among women: a meta-analysis of experimental and correlational studies. Psychol Bull 134(3):460–476

Grogan S (2007) Body image: understanding body dissatisfaction in men, women and children. Routledge, Hove

Gruber A, Pope H, Borowiecki J, Cohane G (1999) The development of the somatomorphic matrix: a bi-axial instrument for measuring body image in men and women. In: Olds T, Dollman J, Norton K (eds) Kinanthropometry VI. ISAK, Sydney, pp 217–231

Kong P, Harris LM (2015) The sporting body: body image and eating disorder symptomatology among female athletes from leanness focused and nonleanness focused sports. J Psychol 149(2):141–160

Krawczyk R, Menzel J, Thompson JK (2012) Methodological issues in the study of body image and appearance. In: Rumsey N, Harcourt D (eds) Oxford handbook of the psychology of appearance (on line). Oxford University Press, Oxford

Kruger J, Lee CD, Ainsworth BE, Macera CA (2008) Body size satisfaction and physical activity levels among men and women. Obesity 16(8):1976–1979

Lai CM, Mak KK, Pang JS, Fong SSM, Ho RCM, Guldan GS (2013) The associations of socio-cultural attitudes towards appearance with body dissatisfaction and eating behaviors in Hong Kong adolescents. Eat Behav 14(3):320–324

Liechty JM (2010) Body image distortion and three types of weight loss behaviors among non-overweight girls in the United States. J Adolesc Health 47(2):176–182

Macfarlane DJ, Lee A, Hume P, Carter L (2016) Development and reliability of a novel iPad-based application to rapidly assess body image: 3776 board# 215. Med Sci Sports Exerc 48(5 Suppl 1):1056

Mutale GJ, Dunn AK, Stiller J, Larkin R (2016) Development of a body dissatisfaction scale assessment tool. New School Psychol Bull 13(2):47–57

Norton KI, Olds T (1996) Anthropometrica: a textbook of body measurement for sports and health courses. University of New South Wales, Sydney

Novella J, Gosselin JT, Danowski D (2015) One size doesn't fit all: new continua of figure drawings and their relation to ideal body image. J Am Coll Heal 63(6):353–360

Olds T, Daniell N, Petkov J, Stewart AD (2013) Somatotyping using 3D anthropometry: a cluster analysis. J Sports Sci 31(9):936–944

Pidgeon AM, McNeil E (2013) Mindfulness, empowerment and feminist identity development as protective factors against women developing body image dissatisfaction. Int J Heal Caring 13(1):1–13

Shibata S (2002) A Macintosh and Windows program for assessing body-image disturbance using adjustable image distortion. Behav Res Methods Instrum Comput 34(1):90–92

Stewart TM, Allen HR, Han H, Williamson DA (2009) The development of the Body Morph Assessment version 2.0 (BMA 2.0): tests of reliability and validity. Body Image 6(2):67–74

Stewart AD, Klein S, Young J, Simpson S, Lee AJ, Harrild K, Crockett P, Benson PJ (2012) Body image, shape, and volumetric assessments using 3D whole body laser scanning and 2D digital photography in females with a diagnosed eating disorder: preliminary novel findings. Br J Psychol 103(2):183–202

Stewart AD, Crockett P, Nevill A, Benson P (2014) Somatotype: a more sophisticated approach to body image work with eating disorder sufferers. Adv Eat Disord Theory Res Pract 2(2):125–135

Stunkard AJ, Sørensen T, Schulsinger F (1983) Use of the Danish Adoption Register for the study of obesity and thinness. Res Publ Assoc Res Nerv Ment Dis 60:115–120

Sundgot-Borgen J, Meyer NL, Lohman TG, Ackland TR, Maughan RJ, Stewart AD, Müller W (2013) How to minimise the health risks to athletes who compete in weight-sensitive sports review and position statement on behalf of the Ad Hoc Research Working Group on Body Composition, Health and Performance, under the auspices of the IOC Medical Commission. Br J Sports Med 47(16):1012–1022

Swami V, Salem N, Furnham A, Tovée MJ (2008) Initial examination of the validity and reliability of the female photographic figure rating scale for body image assessment. Pers Individ Dif 44(8):1752–1761

Thompson JK (2001) Body image, eating disorders, and obesity: an integrative guide for assessment and treatment. American Psychological Association, Washington, DC

Thompson JK (2004) The (mis) measurement of body image: ten strategies to improve assessment for applied and research purposes. Body Image 1(1):7–14

Thompson MA, Gray JJ (1995) Development and validation of a new body-image assessment scale. J Pers Assess 64(2):258–269

Thompson JK, Burke N, Krawczyk R (2012) Measurement of body image in adolescence and adulthood. In: Cash TF (ed) Encyclopedia of body image and human appearance. Elsevier, London, pp 512–520

Tremblay L, Lovsin T, Zecevic C, Larivière M (2011) Perceptions of self in 3–5-year-old children: a preliminary investigation into the early emergence of body dissatisfaction. Body Image 8(3):287–292

Varnes JR, Stellefson ML, Janelle CM, Dorman SM, Dodd V, Miller MD (2013) A systematic review of studies comparing body image concerns among female college athletes and non-athletes, 1997–2012. Body Image 10(4):421–432

Werner A, Thiel A, Schneider S, Mayer J, Giel KE, Zipfel S (2013) Weight-control behaviour and weight-concerns in young elite athletes – a systematic review. J Eating Dis 1:18

Chapter 19
Training and Accreditation Systems and Ethical Considerations

Stephen C. Hollings and Patria A. Hume

Abstract Training and accreditation and quality assurance schemes ensure appropriate levels of professionalism and safety for the public who utilise physique assessment programmes. This chapter describes training and accreditation schemes for both imaging and non-imaging techniques. There are only two international training and certification programmes, for surface anthropometry and ultrasound techniques. Manufacturers training on equipment is provided for 3D scanning, Bod Pod, bioelectrical impedance analysis, dual-energy X-ray absorptiometry, magnetic resonance imaging and computed tomography. In addition, there are several national training and certificate programmes for dual-energy X-ray absorptiometry and magnetic resonance imaging and computed tomography. Ethical considerations in assessing anthropometry profiles for athletes are important. Practitioners need to maintain professional objectivity and integrity and respect the athlete during physique assessment. This chapter also provides guidelines on how to ensure ethical behaviour when conducting physique assessments and when reporting results.

Keywords Training • Accreditation • Quality assurance • Professionalism • Safety Schemes • Imaging techniques • Non-imaging techniques • International training Certification • Surface anthropometry • Ultrasound • Manufacturers training Equipment • 3D scanning • Bod Pod • Bioelectrical impedance • Dual-energy X-ray absorptiometry • Magnetic resonance imaging • Computed tomography • Ethics Integrity • Respect • Behaviour • Reporting

S.C. Hollings (✉)
Auckland University of Technology, Auckland, New Zealand
e-mail: hollings@athletic.co.nz

P.A. Hume
Sport Performance Research Institute New Zealand,
Auckland University of Technology, Auckland, New Zealand
e-mail: patria.hume@aut.ac.nz

© Springer Nature Singapore Pte Ltd. 2018
P.A. Hume et al. (eds.), *Best Practice Protocols for Physique Assessment in Sport*,
https://doi.org/10.1007/978-981-10-5418-1_19

19.1   Introduction

Many organisations involved with the disciplines of sport and exercise science have developed accreditation and quality assurance schemes for professionals working in these fields. These schemes enable professionals to be recognised for their expertise and ensure appropriate levels of measurement quality, operator professionalism and safety for clients who employ their services. In the area of physique assessment in sport, there are many techniques and technologies available. It is essential that the providers of these programmes have the skills, competency and proficiency in using standardised techniques and applications. There exists a requirement to establish accreditation systems so that both professionals and consumers can recognise operator competence at a variety of operator levels. Normally, certification is regarded as the formal recognition of the attainment of specialised knowledge, skills and experience and adoption of best practice and standards for measurement. Successful programmes are built on a foundation of core competencies that are reviewed and updated periodically by experienced practitioners. This chapter describes training and accreditation schemes for techniques and technologies that can be used to assess body physique.

19.2   Techniques/Technologies That Have International Training, Accreditation and/or Quality Assurance Schemes

There are only two international training and certification programmes, for surface anthropometry and ultrasound techniques.

19.2.1   Non-imaging Method: Surface Anthropometry

The International Society for the Advancement of Kinanthropometry (ISAK) approved its initial accreditation scheme for anthropometric assessment in 1996. This scheme was based on the anthropometry section of the Laboratory Standards Assistance Scheme of the Australian Sports Commission. The current ISAK accreditation scheme was approved by the ISAK Executive Council in August 2004. The scheme specifies the requirements for conducting ISAK courses and acts as a significant resource for teaching and examining practitioners. An ISAK textbook is provided to all course participants as part of the course registration fee (Stewart et al. 2011).

The accreditation scheme is based on the concept of a four-level hierarchy. Its foundation principle is the objective maintenance of quality assurance of measurements by requiring that all levels of ISAK practitioner must meet initial technical error of measurement (TEM) criteria.

- Level 1 is designed for the majority of ISAK-accredited anthropometrists who have little ongoing requirement for more than the measurement of height, weight and skinfolds.
- Level 2 is designed for those anthropometrists who wish to offer their participants a more comprehensive range of measurements.
- Level 3 is designed only for those anthropometrists who wish to engage in the training and accreditation of Level 1 and 2 anthropometrists.
- Level 4 is the most senior level. It recognises many years of experience in taking ISAK-approved measurements, a high level of theoretical knowledge, involvement in the teaching and examining of ISAK course participants, involvement in large anthropometric research projects and a significant publication record in a related field. Level 4 is reserved for a small group of internationally recognised anthropometrists (17 in 2016) and carries with it the responsibility to train, examine and re-accredit Level 3 anthropometrists.

The components and requirements for these four accreditation levels are detailed in Table 19.1. Details of the ISAK accreditation scheme can be found on the ISAK website http://isak.global.

19.2.2   Imaging Method: Ultrasound

Training, accreditation and certification of personnel using the ultrasound measurement of physique are undertaken by the International Association for Sciences in Medicine and Sports (IASMS) (www.iasms.org). Basic and advanced level courses are usually conducted together. Participants reach the basic level on the first day of training and the advanced level on the second day. Certificates are issued by IASMS, and the goals and the content for both courses can be found at http://www.iasms.org/COURSES/CERTIFICATIONS/.

Advanced level course participants are required to investigate an additional cohort of participants after the course at their home institute and send the captured images, together with their evaluations, to the course leader who checks the images and gives feedback. The final image evaluations are then sent to Rotosport (www.rotosport.com) to be double-checked by a scientific board member of IASMS. IASMS then sends the advanced level certificate to the participant. The advanced level certification ensures that the participant is competent to acquire quality images using the published technique standards (Müller et al. 2016) and demonstrate competence in the use of the FAT™ software (Rotosport, Austria) to assess subcutaneous adipose tissue. Accredited operators obtain the high accuracy and reproducibility criteria that are possible with this new method.

Table 19.1 Summary of the ISAK accreditation scheme

	Level 1: Technician—restricted profile	Level 2: Technician—full profile	Level 3: Instructor Anthropometrist	Level 4: Criterion Anthropometrist
In course practical hours	18	22	38	-
Theory contact hours	6	10	18	-
Post-course practical hours	16	20	20	-
Independent learning hours	20	28	34	-
Total hours	60	80	110	-
Prerequisites	None	Accreditation at ISAK Level 1 for at least 6 months	(1) Bachelor's degree or equivalent in human movement science, nutrition, sports medicine, medicine, functional anatomy or similar subject. (2) Completion of ISAK Level 2. (3) Significant demonstrable experience in anthropometry, as judged appropriate by a criterion anthropometrist	(1) Hold current Level 3 accreditation. (2) Have many years of experience in taking anthropometric measurements. (3) Have a high level of theoretical knowledge. (4) Be involved in the teaching/examining of ISAK workshops or courses. (5) Have had involvement in large-scale measuring research projects. (6) Have a publication record in anthropometry in international, peer-reviewed journals. (7) Have made a significant contribution to ISAK as an organisation. (8) Be a member in good standing of ISAK

(continued)

Table 19.1 (continued)

	Level 1: Technician—restricted profile	Level 2: Technician—full profile	Level 3: Instructor Anthropometrist	Level 4: Criterion Anthropometrist
Competencies assessed	Adequate precision in two base measures, eight skinfolds, five girths and two breadths of the restricted profile	Competent in the assessment of a full profile: four base measures, eight skinfolds, 13 girths, eight segment lengths, nine breadths	Competent in the assessment of the ISAK full profile and in the teaching and examination of Level 1 and 2 courses	By appointment of ISAK accreditation group
Validity of certification	Certification expires 4 years and 4 months from the practical examination	Certification expires 4 years and 6 months from the practical examination	Accreditation expires 4 years and 6 months from the practical examination	The designation of Level 4 criterion anthropometrist is for 4 years from the letter of approval

19.3 Techniques/Technologies That Have National Training, Accreditation and/or Quality Assurance Schemes

There are several national training and certificate programmes for dual-energy X-ray absorptiometry, magnetic resonance imaging and computed tomography.

19.3.1 Imaging Method: Dual-Energy X-Ray Absorptiometry

In Australia and New Zealand, the group responsible for training courses for practitioners and operators involved with bone densitometry (i.e. dual-energy X-ray absorptiometry) is the Australian and New Zealand Bone and Mineral Society (ANZBMS) (https://www.anzbms.org.au). One such course, the Clinical Densitometry Training course, is intended for both practitioners and technologists. This 2-day course covers the pathophysiology of osteoporosis and the principles and practice of bone density, body composition measurement and aspects of advanced bone measurement techniques. The course is intended for:

- Those with a tertiary education in a science-based course, including nursing, who have not previously received formal training for bone densitometry
- Dual-energy X-ray absorptiometry operators who have not undertaken formal training or who are seeking an advanced update of their work practices

- Medical specialists, or specialist registrars in training, with responsibility for bone density testing and who are seeking deeper knowledge of the technological and quality assurance aspects of bone densitometry measurements and reporting

The course includes the following sections:

- Participants are provided with extensive online course material prior to the commencement of the course and are required to read through all the material before they attend the lecture series.
- Participants then attend a 2-day lecture and workshop series, including interactive sessions allowing use of manufacturer specific dual-energy X-ray absorptiometry software.
- An online multiple-choice examination is held 2 weeks after completion of the lecture series.
- Upon completion of the course and achievement of a pass mark in the examination, participants are awarded a Certificate of Completion in Clinical Bone Densitometry.

Another group involved with training courses for practitioners and operators involved with dual-energy X-ray absorptiometry is the International Society for Clinical Densitometry (ISCD) (http://www.iscd.org). The ISCD certification encompasses clinicians and technologists in bone densitometry through one of three certification programmes: Certified Clinical Densitometrist (CCD), Certified Bone Densitometry Technologist (CBDT) and Certified Densitometry Technologist (CDT). A brief description of the three certification strands is as follows:

- A Certified Bone Densitometry Technologist (CBDT™®) is an accredited professional certification by the National Commission for Certifying Agencies (NCCA), in the field of bone densitometry for technologists who perform bone densitometry scans.
- Certified Clinical Densitometrist (CCD™®) is accredited by the NCCA as a professional designation awarded to clinicians who meet specified knowledge requirements measured through a standardised testing process for the interpretation of bone densitometry.
- Certified Densitometry Technologist (CDT™®) is a professional designation for individuals who have met specified knowledge requirements measured through a standardised testing process in bone densitometry for performing central dual-energy X-ray absorptiometry outside the United States.

Maintenance of Certification (MOC) is a system developed by the ISCD to streamline the requirements of re-certification. MOC provides access to ISCD online education to meet continuing education (CE) requirements. ISCD requires at least seven credits each year to maintain certification. CBDT and CCD are both a 5-year certification requiring 35 h of continuing education to renew. Certification is automatically renewed on the anniversary date, provided that 35 CE/CME credits and annual ISCD membership is current or that the annual MOC agreement is in good standing. An unfortunate consequence of these courses/programmes is that they are heavily focused on the use of dual-energy X-ray absorptiometry to assess bone mineral density and, thus, do not consider the nuances of whole-body physique assessment via dual-energy X-ray absorptiometry.

19.3.2 Imaging Method: Magnetic Resonance Imaging and Computed Tomography

In clinical practice, magnetic resonance imaging and computed tomography scans are generally undertaken by radiographers (radiologic technologists, diagnostic radiographers or medical radiation technologists) that undergo extensive training and accreditation processes. Radiologists (specialist medical doctors) are trained to analyse the generated images for clinical diagnostic purposes. However, other health professionals including sport scientists may be trained to use certain magnetic resonance imaging machines or analyse scans for specialised interpretation. Machines that use radiation require operator and site accreditation and ongoing manufacturer servicing support. Magnetic resonance imaging and computed tomography scanners will have manufacturer-prescribed calibration and quality assurance or quality control processes. Site personnel responsible for the machines will undergo training related to ongoing care, service and software updates.

19.4 Technologies That Have Manufacturers or Organisations Training but No Accreditation or Quality Assurance Schemes

Manufacturers training on equipment is provided for Bod Pod, 3D scanning and bioelectrical impedance; however, there are no international accreditation or quality assurance schemes for the use of these techniques.

19.4.1 Non-imaging Method: Bod Pod

There is no formal accreditation system for operators of the Bod Pod. However, each Bod Pod purchase includes a full day of onsite training on the use of the system, undertaken by the manufacturers of the Bod Pod (www.Bod Pod.com). The training specialists are experts on the Bod Pod and are knowledgeable in related fields such as exercise physiology, nutrition and athletic training. Ongoing support after the initial training is available from the manufacturer. A user's manual that explains how the technology works and the theory behind its application is provided as part of the training. Operators normally issue a fact sheet to each client before they undergo assessment in the Bod Pod. This fact sheet details what happens during the test and lists the requirements for what (and what not) to wear and statements on hydration and fasting status and on prior exercise status. Some institutions have also developed standard Bod Pod operating protocols for pre-use calibration (quality control) with step-by-step instructions for operation.

19.4.2   Non-imaging Method: 3D Scanning

There are no universal training schemes for human 3D scanning, other than the manufacturers' specific guidelines. There are ISO standards which relate to scanning devices, but the nature of the development of the field is so rapid that these standards may date rather quickly.

Consensus is required regarding the standard presentation (e.g. euhydration, fasting, breathing cycle, posture and clothing) of participants when being assessed in the laboratory. At present, there is no international agreement as to what criteria comprise best practice, and, therefore, individual groups have created their own standards in isolation.

The science of metrology can be employed to calibrate scanners by using solid objects of known volume that are placed at various distances from the scanner. This technique will provide in vitro calibration. The specification sheet for individual scanners should contain such information; however, the information is not always presented in a standardised form. A unified approach to the standardisation of the technology and to the training and certification of operatives is urgently needed, but the attractiveness of setting up such systems in a rapidly changing field presents difficulties.

19.4.3   Non-imaging Method: Bioelectrical Impedance

There is no known accreditation system for individuals, or for the equipment, using bioelectrical impedance analysis to assess components of physique. Bioelectrical impedance analysis machines are readily available to individuals and to fitness providers. There are some contraindications for measurement, but the extent of the training is likely to be restricted to a simple reference to the manufacturer's factory warning label for operators not to use on individuals with pacemakers or on pregnant women. Similarly, the reporting of data to the client can be undertaken by an untrained practitioner.

19.4.4   Non-imaging Method: Doubly Labelled Water

The doubly labelled water (DLW) method and standards are overseen by the International Atomic Energy Agency (IAEA) (https://humanhealth.iaea.org). The IAEA undertakes training and sends experts to third-world countries to assist and advise new operators.

The history of attempts to standardise techniques is detailed. Early (pre-1985) papers on human applications of DLW concentrated on theoretical and technical aspects in relation to human nutrition and on the results of new cross-validation studies. Many of the leading groups in the field participated in a methodological workshop during the XIII International Congress of Nutrition at Brighton in 1985. The first biological results were published in the same year. In 1986, several groups from laboratories throughout the world participated in a symposium in Cambridge on stable isotopic methods for measuring energy expenditure. Results from many new studies were presented, and there was a general acceptance by most nutritionists that the method was probably working well.

However, there were two major concerns. The first related to difficulties in making inter-laboratory comparisons of data if each laboratory used a slightly different variant of the technique. The second concern was that new workers in the field may underestimate the complexities of DLW and publish invalid data which could potentially discredit the method. To address these problems, it was decided to convene another workshop to seek a consensus view on the various technical aspects of applying the method. The workshop was held in Clare College, Cambridge, in September 1988. There was a remarkable concurrence of views concerning the causes, consequences and solutions to all the major problems associated with DLW. Following the meeting, views were summarised by several participants whose chapters were re-circulated for comments in order to ensure that the consensus had been fairly represented. The resultant recommendations were published in a report by the working group of the International Dietary Energy Consultancy Group (the doubly labelled water method for measuring energy expenditure—technical recommendations for use in humans—1990). Unfortunately, this report did not stipulate exact rules for how the method should be applied but instead provided a framework of guidelines to ensure that published data were of a high quality. All current and potential users of the doubly labelled water method are strongly encouraged to use these guidelines. Despite this, however, several aspects of the method have not yet been standardised.

19.5 Ethical Considerations in Assessing Anthropometry Profiles for Athletes

19.5.1 What Is Ethical Behaviour?

Ethical behaviour is characterised by honesty, fairness and equity in interpersonal, professional and academic relationships and in research and scholarly activities. Ethical behaviour respects the dignity, diversity and rights of individuals and groups of people. Practitioners need to maintain professional objectivity and integrity and respect the athlete during physique assessment. Applying professional knowledge and skills to all work undertaken will ensure ethical behaviour. Practitioners need to actively seek the advancement of knowledge and respect the cultural environment in which they work.

19.5.2   How Do You Ensure Ethical Behaviour When Measuring Physique of Athletes?

For guidelines on how to uphold professional standards and ethics, see examples such as documented by the Royal Society of New Zealand (http://royalsociety.org. nz/who-we-are/our-rules-and-codes/code-of-professional-standards-and-ethics/ royal-society-of-new-zealand-code-of-professional-standards-and-ethics-in-sci- ence-technology-and-the-humanities/).

It is important to consider who you are assessing, what assessments you will undertake, when the assessments will take place and where you will undertake the measurements.

You need to consider the gender and ethnicity of who you are to measure. Consider how will you measure athletes who do not want their chest marked with + (due to religious reasons), or athletes who do not want the top of their head touched (for cultural reasons), or those who will not allow measurement unless their body is fully clothed. Do you have a screened-off area to measure athletes?

Consider whether your athlete has been measured before and if they are familiar with measurements or whether you need to explain what measurements you want to take. Consider when you will measure the athletes, taking into account their training time and diurnal variances that may affect the measures.

In measuring athlete physique, practitioners must develop, maintain and encour- age a high standard of professional training and competence. Athlete physique prac- titioners need to provide information on their professional qualifications and provide clear descriptions of services to help the public make informed choices of the services.

The practitioner needs to take prime responsibility for the athlete assessment and ensure competent interpretation of the assessment results. It is recommended that consent forms and raw data be kept in a secure place for a period of 6 years from the date of testing. This will enable follow-assessment to have change scores derived.

Do not disclose information without the informed consent of the athlete. Ensure you abide by the Privacy Act for your country.

Be accurate and objective in reporting data or information. Restrict comments to your areas of expertise or refer to other practitioners.

Subject respect must be maintained at all times. Do not exploit a professional relationship with any person. Ensure athletes are fully informed of all aspects of the assessment. Obtain informed consent for the assessment, preferably in writing. Personal space needs to be respected. Be aware of where you put your hands and your body with respect to the athlete.

Requirements must be communicated to the athletes and coach prior to participa- tion as unfamiliarity with the assessment procedures may cause anxiety. Unhurried habituation to the conditions and adequate explanation of the proposed procedures and the objectives should be provided. A quiet, reassuring atmosphere is a pre- requisite for competent assessment in an unfamiliar environment.

Ensure the athlete is in good general health and note any physical and emotional limitations. Know how to operate, maintain and calibrate the equipment. Any isolated area that is used for assessment should have a warning system to alert others in the event of an emergency situation. Ensure a person trained in first aid is available in case of emergency. Ensure you have an emergency action plan.

19.6   Summary

Training and accreditation is available to varying levels for imaging and non-imaging techniques. Future works to develop international programmes for training and certification are warranted to ensure quality provision of body assessment techniques.

Athlete safety and well-being are paramount in assessments. Understand the principles of ethics for anthropometry practice. Understand athlete consent and safety issues for assessment. Ensure the athlete understands all procedures and that consent is gained to conduct the physique assessment. Allow the athlete to habituate to the assessment conditions.

References

Müller W, Lohman TG, Stewart AD, Maughan RJ, Meyer NL, Sardinha LB, Kirihennedige N, Reguant-Closa A, Risoul-Salas V, Sundgot-Borgen J, Ahammer H, Anderhuber F, Fürhapter-Rieger A, Kainz P, Materna W, Pilsl U, Pirstinger W, Ackland TR (2016) Subcutaneous fat patterning in athletes: selection of appropriate sites and standardisation of a novel ultrasound measurement technique: ad hoc working group on body composition, health and performance, under the auspices of the IOC Medical Commission. Brit J Sports Med 50:45–54

Stewart AD, Marfell-Jones MJ, Olds T, de Ridder JH (2011) International standards for anthropometric assessment. ISAK, Lower Hutt

Chapter 20
Resources: YouTube Videos and the JELCKC Website and Archive

Patria A. Hume, Kate Fuller, Kelly R. Sheerin, Gary Slater, Stephen C. Hollings, Timothy R. Ackland, Deborah A. Kerr, Masaharu Kagawa, Kagan J. Ducker, Ava Kerr, Justin W.L. Keogh, Duncan J. Macfarlane, Elaine C. Rush, Greg Shaw, Kristen L. MacKenzie-Shalders, Arthur D. Stewart, Stephven Kolose, Clinton O. Njoku, Helen O'Connor, J. Hans de Ridder, Jacqueline A. Alderson, Wolfram Müller, Alisa Nana, and Anna V. Lorimer

Abstract Additional resources to support the content in *Best Practice Protocols for Physique Assessment in Sport* are available at the J.E. Lindsay Carter Kinanthropometry Clinic and Archive (JELCKCA) website jelckca-bodycomp.com, which links you to the YouTube channel http://tinyurl.com/YouTubeChannel-ProfPatria. YouTube videos include introduction of experts and their background in physique assessment, demonstration of physique assessment procedures and commentary from experts on issues related to physique assessment. The physical kinanthropometry archive is located at the Auckland University of Technology Millennium precinct in Auckland, New Zealand.

Keywords Video • Expert opinion • Demonstration • Best practice • YouTube • Archive

P.A. Hume (✉)
Sport Performance Research Institute New Zealand,
Auckland University of Technology, Auckland, New Zealand
e-mail: patria.hume@aut.ac.nz

K.R. Sheerin • S.C. Hollings • E.C. Rush • A.V. Lorimer
Auckland University of Technology, Auckland, New Zealand
e-mail: kelly.sheerin@aut.ac.nz; hollings@athletic.co.nz; elaine.rush@aut.ac.nz;
anna.lorimer@aut.ac.nz

K. Fuller • G. Shaw
Australian Institute of Sport, Bruce, Australia
e-mail: kate.fuller@ausport.gov.au; Greg.Shaw@ausport.gov.au

G. Slater • A. Kerr
University of the Sunshine Coast, Sippy Downs, Australia
e-mail: gslater@usc.edu.au; akerr@usc.edu.au

T.R. Ackland
School of Sport Science, Exercise and Health, The University of Western Australia,
Crawley, WA 6009, Australia
e-mail: tim.ackland@uwa.edu.au

© Springer Nature Singapore Pte Ltd. 2018   243
P.A. Hume et al. (eds.), *Best Practice Protocols for Physique Assessment in Sport*,
https://doi.org/10.1007/978-981-10-5418-1_20

J.A. Alderson
University of Western Australia, Crawley, WA, Australia
e-mail: jacqueline.alderson@uwa.edu.au

D.A. Kerr
School of Public Health, Curtin University, Perth, West Australia, Australia
e-mail: D.Kerr@curtin.edu.au

K.J. Ducker
Curtin University, Bentley, WA, Australia
e-mail: kagan.ducker@curtin.edu.au

M. Kagawa
Kagawa Nutrition University, Sakado, Japan
e-mail: mskagawa@eiyo.ac.jp

J.W.L. Keogh • K.L. MacKenzie-Shalders
Bond University, Robina, Australia
e-mail: jkeogh@bond.edu.au; kmackenz@bond.edu.au

D.J. Macfarlane
The University of Hong Kong, Pok Fu Lam, Hong Kong
e-mail: djmac@hku.hk

A.D. Stewart
Robert Gordon University, Aberdeen, UK
e-mail: a.d.stewart@rgu.ac.uk

S. Kolose
New Zealand Defence Force, Wellington, New Zealand
e-mail: s.kolose@dta.mil.nz

C.O. Njoku
Ebonyi State University, Ebonyi, Nigeria
e-mail: clinton.njoku@ebsu-edu.net

H. O'Connor
University of Sydney, Sydney, NSW, Australia
e-mail: helen.oconnor@sydney.edu.au

J.H. de Ridder
North-West University, Potchefstroom, NSW, South Africa
e-mail: hans.deridder@nwu.ac.za

W. Müller
Medical University of Graz, Graz, Austria
e-mail: wolfram.mueller@medunigraz.at

A. Nana
Mahidol University, Salaya, Thailand
e-mail: alisa.nan@mahidol.ac.th

20.1   YouTube Videos

It is often easier to appreciate and learn a technique when you can see an expert using the technique and providing explanations on key points. We have provided videos of several of our experts demonstrating the techniques and also commenting on issues related to the techniques. YouTube videos include introduction of experts and their background in physique assessment, demonstration of physique assessment procedures and commentary from experts on issues related to physique assessment. Find the information via the link at jelckca-bodycomp.com or go to http://tinyurl.com/YouTubeChannel-ProfPatria.

Identify the videos in the series with the logo.

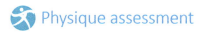 Physique assessment

20.1.1   Physique Assessment Experts

Figure 20.1 shows the YouTube physique assessment experts who share some of their background in physique assessment in the YouTube videos. Table 20.1 provides the links for the experts YouTube videos.

20.1.2   Physique Assessment Technique Demonstrations

Figure 20.2 shows the YouTube physique assessment technique demonstrations start screen that appears for the videos of the experts demonstrating physique assessment procedures videos. Table 20.2 provides the links for the physique assessment experts' technique demonstration YouTube videos.

20.1.3   Experts Commentary on Issues Related to Physique Assessment

Professor Patria Hume posed questions to experts. Figure 20.3 shows the YouTube physique assessment expert commentary start screen that appears for the videos of some of the experts providing commentary on questions commonly asked regarding physique assessment. Table 20.3 provides the links for the physique assessment experts' commentary on issues related to physique assessment YouTube videos.

A selection of quotes from some of the questions posed is provided in this chapter so readers can appreciate the nature of the content available in the videos related to the book chapters.

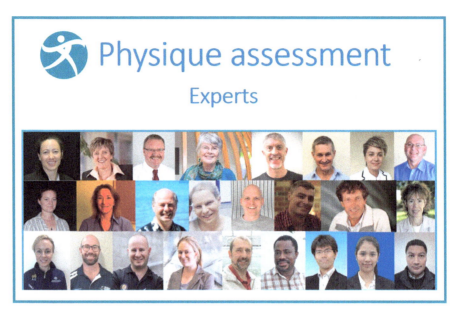

Fig. 20.1 YouTube physique assessment experts start screen

20.1.3.1   Part I: Why Measure Physique?

Why would a health-care practitioner consider monitoring the body composition of a client?

- "The monitoring of physique traits affords a practitioner the opportunity to further personalise their interventions (training and/or diet) for clients based on adaptations. Personally, I think it is unprofessional if you are not monitoring adaptations of clients when working with them to manipulate body composition. How else can you know if your intervention/s are having a favourable impact?" Associate Professor Gary Slater
- "For a variety of reasons. Many factors relating to your body composition are related to health outcomes (e.g. bone density and osteoporosis, visceral fat and risk of CV disease etc.). If you then choose to change these to positively affect risk factors, you need to be able to monitor body composition to see how things are changing". Dr. Kagan Ducker
- "It is because body composition variables such as fat mass and fat-free mass are known to be associated with a number of health risks, physical performance and appropriate growth and development". Associate Professor Masaharu Kagawa

What benefits would an individual gain from having their physique assessed?

- "Aside from facilitating further personalisation of interventions based on how the client responds, physique assessment provides invaluable motivation for clients, confirming the lifestyle (or other) changes they have made are resulting in favourable adaptations". Associate Professor Gary Slater

Table 20.1 Links for the physique assessment experts YouTube videos

Physique assessment expert	YouTube link
Professor Patria **Hume** PhD, MSc (Hons), BSc, ISAK4, DipCoachNZG, FISBS (Auckland University of Technology)	http://tinyurl.com/ PA-Expert-Patria-Hume
Associate Professor Deborah **Kerr** PhD, MSc, GradDipDiet, BAppSc, APD, ISAK4 (Curtin University)	https://tinyurl.com/ PA-Expert-Deborah-Kerr
Professor Tim **Ackland** PhD, FASMF, FRSB (University of Western Australia)	https://tinyurl.com/ PA-Expert-Tim-Ackland
Associate Professor Jacqueline **Alderson** PhD, FISBS (University of Western Australia)	https://tinyurl.com/ PA-Expert-Jacqueline-Alderson
Professor J. Hans **de Ridder** PhD, ISAK4 (North-West University)	https://tinyurl.com/ PA-Expert-Hans-De-Ridder
Dr Kagan **Ducker** PhD, BSc (Hons), ESSAM, AES, ASpS2, ISAK3 (Curtin University)	https://tinyurl.com/ PA-Expert-Kagan-Ducker
Dr Stephen **Hollings** PhD, DipEd, DipSpEd, AdvDipTchg, ISAK3 (Auckland University of Technology)	https://tinyurl.com/ PA-Expert-Stephen-Hollings
Associate Professor Masaharu **Kagawa** PhD, BSc (Hons), RPHNutr, ISAK3 (Kagawa Nutrition University)	https://tinyurl.com/ PA-Expert-Masaharu-Kagawa
Associate Professor Justin **Keogh** PhD, BHMS (Hons), BHSc (Ex & Sp Sci), FAAG, FISBS (Bond University)	https://tinyurl.com/ PA-Expert-Justin-Keogh
Ms Ava **Kerr** BSc., MSc, AES, CSCS, ISAK3 (University of the Sunshine Coast)	https://tinyurl.com/PA-Expert-Ava-Kerr
Mr Stephven **Kolose** MSc, PGDipErg, BSc, ISAK2 (Auckland University of Technology)	https://tinyurl.com/ PA-Expert-Stephven-Kolose
Dr Anna **Lorimer** PhD, BSc (Hons), ISAK3 (Auckland University of Technology)	https://tinyurl.com/ PA-Expert-Anna-Lorimer
Associate Professor Duncan **Macfarlane** DPhil Oxon, BSc (Hons), BPhEd, FACSM, ISAK3 (The University of Hong Kong)	https://tinyurl.com/ PA-Expert-Duncan-Macfarlane
Dr Kristen **MacKenzie-Shalders** PhD, APD, Adv Sports Dietitian, Acc. Sports Scientist, ISAK3 (Bond University)	https://tinyurl.com/ PA-Expert-Kristen-MacKenzie-Sh
Professor Wolfram **Müller** PhD, Mag.rer.nat. (Medical University of Graz)	https://tinyurl.com/ PA-Expert-Wolfram-Muller
Dr Alisa **Nana** PhD, APD, ASD (Mahidol University)	https://tinyurl.com/PA-Expert-Alisa-Nana
Mr Clinton **Njoku** MSc (Hons), BSc (Ebonyi State University, Abakaliki)	https://tinyurl.com/ PA-Expert-Clinton-Njoku
Associate Professor Helen **O'Connor** PhD, DipND, BSc., ISAK3, APD, Adv. SD (University of Sydney)	https://tinyurl.com/ PA-Expert-Helen-OConnor
Professor Elaine **Rush** MNZM, PhD, MSc (Hons), Registered Nutritionist, FCT (Auckland University of Technology)	https://tinyurl.com/ PA-Expert-Elaine-Rush

(continued)

Table 20.1 (continued)

Physique assessment expert	YouTube link
Mr Greg **Shaw** BHSc (Nutr & Diet), IOC Diploma in Sports Nutrition, ISAK3 (Australian Institute of Sport)	https://tinyurl.com/PA-Expert-Greg-Shaw
Mr Kelly **Sheerin** MHSc (Hons), BHSc, BSc, ISAK3 (Auckland University of Technology)	https://tinyurl.com/PA-Expert-Kelly-Sheerin
Associate Professor Gary **Slater** PhD, MSc, BSc, APD, Adv ASD, ISAK3 (University of the Sunshine Coast)	https://tinyurl.com/PA-Expert-Gary-Slater
Dr Arthur **Stewart** PhD, ISAK4 (Robert Gordon University)	https://tinyurl.com/PA-Expert-Arthur-Stewart
Ms Kate **Fuller** BSc, HMS, ISAK3 (Australian Institute of Sport)	https://tinyurl.com/PA-Expert-Kate-Fuller

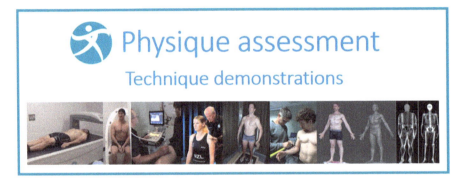

Fig. 20.2 YouTube physique assessment technique demonstration start screen

- "By their physique and body composition being assessed, individuals have better understanding of their current body size, proportion and adiposity or muscularity that is allows them to increase awareness of themselves and provide an opportunity to look at their lifestyle as a whole". Associate Professor Masaharu Kagawa

When do you use anthropometry?

- "I use anthropometry before and after specific periods of training to assess any changes. I also monitor skinfold measurements periodically throughout extensive periods of training to assess whether the changes, if any, are the direct result of the type of middle-distance training that has been undertaken". Dr. Stephen Hollings
- "I have used anthropometry on a number of occasions to compare groups of a diverse range of ethnic and cultural backgrounds, including for health screening, assessment of health risks, monitoring young athletes, and a tool to assess one's body image". Associate Professor Masaharu Kagawa

Table 20.2 Links for the physique assessment experts' technique demonstration YouTube videos

Bod Pod demonstration	
Associate Professor Gary Slater demonstrates Bod Pod body composition assessment	https://tinyurl.com/PA-Demo-GS-Bod-Pod
Dual-energy X-ray absorptiometry (DXA) demonstrations	
Associate Professor Gary Slater demonstrates DXA body composition assessment	https://tinyurl.com/PA-Demo-GS-DXA
Professor Tim Ackland demonstrates DXA body composition assessment	https://tinyurl.com/PA-Demo-TA-DXA
Ultrasound demonstration	
Professor Tim Ackland demonstrates ultrasound body composition assessment	https://tinyurl.com/PA-Demo-TA-Ultrasound
Bioelectrical impedance analysis (BIA) demonstration	
Dr Kagan Ducker demonstrates BIA measurement	https://tinyurl.com/PA-Demo-KD-BIA
Surface anthropometry (ISAK) demonstrations	
Landmarking	
Associate Professor Gary Slater demonstrates acromiale landmarking	https://tinyurl.com/PA-Demo-GS-Acromiale-landmark
Associate Professor Gary Slater demonstrates radiale landmarking	https://tinyurl.com/PA-Demo-GS-Radiale-landmark
Associate Professor Gary Slater demonstrates mid-acromiale landmarking	https://tinyurl.com/PA-Demo-GS-MidAcromRad-landmark
Skinfolds	
Associate Professor Gary Slater demonstrates sub-scapula skinfold marking and measurement	https://tinyurl.com/PA-Demo-GS-Subscapula-Skinfold
Associate Professor Gary Slater demonstrates biceps skinfold marking and measurement	https://tinyurl.com/PA-Demo-GS-Biceps-Skinfold
Associate Professor Gary Slater demonstrates triceps skinfold marking and measurement	https://tinyurl.com/PA-Demo-GS-Triceps-Skinfold
Associate Professor Gary Slater demonstrates iliac crest skinfold marking and measurement	https://tinyurl.com/PA-Demo-GS-Iliaccrest-Skinfold
Associate Professor Gary Slater demonstrates supraspinale skinfold marking and measurement	https://tinyurl.com/PA-Demo-GS-Supraspinale-Skinfold
Associate Professor Gary Slater demonstrates abdominal skinfold marking and measurement	https://tinyurl.com/PA-Demo-GS-Abdominal-Skinfold
Associate Professor Gary Slater demonstrates front thigh skinfold marking and measurement	https://tinyurl.com/PA-Demo-GS-Front-thigh-Skinfold
Associate Professor Gary Slater demonstrates calf skinfold marking and measurement	https://tinyurl.com/PA-Demo-GS-Calf-Skinfold
Associate Professor Gary Slater demonstrates all skinfold measurements	https://tinyurl.com/PA-Demo-GS-All-Skinfolds
Associate Professor Gary Slater explains skinfold measurement process	https://tinyurl.com/PA-Demo-GS-Skinfold-process
Associate Professor Masaharu Kagawa demonstrates calf skinfold measurement	https://tinyurl.com/PA-Demo-MK-Calf-Skinfold

(continued)

Table 20.2 (continued)

Associate Professor Masaharu Kagawa demonstrates Japanese skinfold caliper jaw calibration	https://tinyurl.com/PA-Demo-MK-Caliper-calibrate
Girths	
Our physique assessment experts Associate Professors Deborah Kerr and Masaharu Kagawa demonstrate calf girth measurement	https://tinyurl.com/PA-Demo-DKMK-Calf girth
Associate Professor Masaharu Kagawa demonstrates head girth measurement	https://tinyurl.com/PA-Demo-MK-Head-girth
Associate Professor Masaharu Kagawa demonstrates Japanese tape for girth measurements	https://tinyurl.com/PA-Demo-MK-Japan-girth-tape
Breadths	
Our physique assessment experts Associate Professors Deborah Kerr and Masaharu Kagawa demonstrate humerus bone breadth measurement	https://tinyurl.com/PA-Demo-DKMK-Humerus
Our physique assessment expert Associate Professor Masaharu Kagawa demonstrates femur bone breadth measurement	https://tinyurl.com/PA-Demo-MK-Femur
Our physique assessment experts Associate Professors Deborah Kerr and Masaharu Kagawa demonstrate bi-acromiale bone breadth measurement	https://tinyurl.com/PA-Demo-DKMK-Biacromiale
Lengths	
Associate Professor Masaharu Kagawa demonstrates foot length measurement	https://tinyurl.com/PA-Demo-MK-Foot-length
Associate Professor Masaharu Kagawa demonstrates tibiale-laterale length measurement	https://tinyurl.com/PA-Demo-MK-Tibiale-laterale
Basics	
Associate Professor Masaharu Kagawa demonstrates standing height measurement	https://tinyurl.com/PA-Demo-MK-Standing-height
Associate Professor Masaharu Kagawa demonstrates sitting height measurement	https://tinyurl.com/PA-Demo-MK-Sitting-height

- "I have used anthropometry throughout my career as a sports performance focused dietitian. I completed my Level 1 course some 20 years ago and there's not a week goes by where I'm not using anthropometry to monitor clients. Why is it so good… very economical, easily portable and robust, impacted by few if any of the factors that influence other physique assessment techniques reliability such as hydration status, acute food and fluid intake etc. What it demands though is highly skilled practitioners". Associate Professor Gary Slater
- "I use it to assess changes in an athlete's body composition in response to the training that they are completing or when there is a change in a factor that may affect their body composition, e.g. change in diet, travel to altitude, etc. The key point is that we may monitor regularly over time so that we have some on-going baseline data but mostly it's to be used when we expect a change". Dr. Kagan Ducker

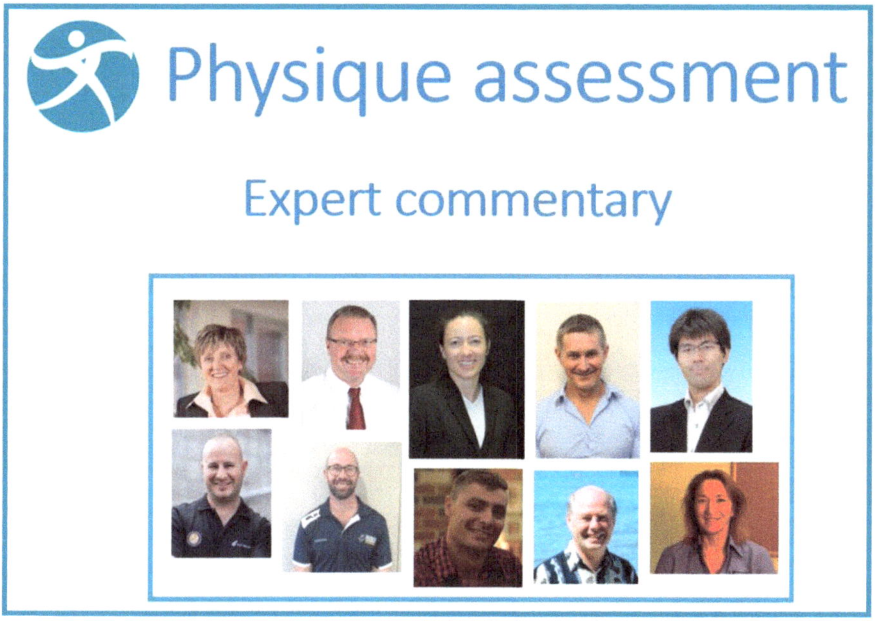

Fig. 20.3 YouTube physique assessment technique expert commentary start screen

Chapter 1: Physique Assessment in Youth Sports for Talent Identification and Development

Why do you measure body size and shape for talent identification and development?

- "There is application of physique assessment for talent identification in sports where specific traits may predispose an athlete to competitive success. This can extend beyond body composition to broader physique traits. For example, longer levers provide a biomechanical advantage to rowers". Associate Professor Gary Slater

- "We know that certain body sizes/shapes and compositions are beneficial for certain sports (e.g. weightlifters having a low crural and brachial index, long distance runners being lean), which can help us with talent identification and developing our athletes to excel in their sports. Assessing their size/shape and composition can help us to monitor changes that are occurring in their body that we may or may not have been trying to elicit (e.g. measuring changes in muscle size when an athlete is progressing through a resistance training program that we have written)". Dr. Kagan Ducker

Table 20.3 Links for the physique assessment experts' physique assessment experts' commentary on issues related to physique assessment YouTube videos.

Chapter and questions	YouTube link
Why is the Physique Assessment book useful?	https://tinyurl.com/ PA-Q-DK-Book-useful-why
Part I: Why Measure Physique?	
Why would a health-care practitioner consider monitoring the body composition of a client?	https://tinyurl.com/ PA-Q-expert-Why-monitor-body
What benefits would an individual gain from having their physique assessed?	https://tinyurl.com/ PA-Q-Benefit-physique-assess
When do you use anthropometry?	https://tinyurl.com/ PA-Q-expert-When-anthropometry
Chapter 1: Physique Assessment in Youth Sports for Talent Identification and Development	
Why do you measure body size and shape for talent identification and development?	https://tinyurl.com/ PA-Q-expert-Body-size
Chapter 2: Anthropometry and Health for Sport	
Does body composition influence health?	https://tinyurl.com/ PA-Q-expert-Bodycomp-Health
How do you use growth charts and normative data sets?	https://tinyurl.com/ PA-Q-expert-Growth-chart
What variables are you interested in for determining appropriate growth?	https://tinyurl.com/ PA-Q-expert-Growth-vars
How do you use physique assessment to understand growth changes?	https://tinyurl.com/ PA-Q-expert-Growth-changes
What variables are you interested in for determining malnourishment?	https://tinyurl.com/ PA-Q-expert-Malnourishment
What variables are you interested in for determining obesity and related health problems?	https://tinyurl.com/ PA-Q-expert-Obesity-vars
Chapter 3: Optimising Physique for Sports Performance	
How do you work with coaches to plan athlete assessment?	http://tinyurl.com/ PA-Q-expert-Coach-work
What are your clinical considerations in assessment of nutrition status of athletes?	https://tinyurl.com/ PA-Q-expert-Clinical-consider
Does where you store body fat provide insight into the type of diet you should follow?	https://tinyurl.com/ PA-Q-expert-Store-body-fat
What do you consider an ideal body fat level for an athlete?	https://tinyurl.com/ PA-Q-GS-Body-fat-ideal
Chapter 4: Physique Assessment for Sports Equipment Design, Fit and Performance Optimisation	
How is physique assessment important for ergonomics in sports?	https://tinyurl.com/ PA-Q-expert-Paralympic
Part II: How to Use the Selected Method and Report the Data	
What is the best method for assessing body composition?	https://tinyurl.com/ PA-Q-expert-Best-method
Is there a gold standard method of assessing body composition?	https://tinyurl.com/ PA-Q-expert-Gold-std

(continued)

Table 20.3 (continued)

Chapter and questions	YouTube link
Why do you assess body size, shape and composition for athletes?	https://tinyurl.com/PA-Q-expert-Why-assess-body-sz
What are your key tips for body composition assessment for athletes?	https://tinyurl.com/PA-Q-expert-Key-tips-bodycomp
As a health-care practitioner, should I consider purchasing equipment to monitor the body composition of my clients? If so, what should I use?	http://tinyurl.com/PA-Q-expert-Equipment-purchase
Chapter 5: Athlete Considerations for Physique Measurement	
Does what I do prior to a scan influence results?	http://tinyurl.com/PA-Q-expert-Prior-scan
Chapter 6: Non-imaging Method: Surface Anthropometry	
In the modern age of body scanning, does surface anthropometry still have a role to play?	https://tinyurl.com/PA-Q-expert-Surface-anthro-role
Is surface anthropometry still worthwhile given all the new technology available?	https://tinyurl.com/PA-Q-expert-Anthro-worth
Is surface anthropometry actually accurate?	https://tinyurl.com/PA-Q-expert-Anthro-accurate
I measured myself on some scales and they told me I had 9% body fat. Will your results be able to compare to these?	https://tinyurl.com/PA-Q-expert-Fat-scales
Chapter 7: Non-imaging Method: 3D Scanning	
What is 3D scanning useful for?	http://tinyurl.com/PA-Q-expert-3D-body-scanning
Chapter 8: Non-imaging Method: Air Displacement Plethysmography (Bod Pod)	
What is air displacement plethysmography or Bod Pod useful for?	https://tinyurl.com/PA-Q-expert-Bod-Pod-use
Chapter 9: Non-imaging Method: Bioelectrical Impedance Analysis (BIA)	
What is bioelectrical impedance useful for?	https://tinyurl.com/PA-Q-expert-BIA
Chapter 10: Non-imaging Method: Doubly Labelled Water	
Why is the doubly labelled water technique not commonly used for athletes?	https://tinyurl.com/PA-Q-expert-Double-label-water
Chapter 11: Imaging Method: Ultrasound	
What is ultrasound useful for?	https://tinyurl.com/PA-Q-expert-Ultrasound
Chapter 12: Imaging Method: Computed Tomography (CT) and Magnetic Resonance Imaging (MRI)	
What is magnetic resonance imaging useful for?	https://tinyurl.com/PA-Q-expert-MRI-use
Chapter 13: Imaging Method: Dual-Energy X-Ray Absorptiometry (DXA)	
What is dual-energy X-ray absorptiometry useful for?	https://tinyurl.com/PA-Q-expert-DXA
How do you assess skeletal size, shape and bone mineral density?	https://tinyurl.com/PA-Q-expert-Skeletal-size

(continued)

Table 20.3 (continued)

Chapter and questions	YouTube link
How do you assess muscle tissue changes?	https://tinyurl.com/ PA-Q-expert-Msucle-change
What is the effect of client presentation on DXA assessment?	https://tinyurl.com/ PA-Q-GS-DXA-client-present
Chapter 14: Imaging Method: Technological and Computing Innovations	
What is new for imaging physique given technology developments?	https://tinyurl.com/ PA-Q-expert-Tech-developments
Part III: Application of Physique Assessment in Athletes	
Chapter 15: Physique Assessment in Practice	
Do you have an example of when and how you measure physique of athletes?	http://tinyurl.com/ PA-Q-expert-Example-athlete
How often should body composition be assessed?	https://tinyurl.com/ PA-Q-expert-How-often
Why do you use multicomponent models of body composition?	https://tinyurl.com/ PA-Q-expert-Multi-models
What variables are you interested in when tracking clients longitudinally?	http://tinyurl.com/ PA-Q-expert-Track-variables
Is it important to include other data when interpreting body composition data for athletes?	https://tinyurl.com/ PA-Q-DK-Interpret-data
Can body composition variables be compared in cross-ethnic settings without problems?	https://tinyurl.com/ PA-Q-expert-Ethnic-diffs
Are there any issues with anthropometry measurement protocols and data in Japan?	https://tinyurl.com/ PA-Q-expert-Japan-prot-issue
What are examples of different protocols available in Japan, and how are they different to each other?	https://tinyurl.com/ PA-Q-expert-Japan-prot-diffs
Chapter 16: Recommendations for Conducting Research on Athletes	
How do you report results back to clients?	http://tinyurl.com/ PA-Q-expert-Report-result
What large-scale anthropometry projects have you been involved in?	https://tinyurl.com/ PA-Q-DK-What-large-projects
Chapter 17: Physique Characteristics Associated with Athlete Performance	
What types of physique characteristics are related to the expression of muscular strength?	https://tinyurl.com/ PA-Q-expert-Muscle-Strength
Chapter 18: Body Image for Athletes	
Does body composition assessment create unnecessary anxiety for clients?	http://tinyurl.com/ PA-Q-expert-Anxiety-physique
What variables are you interested in for examining body image in your study group?	https://tinyurl.com/ PA-Q-expert-Body-image-vars
What is the SomatoMac app used for?	https://tinyurl.com/ PA-Q-expert-Somatomac
Why is physique assessment important for aesthetic sports?	https://tinyurl.com/ PA-Q-GS-Aesthetic-sport
Chapter 19: Training and Accreditation Systems and Ethical Considerations	

(continued)

Table 20.3 (continued)

Chapter and questions	YouTube link
Why are standardised protocols and valid and reliable measures needed for assessment?	http://tinyurl.com/ PA-Q-expert-Valid-std
Why is precision in body composition measurement techniques important?	https://tinyurl.com/ PA-Q-expert-Precision
Does it matter if I am assessed by different people on different equipment?	https://tinyurl.com/ PA-Q-expert-Diff-people
Where do I go to get my body composition assessed?	https://tinyurl.com/ PA-Q-expert-Where-assessed
How do you gain consent to conduct measurements of athletes?	http://tinyurl.com/PA-Q-expert-Consent
How do you maintain confidentiality when assessing body composition, especially in a team sport environment?	https://tinyurl.com/ PA-Q-expert-Confidentiality
How do you store athlete information?	https://tinyurl.com/ PA-Q-expert-Store-information
If I have concerns about body composition assessment, where do I go for information?	http://tinyurl.com/ PA-Q-expert-Concerns
Why is certification for physique assessment important?	https://tinyurl.com/ PA-Q-KD-Why-certification

Chapter 2: Anthropometry and Health for Sport

Does body composition influence health?

- "Population data suggests being overfat increases the risk of developing lifestyle related diseases. However, it's understanding the distribution of that fat which may be most important… subcutaneous vs visceral fat mass. In contrast, being under muscled may also have adverse effects. Within the older population this is known as sarcopenia (age related loss of lean mass) which is also associated with impaired ability to maintain activities of daily living and thus need for care or ability to live independently". Associate Professor Gary Slater
- "Yes. Numerous studies have reported that increased fat mass, particularly visceral and ectopic fat tissues, influence risk of developing obesity and related diseases. Low fat-free mass, including bone mineral content and muscle tissues, increases risk of frailty and osteoporosis for elder populations". Associate Professor Masaharu Kagawa

How do you use growth charts and normative data sets?

- "As a brief comparison for growth, acknowledging individual variability in growth". Associate Professor Masaharu Kagawa
- "It is important to keep in mind that for individuals less than 20 years of age, normative data comes from growth charts and thus it is inappropriate to use normative adult data. Growth charts exist for several variables including weight for age, stature for age, BMI for age, head circumference for age charts". Associate Professor Gary Slater

What variables are you interested in for determining appropriate growth?

- "Body mass, length/height, sitting height for general growth and circumferences and skinfolds for better understanding muscle and adipose tissue accumulations". Associate Professor Masaharu Kagawa

How do you use physique assessment to understanding growth changes?

- "Regular assessments on body size allow us to plot an individuals' growth that we can compare with the norms. Both regular assessments of body size and somatotype of children allows us to depict timing of puberty, including timing of peak velocities for height, body mass, and leg length. Tracking information on both genders allows us to observe gender differences". Associate Professor Masaharu Kagawa

What variables are you interested in for determining malnourishment?

- "Height, body mass, upper-arm circumferences etc…". Associate Professor Masaharu Kagawa

What variables are you interested in for determining obesity and related health problems?

- "Body mass, length/height to determine overall body size, whereas skinfolds, waist circumference and waist-to-height ratio for fat accumulation and distribution patterns". Associate Professor Masaharu Kagawa

Chapter 3: Optimising Physique for Sports Performance

How do you work with coaches to plan athlete assessment?

- "I usually work in conjunction with the coach to determine a schedule for when assessments take place". Dr. Stephen Hollings
- "It's always dealt with as part of planning the yearly program with coaching and sport science staff. This gives us our regular data points that form the basis of our testing program and aligns us with when we expect to see changes in certain variables. The testing can be repeated for individuals who need to be monitored more closely due to issues with weight management or when we are intensively trying to make changes to their body composition". Dr. Kagan Ducker
- "Physique assessment is usually scheduled during planning prior to the pre-season. At this point in time we will identify what physique assessment techniques we will use and when assessments will be scheduled. Assessments are usually scheduled according to the training cycle, which varies markedly depending on the sport. However, as a minimum, assessments would be undertaken at the start and end of the pre-season, plus end of season. Additional assessments will be scheduled for athletes I am working with to manipulate their body composition, or for those who experience an injury or other event likely to impact body composition". Associate Professor Gary Slater

What are your clinical considerations in assessment of nutrition status of athletes?

- "As a sports physiologist my part is knowing the training load that I am imparting and knowing what adaptations I am trying to stimulate. Then I can work with the sports dietitian so that they can ensure that the nutrition planning for the athlete is spot on". Dr. Kagan Ducker

Does where you store body fat provide insight into the type of diet you should follow?

- "Within the fitness industry a program has gained popularity for that very reason. It claims that distribution of body fat provides insight into perturbations in specific hormones such as cortisol and growth hormone. For example, the iliac crest skinfold offers insight into 'carbohydrate tolerance or management of blood glucose levels', while the abdominal skinfold is an indirect measure of cortisol levels and the ability to manage stress. Furthermore, this program claims that dietary adjustments and strategic supplementation can help to manipulate these hormones and with this, reductions in site specific body fat. While fat distribution is clearly impacted by an array of hormones, the impact of specific dietary adjustments to influence targeted fat deposits remains a hypothesis to be tested. Thus other factors such as training loads and associated specific sporting and body composition goals, underlying medical conditions, existing diet and other factors, including social issues like cost and convenience should take precedence when planning the dietary intake of clients". Associate Professor Gary Slater

Chapter 4: Physique Assessment for Sports Equipment Design, Fit and Performance Optimisation

How is physique assessment important for ergonomics in sports?

- "The importance of quantifying the individual Paralympic athletes' anthropometry to maximise the potential benefit of their assistive technology may be observed in the selection and fitting of the appropriate prosthesis (prosthetic limb) for running and cycling athletes". Associate Professor Justin Keogh

20.1.3.2   Part II. How to Use the Selected Method and Report the Data

What is the best method for assessing body composition?

- "That partly depends on what you have access to and what you want the information for. At the end of the day that will guide what your best method is. A combination of measurements is likely to be best". Dr. Kagan Ducker
- "This really depends on what outcome measures you are after and resources available. For example, will changes in skinfold sum in conjunction with body mass changes provide sufficient insight into body composition change or do you

require an absolute estimate of fat and fat free mass or their change over time. Furthermore, consideration must be given to the validity, reliability, availability, expertise required and cost effectiveness of available techniques, especially given the fact that most practitioners will be undertaking assessments on clients periodically over time". Associate Professor Gary Slater

Is there a gold standard method of assessing body composition?

- "The one true reference or gold standard method is cadaver analysis so it's not something I would encourage with your clients! However a combination of techniques in what we call a 4-compartment model is something we use for any study in which changes in body composition are a key outcome variable. In this instance we use a combination of techniques. The Bod Pod measures body density, while dual energy X-ray absorptiometry measure bone mineral content and deuterium dilution measures total body water. Measuring bone and water content, rather than estimating these variables (as occurs when Bod Pod is used in isolation), significantly enhances the validity and precision of measurement". Associate Professor Gary Slater
- "Ultimately if we have access to you as a cadaver that we can break you down into smaller and smaller components until we figure out what you're made of. In a practical sense it's likely to be a combination of several assessments to increase the number of compartments we're assessing e.g., dual energy X-ray absorptiometry and Bod Pod". Dr. Kagan Ducker

Why do you assess body size, shape and composition for athletes?

- "Physique assessment is generally undertaken to monitor the impact of training and/or diet on body composition. The association between physique traits and competitive success varies markedly from sport to sport and our assessments should reflect this. Routine monitoring may be undertaken for sports in which physique traits are associated with competitive success, but clearly less regularly in those in which there is little or no association". Associate Professor Gary Slater.

What are your key tips for body composition assessment for athletes?

- "Firstly, identify what outcome variables you are after. Understand the time and resources that are available, plus frequency of assessment required. It's equally important to understand the precision of your method as knowing this helps to infer what is a real change in composition versus noise in the test. Understanding what factors influence the reliability of your measure will help to establish testing protocols that can be implemented at each assessment period. Finally, never assume an athlete has had their body composition assessed before. As such, explain the procedures to be undertaken in advance and why the assessment is to be undertaken. Timely feedback on the assessment is also critical". Associate Professor Gary Slater
- "Know the accuracy of your methods and be sure that you know that what you're measuring is meaningful and represents a real change. Recognise the right time

to present results. Be sure to remember that the results are confidential". Dr. Kagan Ducker

- "Ensure that the athlete is in the same nutritional, hydration, and pre-exercise state before each assessment". Dr. Stephen Hollings

As a health-care practitioner, should I consider purchasing equipment to monitor the body composition of my clients? If so, what should I use?

- "This is a question I am often asked by practitioners. When considering such an investment, the practitioner really needs to understand the technique and its associated assumptions plus outputs, including which of those that have been validated. There is also a need to give consideration to equipment maintenance and servicing to ensure the results don't drift over time. For most practitioners, this is a time consuming and expensive process. There are also practical issues to address like cost implications. In general, this often means limiting in-house assessment to surface anthropometry. If an absolute estimate of body composition is required, a practitioner should explore partnering with a group that has expertise in body composition assessment. Entrusting the interpretation of the effectiveness of your interventions is not a decision that should be taken lightly so due diligence is encouraged. For example, machine specific precision error should be made available to you, plus detailed advice on client presentation that can be forwarded to clients in advance of assessment". Associate Professor Gary Slater

- "It always depends on your budget. If you only have money for anthropometric measures then stick with that equipment (suppliers on the ISAK website). If you have money for more expensive tools (e.g. bioelectrical impedance analysis, Bod Pod, dual energy X-ray absorptiometry) just be aware of what the limitations are of that equipment. Sometimes the expensive tools aren't as good as a qualified and experienced professional. More importantly you should consider the training that you need to use the techniques effectively". Dr. Kagan Ducker

Chapter 5: Athlete Considerations for Physique Measurement

Does what I do prior to a scan influence results?

- "Absolutely. We have recently completed a six month study which clearly illustrated that if client presentation is not standardised, you can get a completely different interpretation of changes on body composition. This was true for almost all techniques we tracked, including bioelectrical impedance analysis, Bod Pod, dual energy X-ray absorptiometry and various combinations of these. The exception was surface anthropometry, which seems to be a very robust measure. As such, we now provide detailed advice to clients well in advance of assessments that aims to ensure they present overnight fasted, bladder voided, in a rested, euhydrated and glycogen replete state while wearing suitable clothing". Associate Professor Gary Slater

- "Most certainly. Things like whether you've eaten, hydration status, prior exercise (especially swimming) may influence the results of the scan. It's important to standardise some factors". Dr. Kagan Ducker

Chapter 6: Non-imaging Method: Surface Anthropometry

In the modern age of body scanning, does surface anthropometry still have a role to play?

- "Scanning techniques including dual energy X-ray absorptiometry, computed tomography and magnetic resonance imaging are becoming increasingly used in hospital and research settings compared to surface anthropometry. However, while these techniques provide detailed anthropometric and morphological characteristics of a variety of body tissues, they still have limitations based on ease of access, training required to perform the scans and cost. On this basis, I believe surface anthropometry still has an important role to play for many more years". Associate Professor Justin Keogh

Is surface anthropometry still worthwhile given all the new technology available?

- "Yes, certainly. The benefit of surface anthropometry is its portability and the fact that you can test athletes at their training or competition venues with minimal disruption to their normal routines". Mr. Kelly Sheerin

Is surface anthropometry actually accurate?

- "As long as the measurer is appropriately trained, regularly measures, and follows the ISAK guidelines, accurate results can be obtained".

I measured myself on some scales and they told me I had 9% body fat. Will your results be able to compare to these?

- "Body fat percentage results are estimates that are calculated via one of a range of regression equations. There are a number of assumptions and limitations associated with the use of such equations. The foundation of these equations are neither valid nor reliable, the value of such variables is highly questionable. Sticking with the raw scores provided by surface anthropometry is a much better approach". Mr. Kelly Sheerin

Chapter 7: Non-imaging Method: 3D Scanning

What is 3D scanning useful for?

- "Three-dimensional scanning is a reference method for measuring body volume and surface area. There is limited research validating its use to track changes in body composition to date. However the technique has been used in large scale observational studies to easily collect information on body circumference and length measures in a timely manner". Associate Professor Gary Slater

• "Probably not so much for body composition just yet, but it is quite useful for body shape and volume. Three-dimensional scanning is used a lot within textiles and ergonomics applications". Dr. Kagan Ducker

Chapter 8: Non-imaging Method: Air Displacement Plethysmography (Bod Pod)

What is air displacement plethysmography or Bod Pod useful for?

• "This is the new age version of underwater weighing, providing a best practice measure of body volume and density based on displacement of air from an enclosed chamber. Unfortunately, the technique still relies on equations from 50s and 60s to convert to density into composition estimates, that fail to account for biological variability in the density of fat free mass components, resulting in errors of as much as 4%". Associate Professor Gary Slater

• "Considering the downsides of underwater weighing, it's a useful technique to assess body density and volume. It is now relatively common place, so access is good". Dr. Kagan Ducker

Chapter 9: Non-imaging Method: Bioelectrical Impedance

What is bioelectrical impedance useful for?

• "This is a measure of resistance to flow. This impedance measure is then converted into composition estimates based on one of many regression equations. It is the most readily available technique commercially but also tends to be one impacted the most by client presentation, with estimates of fat and fat free mass both potentially increasing and decreasing depending on individual client nuances in their presentation". Associate Professor Gary Slater

• "Bioelectrical impedance analysis devices are now relatively cheap and access is good. If standardised procedures are used it could add another method to estimate body composition from body water". Dr. Kagan Ducker

Chapter 10: Non-imaging Method: Doubly Labelled Water

Why is the doubly labelled water technique not commonly used for athletes?

• "The use of doubly-labelled water (commonly known as deuterium dilution) amongst athletic populations is uncommon due to the technical nature, cost and lack of availability of the assessment". Professor Elaine Rush

Chapter 11: Imaging Method: Ultrasound

What is ultrasound useful for?

* "The ultrasound technique allows us to visualize subcutaneous adipose tissue for participants. Unlike skinfolds that measure a double fold of skin and subcutaneous adipose tissue, ultrasound provides a single layer of skin and the underlying subcutaneous adipose tissue, therefore it may be easier for athletes to understand the results". Associate Professor Masuhara Kagawa
* "Research on ultrasound is really starting to emerge again after initial interest in the 80s. The technique carries with it many of the strengths of surface anthropometry but without the same degree of technical issues. For me, it's a watch this space". Associate Professor Gary Slater
* "The ultrasound technique for physique assessment is new. It could be the new common, quick, accurate and relatively cheap method of assessment to replace skinfolds". Dr. Kagan Ducker

Chapter 12: Imaging Method: Computed Tomography and Magnetic Resonance Imaging

What is magnetic resonance imaging useful for?

* "Magnetic resonance imaging is an excellent tool for visceral fat assessment, plus tracking relative change in a specific region of interest. While it does not provide is an absolute measure of fat or lean mass within a particular region, the cross sectional area information is invaluable". Associate Professor Gary Slater
* "I consider magnetic resonance imaging mostly a research tool for relatively accurate assessment of the body composition at particular sites/slices. It is good for seeing into any part of the tissues rather than being stuck closer to the surface or not having a good idea of the breakdown of the tissue in an area". Dr. Kagan Ducker

Chapter 13: Imaging Method: Dual-Energy X-Ray Absorptiometry

What is dual-energy X-ray absorptiometry useful for?

* "Dual energy X-ray absorptiometry provides insight into a range of different variables, including whole body but also regional composition, invaluable when exploring issues of symmetry or regional composition changes such as tracking a client following injury. It has been validated to provide an index of visceral fat mass without the cost or high radiation exposure of magnetic resonance imaging and computed tomography respectively. It is also reference technique for assessment of bone health". Associate Professor Gary Slater

- "Dual energy X-ray absorptiometry allows us to get an idea about the body composition of the whole body and in different regions relatively quickly and accurately. It is a typical method for assessing bone health". Dr. Kagan Ducker

How do you assess skeletal size, shape and bone mineral density?

- "Skeletal size and shape we would typically measure using anthropometry. Bone mineral density is typically measured using dual energy X-ray absorptiometry". Dr. Kagan Ducker
- "Surface anthropometry derived length measures become particularly pertinent to assist in quantifying skeletal size. However when a measure of bone mineral density is sought, a dual energy X-ray absorptiometry scan would be required". Associate Professor Gary Slater

How do you assess muscle tissue changes?

- "My test of choice to track changes in muscle mass is generally dual energy X-ray absorptiometry because it also provides insight into symmetry, something that is particularly pertinent following an injury when an athlete is vulnerable to disuse atrophy. However, if dual energy X-ray absorptiometry is not available, other measures like skinfold corrected girths may offer some insight into regional changes in muscle mass". Associate Professor Gary Slater
- "Dual energy X-ray absorptiometry is probably the easiest global measure to use. On a regular basis I tend to use anthropometry. The combination of body-mass, skinfolds and girths is quite handy". Dr. Kagan Ducker

Chapter 14: Imaging Method: Technological and Computing Innovations

What is new for imaging physique given technology developments?

- Three-dimensional body scanning systems integrated with other imaging modalities to create multi-faceted digital human profiles, and artificial intelligence techniques such as deep learning and artificial neural networks, are set to revolutionise the physique assessment landscape over the coming decade". Professor Jacqueline Alderson

20.1.3.3   Part III: Application of Physique Assessment in Athletes

Chapter 15: Physique Assessment in Practice

Do you have an example of when and how you measure physique of athletes?

- "See my YouTube Physique Assessment series of videos where I demonstrate measurements using dual energy X-ray absorptiometry, Bod Pod and surface anthropometry". Associate Professor Gary Slater

- "I commonly measure physique of athletes for talent identification. We know that some factors are important for success in a sport so we monitor those. I mostly use surface anthropometric techniques and dual energy X-ray absorptiometry". Dr. Kagan Ducker

How often should body composition be assessed?

- "Depends on 2 things…1. Client and goal they are trying to achieve, and 2. Method of assessment and its reliability. Highly precise or reliable techniques allow more regular assessments. While I may skinfold an athlete I am working with to change body composition every three to four weeks, other techniques like DXA or BOD POD would not be implemented more frequently than every two to three months". Associate Professor Gary Slater
- "The main question is how often are you expecting to see a change? We do need to collect regularly so that we have a "normal" reference point and tracking over time, but mostly we want to know if things are changing when we know that factors may affect body composition (training, diet, external factors)". Dr. Kagan Ducker

Why do you use multicomponent models of body composition?

- "All 2-compartment models make assumptions. By combining results from various techniques you can omit assumptions. For example, the Bod Pod assumes a certain amount of bone and water within the far free mass. Rather than accepting this assumption, bone can be measured via dual energy X-ray absorptiometry while total body water can be measured using deuterium dilution. This multicompartment model offers a more accurate measure of body composition but is resource heavy, including cost and time commitment required for assessment". Associate Professor Gary Slater
- "The more compartments that you can accurately assess, the better of an idea you can get about the breakdown of the composition of the body. Given that we're estimating body composition from these techniques it's important that we give ourselves the best chance of making an accurate assessment by maximising the compartments in our model". Dr. Kagan Ducker

What variables are you interested in when tracking clients longitudinally?

- "Mainly skinfolds for the middle-distance athletes that I work with". Dr. Stephen Hollings
- "Height, body mass, skinfolds, circumferences". Associate Professor Masaharu Kagawa
- "Changes in body mass are quite noisy and offer little insight into body composition. As such, I'm most interested in tracking changes in absolute fat and fat free mass. While athletes get caught up in their body fat percentage, it's important to recognise this is a derived variable and as such, is impacted just as much by changes in fat free mass as it is fat mass. If absolute estimates of fat and fat free mass are not required, simply tracking changes in raw skinfold data in conjunc-

tion with body mass changes often provides me all the information I need". Associate Professor Gary Slater

- "Typically I will track the core variables such as height and body-mass, but in sports physiology we're most interested in tracking changes in body composition associated with athletic adaptations. So muscle and body fat. Therefore, skinfolds and girths are the core of my work". Dr. Kagan Ducker

Can body composition variables be compared in cross-ethnic settings without problems?

- "Sometimes requires consideration of differences in body size". Associate Professor Masaharu Kagawa

Are there any issues with anthropometry measurement protocols and data for in Japan?

- "Yes, many different protocols exist and therefore we are unable to compare the reported values". Associate Professor Masaharu Kagawa
- "Lack of reliability in reported data". Associate Professor Masaharu Kagawa

What are the examples of different protocols available in Japan and how are they different to each other?

- "National School Health Survey, and Japan Anthropometric Reference Data. They use different definitions for measurement sites, subject position and equipment". Associate Professor Masaharu Kagawa

Chapter 16: Recommendations for Conducting Research on Athletes

How do you report results back to clients

- "Written reports that present the raw and important data, but with explanations of what it all means. It's often best to include some information to give context to the data e.g. comparisons to norms and conversion to other variables that are more intuitive such as somatotypes and ratios". Dr. Kagan Ducker

Chapter 17: Physique Characteristics Associated with Athlete Performance

What types of physique characteristics are related to the expression of muscular strength?

- "The ability to accumulate large amounts of muscle mass in the primary agonist muscles per unit of height is perhaps the key anthropometric determinant of absolute muscular strength". Associate Professor Justin Keogh
- "Weightlifting, powerlifting and strongman athletes may be the strongest athletes in the world. Weightlifting and powerlifting, even at the highest level have body weight classes allowing lighter and heavier individuals to compete on an equal

basis with athletes of their own body mass. The most successful athletes within their weight classes may be shorter in stature and possess short limbs then their less successful counterparts. Certain segment length proportions may also provide some advantage, with longer arms advantageous in the deadlift but disadvantageous in the bench press and overhead lifts". Associate Professor Justin Keogh

Chapter 18: Body Image for Athletes

Does body composition assessment create unnecessary anxiety for clients?

- "Certainly body composition assessment has the potential to cause anxiety if not planned appropriately. Clients should be informed well in advance what to do the 24 h or so prior to scan, what to wear and what procedures will be undertaken. Dialogue should also be undertaken on the rationale for assessment and what outputs the athlete will obtain. During an assessment, the clients' safety and comfort should be your highest priority, with assessments undertaken accordingly, giving consideration to privacy issues". Associate Professor Gary Slater
- "For sure, particularly in athletes where they are often essentially made to do the testing as part of their organisation's testing procedures. This often stems from negative feedback following the assessment, like when results are released to be seen by all members of a training group, or when they are part of selection procedures. These are some of the many reasons that these practices are discouraged". Dr. Kagan Ducker

Chapter 19: Training and Accreditation Systems and Ethical Considerations

Why are standardised protocols and valid and reliable measures needed for assessment?

- "This ensures you minimise the noise inherently in all body composition assessment techniques so that you can more easily track the true changes in composition. That noise can be either technical or biological so there is a need for standardisation in what the technician does but also the client presentation. Ensuring a client presents rested and in a well hydrated state can really enhance the reliability of most assessment techniques. When protocols are implemented that recognise and control for the technical and biological error in valid techniques, we have an opportunity to identify small but potentially important changes in body composition. This can be especially important for athletic groups". Associate Professor Gary Slater
- "They are vital. If you don't standardise everything you will struggle to pick up a change from the "noise" of your measurement. With athletes we are often chasing small changes and we need to know that the measures that we have are real and meaningful in some way. Standardisation means that we can assess change over time accurately". Dr. Kagan Ducker

Why is precision in body composition measurement techniques important?

- "Read the paper by Professor Patria Hume about how important it is to measure skinfolds at the correct site". Dr. Stephen Hollings
- "If you have the best training and/or dietary intervention in the world, you won't know really how effective it is unless the measurement obtained by body composition methods can identify real change. If the 'noise' in the measurement is greater than the change in physique, then an opportunity is lost. This may result in a frustrated athlete or client who loses faith in your professional skills for obtaining successful changes in physique. The athlete won't blame the machine or its' findings, they'll blame you for not implementing a good training and/or diet regime". Ms. Ava Kerr

Does it matter if I am assessed by different people on different equipment?

- "Absolutely. There is little value in having repeat measures taken if assessed by different technicians and/or different equipment. Research shows that even the same model of equipment can give different results". Associate Professor Gary Slater
- "100% yes! For anthropometry definitely, that's the reason that ISAK exists, to standardise techniques. The difference between people and equipment can be vast. We know that there are differences between things like dual energy X-ray absorptiometry scanners, but if we take something like anthropometry, ISAK exists to standardise techniques and calibration methods to ensure a relatively known level of intra and inter-rater TEM". Dr. Kagan Ducker

Where do I go to get my body composition assessed?

- "Accredited practicing dietitians or accredited exercise physiologists are professionals who often have expertise in the assessment of body composition. Check if your dietitian or physiologist has training through the International Society for the Advancement of Kinanthropometry. If you are interested in having a DXA, BOD POD or bioelectrical impedance assessment, your dietitian or physiologist may be best placed to advise you on a group who specialise in the use of these techniques to provide an accurate measure of body composition". Associate Professor Gary Slater
- "Your local sports physiologist or accredited practicing dietitian may be your best bets. Be sure to check that they are ISAK accredited so that you know that they meet a certain standard of reliability and training. Having said that, many health professionals including nutritionists, Exercise and Sports Science Australia (ESSA) accredited exercise scientists, accredited sports scientists and accredited exercise physiologists may hold an ISAK accreditation. Be sure to check". Dr. Kagan Ducker

How do you gain consent to conduct measurements of athletes?

- "As with any technique, we must obtain consent prior to assessment, whether that be in writing as part of a research activity or verbally as part of day to day monitoring of clients. It is critical to explain what is going to occur using terminology clients understand". Associate Professor Gary Slater

- "This depends on the situation in which they are collected. Many athletes sign off an agreement as part of training with a group or team. The consent process can be obtained there, otherwise an individual consent form should be signed off by the athletes in writing. Following the Australian health and medical research council guidelines that academics follow for research would be ideal". Dr. Kagan Ducker

How do you maintain confidentiality when assessing body composition, especially in a team sport environment?

- "Confidentiality is a key concern. The primary way is to avoid posting group results as has been the common practice of many team environments. Typically team-sport athletes should have signed off something with their team to say that their testing results can be shared with club coaching, medical and sports science staff before any information is shared. The scientist (dietitian or sports scientist) should consider whether the information is pertinent right at that moment and then the results should be shared with the athlete, or potentially with the athlete and coaches/medical/sports science staff in the confidential team meeting". Dr. Kagan Ducker

How do you store athlete information?

- "Hard copies are always in locked cabinets and electronic copies are always stored on password secured hard drives. The information is confidential". Dr. Kagan Ducker

If I have concerns about body composition assessment, where do I go for information?

- "Professionals with training in body composition assessment include accredited practising dietitians and accredited exercise physiologists. The respective professional governing bodies of these health practitioners provide links to professionals in your region". Associate Professor Gary Slater
- "Your Dietitians Associate of Australia accredited practicing dietitian or ESSA accredited exercise scientist/sports scientist/exercise physiologist should be able to help you, or will know someone with the skills and experience who can". Dr. Kagan Ducker

20.2   J.E. Lindsay Carter Kinanthropometry Clinic and Archive

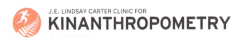

The J.E. Lindsay Carter Kinanthropometry Clinic and Archive (JELCKCA) is available at jelckca-bodycomp.com. The JELCKCA provides a database of previous research in the field of kinanthropometry. Published papers and books, teaching material and other related resources are available to the international community in order to facilitate expansion of research around the globe. Physical resources are stored in the J.E. Lindsay Carter Kinanthropometry Clinic in New Zealand and can be searched electronically in the online archive. Most resources are available electronically for download via the website.

In scientific fields investigating humans, change over time is often an important factor, which can shed light on the findings for the current population. However, keeping track of historical data can be problematic. In the relatively new field of kinanthropometry, we are fortunate to have access to the research of some of the earliest experts in the field and are now making them available internationally. It is envisioned that the archive will continue to grow as people continue to contribute their research and data. Data from studies of athletes, growth and development, special populations and different ethnic groups are collected in the database. Researchers will be able to study larger population groups from within the database, while individuals will be able to compare their anthropometric profile to a selected reference population.

Some content housed in the database are not available to individuals without an ISAK level 2 or higher accreditation. If you have an ISAK level 2 or higher accreditation, you need to register in order to unlock this content. From the main page, click on the JELCK archive search link found in the menu on the left of the page. You will be taken to the main search page where there is the option to login. Below the login box, there are links to reset your password or to register. Click on the register link. Fill in the details requested. In the box labelled ISAK number, please enter your level (i.e. 2 for ISAK level 2) and the year you received this accreditation. Once you click *save*, a message will be sent to the archive administrator who will then unlock the material specific to your level. You will need to login in order to search and view this material in future. The locked material is material relevant to the measurement, recording, assessment and teaching of ISAK specific content.

20.3 Summary

See jelckca-bodycomp.com and http://tinyurl.com/YouTubeChannel-ProfPatria for additional resources for *Best Practice Protocols for Physique Assessment in Sport.*

Index

© Springer Nature Singapore Pte Ltd. 2018   271
P.A. Hume et al. (eds.), *Best Practice Protocols for Physique Assessment in Sport*,
https://doi.org/10.1007/978-981-10-5418-1

Printed by Printforce, the Netherlands